Dyslexia in Practice
A Guide for Teachers

Edited by

Janet Townend and Martin Turner

The Dyslexia Institute
Staines, United Kingdom

Kluwer Academic/Plenum Publishers
New York, Boston, Dordrecht, London, Moscow

Library of Congress Cataloging-in-Publication Data

Dyslexia in practice: a guide for teachers/edited by Janet Townend and Martin Turner.
    p. cm.
    Includes bibliographical references and index.
    ISBN 0-306-46251-6 (hard)—ISBN 0-306-46252-4 (pbk.)
     1. Dyslexic children—Education—Great Britain. 2. Dyslexics—Education—Great Britain.
3. Dyslexia—Great Britain. I. Townend, Janet. II. Turner, Martin, 1948–

LC4710.G7 D94 1999
371.91'44 21—dc21

                                        99-043454

ISBN 0-306-46251-6 (hardback)
ISBN 0-306-46252-4 (paperback)

©2000 Kluwer Academic/Plenum Publishers, New York
233 Spring Street, New York, New York 10013

http://www.wkap.nl

10 9 8 7 6 5 4 3 2

A C.I.P. record for this book is available from the Library of Congress.

Printed in the United States of America

Contributors

Caroline Borwick, The Dyslexia Institute, 133 Gresham Road, Staines, Middlesex, TW18 2AJ, UK

Pauline Clayton, Furzewood Bungalow, East Street, Turners Hill, Crawley, Sussex RH10 4QQ, UK

Jennifer Cogan, Westminster School, 17 Dean's Yard, Westminster, London SW1P 3PF, UK

Clare Elwell, Joules Lodge, London Road, Sunninghill, Ascot, Berkshire, SL5 7SB, UK

Christine Firman, SpLD Service, Education Division, The Mall, Floriana, Malta

Mary Flecker, 34 Burnaby Street, London SW10 OPL, UK

Wendy Goldup, The Dyslexia Institute, 32 Avebury Avenue, Tonbridge, Kent, TN9 1UA, UK

Jenny Lee, Education Department, Community Education Service, LEAP Adult Basic Education, The LEAP Office, Witham Hall, Barnard Castle, Co. Durham DL12 8BG, UK

Helen Moss, The Dyslexia Institute, The Huntingdon Centre, The Vineyards, The Paragon, Bath BA1 5NA, UK

Angela Nicholas, The Dyslexia Institute, 133 Gresham Road, Staines, Middlesex, TW18 2AJ, UK

Christine Ostler, The Garden Flat, Cobham Hall, Cobham, Kent DA12 3BL, UK

Margaret Rooms, The Dyslexia Institute, 2 Grosvenor Gardens, London SW1W ODH, UK

Janet Townend, The Dyslexia Institute, 133 Gresham Road, Staines, Middlesex, TW18 2AJ, UK

Martin Turner, The Dyslexia Institute, 133 Gresham Road, Staines, Middlesex, TW18 2AJ, UK

Jean Walker, The Dyslexia Institute, 53 Queen Street, Sheffield S1 1UG, UK

Foreword

It is now widely recognized that dyslexia falls on the spectrum of language disorders and affects individuals across the lifespan. Dyslexia is characterized by a deficit in phonological (speech) processing, but its behavioral manifestations are varied. Knowledge of the cardinal symptoms of reading and spelling difficulty has increased in recent years, yet there is still relatively little awareness of the other problems that dyslexic readers experience. These range from problems of written expression, to aspects of mathematics, verbal memory, and organizational skills. This book should clarify what these problems are and explain how they can be approached.

Collectively, these chapters provide a synthesis of current practice by focusing on how to assess and treat the symptoms of dyslexia, guided by a proper understanding of the cognitive and linguistic weaknesses that underpin the condition. This book makes clear that the backbone of intervention for dyslexia is a highly structured multisensory approach that teaches reading and spelling skills at the appropriate rate. Such a program must be delivered with due attention to individual differences in the other cognitive skills that contribute to literacy development, and take account of the learner's style, interests, as well as their confidence and self-esteem.

This book is meant to be an important resource for teachers who wish to become competent in the skills required for the assessment, teaching, supporting, and counseling of dyslexic people in a variety of settings. We hope it will reach many teachers and in turn, their students and families.

Margaret J. Snowling
University of York

Preface

1. THE GROWTH OF DYSLEXIA AWARENESS

There has been a dyslexia awareness movement for thirty years in Britain. Not so long gone are the days of battling mothers in the provinces, who took on education officials, and got little support other than that from other parents or the occasional avuncular academic. Some of the heroic pioneers from this era are still with us. Some, alas, are gone. Certain things remain the same: The uphill struggle faced by families with a dyslexic child in the maintained system, though perhaps easier than in earlier years, is still very difficult. But other things are different, too. The acrid fumes of controversy have lessened, as the level of public awareness and understanding has increased. Dyslexia may still be considered controversial among educational psychologists, but that is not the same thing as to say it *is* controversial.

The pioneers in the world of the British university were the University of North Wales at Bangor and the University of Aston in Birmingham. At present, there are many such centers of research endeavor and dyslexia studies that bring together the many contributing disciplines of the cognitive neurosciences. Dyslexia is thus a matter established in scientific research, law, public policy, and in the efforts of many teachers, as well as, long since, a fact as ineluctable in the life of a family as a failing child.

2. DEFINITIONS

Yet dyslexia has long been established in the language, too, as an acceptable lay term. The first English language author cited for the term *dyslexia* by the 1928 *Oxford English Dictionary* is W.R. Gowers in *A Manual of Diseases of the Nervous System 1886–1888* (1893). He noted dyslexia to be a

> cerebral symptom . . . a peculiar intermitting difficulty in reading.

The term is therefore almost as old as the *Oxford English Dictionary* itself. The Supplement of 1933 records the still earlier usage from R. Berlin (1883) in *Med.*

Correspondenz-Blatt des Württemburg, though with "earlier and later examples."
Today, the Chambers dictionary describes *dyslexia* as

> word-blindness, great difficulty in learning to read or spell, unrelated to intellectual
> competence and of unknown cause.

Any dictionary may provide at best a slow way of learning about the world, but we
immediately recognize *word-blindness* as an outdated usage and suppose the cause
to be no longer entirely unknown. Perhaps, indeed, it is true to say that, in the great
jigsaw which is scientific research into dyslexia, there are more pieces identified
and fitted together correctly than there are pieces, parts of some vague sky or mass
of pleasing but undifferentiated trees, that are remaining to be explained.

In November 1994, the Research Committee of the Orton Dyslexia Society
(O.D.S., now the International Dyslexia Association) consolidated what appeared
to be a new consensus by proposing a new definition of this "most common and
best defined" learning disability:

> Dyslexia is one of several distinct learning disabilities. It is a specific language-based
> disorder of constitutional origin characterised by difficulties in single word decoding,
> usually reflecting insufficient phonological processing abilities. These difficulties in
> single word decoding are often unexpected in relation to age and other cognitive and
> academic abilities; they are not the result of generalised developmental disability or
> sensory impairment. Dyslexia is manifested by variable difficulty with different forms
> of language, often including, in addition to problems reading, a conspicuous problem
> with acquiring proficiency in writing and spelling (O.D.S., 1994).

In March 1996, the Dyslexia Institute, following extensive consultation,
launched its own revised definition:

> Dyslexia is a specific learning difficulty that hinders the learning of literacy skills. This
> problem with managing verbal codes in memory is neurologically based and tends to
> run in families. Other symbolic systems, such as mathematics and musical notation,
> can also be affected. Dyslexia can occur at any level of intellectual ability. It can ac-
> company, but is not a result of, lack of motivation, emotional disturbance, sensory im-
> pairment or meagre opportunities. The effects of dyslexia can be alleviated by skilled
> specialist teaching and committed learning. Moreover many dyslexic people have vi-
> sual and spatial abilities which enable them to be successful in a wide range of careers.

3. THE INITIAL TEACHING OF LITERACY

During the early 1990s, public concerns mounted about the initial teaching of literacy in primary schools. For the first time the deleterious habits of dyslexic children—guessing at words from context and picture cues—had been elevated as a
model to which all children should aspire. (That children should learn to read
more slowly is claimed, by the Whole Language movement, as one of its outcomes.) When it became clear that, as a result, children were failing to learn to
read in increasing numbers (Turner, 1990; Brooks, et al., 1994), a series of gov-

ernment-backed reforms was instituted to restore the place of phonics in initial literacy teaching. These reforms have continued, indeed intensified, under the Labour Government (elected in 1997), showing that concern about the teaching of reading transcends party divisions.

Traditional knowledge about phonics, literacy teaching, grammar, and spelling may have gradually disappeared from teacher training institutions, but there remained a reservoir of such traditional knowledge in the dyslexia community, especially in the teaching programs evolved over sixty years (e.g., Augur and Briggs, 1992; Walker and Brooks, 1993) and the courses of training for teachers that supported them. An almost monastic reverence for the written word had secured this knowledge from the marauders' attention.

4. FROM THEORY INTO PRACTICE

This book fulfills manifold needs. Over the years the practice of multisensory teaching did not wait on theory, but evolved as a gathering tradition in the hands of seasoned experts who directly passed on their knowledge. Because much of this knowledge concerns the alphabetic code, it now has a wider prestige and shortage value. The special educator's teaching skills have grown and accommodated many new areas, while stabilizing, as happens with any tradition, across differing interpretations. There is thus a profound commonality among dyslexia teaching traditions, even while practitioners argue about differences of emphasis and preference.

Nowadays, however, with the success of much research investigation, there has been an unprecedented cross-fertilization between the study of dyslexia and the practice of special education. It is this interface that this book seeks to occupy. Moreover the practice of teaching and the practice of assessment have drawn closer together because practitioners have allowed their *understanding* of dyslexia to influence their search for its defining features. The implications of both for teaching have become clearer.

5. THEMES OF THE BOOK

Almost all the contributors to this book are associated in some way with the Dyslexia Institute. The institute is an independent organization in the voluntary sector that has innovated and developed its intellectual property over twenty-six years, finding room for innumerable tests, teaching procedures, lore, and custom that will never all see the light of day.

With the rise of the phonological account of the central language processing problem in dyslexia, research has highlighted the importance of developmental foundations. Janet Townend opens this book by outlining the progress of the in-clinations that become skills, and the skills that become habits. She explores some strategies to employ when this progress fails to happen. These skills consist largely, but by no means exclusively, of the development of spoken language: at-tending and responding to speech, with a growing analytic awareness of the fine acoustic grain of language.

This theme continues in Chapter 2, where Caroline Borwick elaborates on the stages of linguistic development to provide a hospitable context for the exer-cise of the most sophisticated literacy skills. She gives an account of assessment resources relevant to language and offers teaching procedures that address identi-fied deficits.

What of the bilingual or multilingual child, who has a greater learning burden? In Chapter 3 Christine Firman draws on her Maltese experience to illustrate in con-crete ways the confusions over words that can result. This chapter addresses a set of issues that is currently coming to the forefront of professional interest. Firman wisely concludes that languages are different, rather than "equal," and that in spite of children's celebrated ability to *code-switch*, they need a patient teacher, skilled in both languages, who can handle the interference set up between languages.

Martin Turner and Angie Nicholas show in Chapter 4 how theory evolves gracefully into practice when assessment is used to construct a teaching program. The scope of the special education teacher's assessment has greatly increased. This chapter discusses the main terms of an assessment, what features it inter-prets, and how a profile can be built up.

This leads us to a consideration of the principles of special education. In Chapter 5, Jean Walker integrates all the many strands that are drawn upon in the teaching of reading and spelling. She carefully explains the interaction between the *structure* of English words and the *memory* characteristics of dyslexic learn-ers. She provides a detailed account of dyslexia literacy teaching programs within the context of a helpful theoretical understanding.

Wendy Goldup considers the acquisition of writing skills in Chapter 6. Dis-tinguishing between mechanical and communication aspects of writing, she draws out the process of writing from its motor beginnings, discussing cursive (joined-up) script, to word-processing, e-mail, composition and artistic control. She sup-plies a generous profusion of teaching ideas and uses the National Curriculum and the National Literacy Strategy (NLS) as a background.

Helen Moss addresses, in Chapter 7, the dilemmas facing the user of any lit-eracy program. The special education teacher needs to manage an extenuated process from assessment through to evaluation, with students whose ages range from infant to adult. Moss illustrates this process with examples of actual students and teaching programs, the latter respected rather than "adapted."

In Chapter 8, Clare Elwell and Janet Townend look at the needs of more ad-vanced learners who may, nevertheless, exhibit the familiar problems. They ad-dress spelling by way of morphology and comprehension through cognitive apprenticeship and scaffolding. They review a range of strategies and study skills and take in many higher order skills of reading and writing.

Chapter 9, by Mary Flecker and Jennifer Cogan, explores the usefulness of strategies and metacognition. Their chapter is rich in practical teaching ideas and methods which address a great variety of situations, including memorization, note-taking, mind-mapping, as well as the learning of formulae, sequential information, or a foreign language.

Dyslexic students face particular problems when learning mathematics. Pauline Clayton addresses this issue in Chapter 10. Clayton, herself, was instrumental in developing the Dyslexia Institute Mathematics Programme (DIMP). She follows the assessment of number skills with advice for patient teaching using structured, multisensory, cumulative methods and involving both special education teacher and parents.

Margaret Rooms, in Chapter 11, reviews the fast-moving world of Information and Communication Technology (ICT) which offers many opportunities for the dyslexic learner. She reviews hardware, software, voice technology in a way that will not intimidate the general reader. Keyboard skills are related to spelling and literacy aids. Some of the possibilities of e-mail and the Internet are lightly sketched in.

Jenny Lee gives sympathetic consideration to the distinctive needs of adults. In Chapter 12, she records how the individuals describe their own difficulties. She shows how assessment and teaching strategies must be carefully adapted to the needs and sensitivities of adults, for whom the objective of functional literacy may be appropriate. She discusses school and work dyslexia policies. She also includes sample learning plans together with a multisensory spelling program for priority words and an essential guide to suffixes.

In this book's final chapter, Wendy Goldup and Christine Ostler look at the many possible emotional problems the dyslexic student may encounter at home and school. They suggest many helpful strategies to increase teacher sensitivity, and discuss parents' worries in a sensible, problem-solving way that can only make home–school communication and the homework nightmare more manageable. They include a useful appendix which outlines the procedures contained in the Special Educational Needs Code of Practice in England and Wales.

This book represents a full, if far from definitive, statement of the best practice to be found in the many kinds of intervention that are conducted with dyslexic students. It addresses some fundamental questions that are seldom asked. Much of what the skilled teacher knows and does is here set down in print for the first time.

6. ACKNOWLEDGMENTS

We thank the contribution of the many colleagues whose work is represented only indirectly in these pages; the parents who bore patiently with experiment and repetition, when positive outcomes seemed for a long time far from assured; and the students themselves who gave us their commitment when, after so many setbacks, it seemed no one had the right to ask it of them, and whose steady progress has been the greatest reward for those who teach them.

Martin Turner, Janet Townend

REFERENCES

Augur, J., & Briggs, S. (eds.). (1992). *The Hickey Multisensory Language Course*, second edition. London: Whurr.

Brooks, G., Foxman, D., & Gorman, T. (1995). *Standards In Literacy and Numeracy: 1948–1994*. London: National Commission on Education (Paul Hamlyn Foundation).

Orton Dyslexia Society. (1994). A new definition of dyslexia. *Bulletin of the Orton Dyslexia Society*.

Turner, M. (1990). *Sponsored Reading Failure*. Warlingham Park School, Warlingham, Surrey: IPSET, September 1990.

Walker, J., & Brooks, L. (1993). *Dyslexia Institute Literacy Programme*. London: James and James.

Contents

Dyslexia in Practice

A Guide for Teachers

1

Phonological Awareness and Other Foundation Skills of Literacy

Janet Townend

1. INTRODUCTION

This chapter looks at some of the skills which underpin the development of literacy: phonological awareness; attention and listening; and spoken language, including vocabulary (see Chapter 2). Visual perception (particularly letter recognition), directionality, memory, sequencing, and fine motor control are also considered. These areas of development are sometimes referred to as early skills, which may be misleading because many dyslexic individuals acquire them rather late.

Particular attention is paid to those skills which have been most extensively researched in recent years, namely language and phonological awareness. They have been shown to be the most important factors in literacy development. We will also look at recent memory and dyslexia research. However, we cannot ignore the other skills with which we see our pupils struggle: sequencing; handwriting; and direction. This chapter will consider how these difficulties fit into the overall picture and how they may be addressed.

The acquisition of spoken language, phonological awareness, and fine motor control take place in a sequence that has been well documented. Progress

Janet Townend, The Dyslexia Institute, 133 Gresham Road, Staines, Middlesex, TW18 2AJ, United Kingdom

tends to occur within broadly predictable age bands. This means there is an optimum time for the acquisition of any developmental skill, though there is no age beyond which improvement becomes impossible. The obvious implication is that, for children whose development of these skills is late, early identification and intervention will be of greater benefit than later intervention.

2. DEFINING THE TERMS

2.1. Foundation Skills

There is a surprising degree of consensus among recent research papers looking at the factors which influence literacy development. We will call those factors the *foundation skills*. The early indicators of future literacy success are all language based: spoken language, attention and listening, and most important, phonological awareness. Some aspects of memory are also believed to play a part in literacy. Phonological awareness, the awareness of sounds in words, is more closely related to reading than is general intelligence, listening comprehension, or "reading readiness" (Jager Adams, 1990). The theoretical and practical importance of phonological skills form the largest part of this chapter.

2.2. Early Skills

We use *early skills* to refer to the early developmental skills which are associated by function with literacy: visual perception, directionality, sequencing, and fine motor control. There is little research evidence to indicate a skill deficit in any of these areas would predict later literacy failure, yet it is well known that children who struggle to learn to read and write often have difficulty in one or more of these areas.

2.3. Phonological Awareness

Phonological awareness is the accurate perception of all the individual sounds, or phonemes, within a spoken word. This definition also includes the perception of relationships between sounds, such as rhyme.

2.4. Attention and Listening

Attention is the skill of focusing selectively and exclusively on a stimulus; *listening* is attending to an auditory stimulus. It is more active than hearing. The ability to listen to the spoken word is the aspect of listening which is most relevant to literacy.

2.5. Spoken Language

This includes comprehension, which is the understanding of the spoken word and expressive language, which is the sounds, words and sentences used in speaking. Vocabulary is probably the aspect of spoken language which is most important in literacy. This chapter will touch on it briefly, but Chapter 2 will cover it in depth.

2.6. Phonological Memory

Specifically, *phonological memory* is the short-term memory for speech sounds. This can be tested by using sounds without meaning or context, such as nonwords.

2.7. Visual Perception

Visual perception is the ability to recognize and comprehend incoming visual information. Letter recognition is an important skill in literacy development.

2.8. Directionality

In this context *directionality* is the ability of the eye for reading and the hand for writing to move from left to right and from the top of the page to the bottom.

2.9. Sequencing

Sequencing is the ability to perceive and control serial groups, such as the alphabet, a series of verbal instructions, letter order when spelling a word, and sound order when pronouncing a word.

2.10. Fine Motor Control

Fine motor control means the ability to use the hands and fingers to manipulate tools (scissors, pencil, a knife and fork). It has obvious implications for handwriting.

3. THE RESEARCH BACKGROUND

It is important at the outset to be really clear about the distinction between the status of early skills and foundation skills. Spoken language skills, although not actually prerequisites of literacy, tend to precede literacy and play an important part in its development. Any child who exhibits a disability or late development in one or more of these areas could be at risk for later literacy failure. There is now an overwhelming body of evidence to support a linguistic–phonological basis for dyslexia. These theories of dyslexia have been gaining ascendancy since the publication of Vellutino's (1979) review of the research. A leading optometrist (Evans, 1997) believes visual problems may contribute to dyslexia but they are not its major cause. We include letter recognition in this group; it is the only skill involving visual perception which has been found to be a useful predictor of literacy acquisition. However, it is important to remember that students demonstrate letter recognition by naming, which is a language skill. So, these skills can be considered from the top to the bottom, so to speak. How can the research shed light on the early development of literacy, and how can it inform our practice as we teach those who struggle with literacy?

Although there is an extensive body of research on memory skills and dyslexia, we will confine ourselves to a small number of recent studies of memory skills and emerging literacy.

Sequencing, directionality, and fine motor control are included in our list because many dyslexic children have difficulties in these areas. A survey of the current literature on dyslexia reveals very little research data on any of these areas, though motor skills are well covered in the dyspraxia literature. There have been some attempts to present an integrated theory of dyslexia, to take into account the whole span of observed difficulties (see Frith, 1997 for a review of some of these). We must take a pragmatic, from the bottom–up approach to handskills, sequencing, and directionality and focus on their implications for teaching and learning.

3.1. Phonological Processing Difficulties in Dyslexia

Many studies have shown dyslexic children struggle with processing phonological information, such as rhyme (Bryant and Bradley, 1985), sound blending (Stackhouse and Wells, 1997), and nonword repetition (Snowling, 1981). These findings have been replicated elsewhere (see for example Snowling and Nation, 1997; Snowling, 1995). Goswami and Bryant (1990) have a review of the literature.

3.2. The Effectiveness of Training in Phonological Awareness

Hatcher, Hulme, and Ellis (1994) looked at the effect of phonological skill training on reading development. They divided their subjects into four groups. The first group had a reading experience program; the second group had a phonological awareness program; the third group had a combination of both; and the fourth, the control group, had no intervention. The first three groups made gains in reading: the reading only group made the smallest gain; the phonological awareness only group did better; and the children who were taught phonological skills in partnership with reading practice showed the greatest improvement.

In the study by Wise et al, (1997), over 200 second to fifth grade (Key Stage 2; ages 7–11) children participated in small-group instruction and individual computer-based work, in either phonological skills or comprehension strategies. The phonological group made very significant gains in nonword reading and phonemic awareness, much larger than those made by the comprehension group. The comprehension group did slightly better on timed word recognition. One year after direct instruction had ceased, the phonology group had retained their lead in phonological skills and caught up the comprehension group in untimed word recognition. However, in the absence of direct instruction, all of the children's progress had slowed. This clearly has implications for teaching at several levels and indicates that appropriate direct instruction is efficacious.

Lindamood (1985) demonstrated that students' weak phonological awareness could be substantially improved by using an intensive phonemic awareness program that supplied precise articulatory feedback. This program is called The Auditory Discrimination in Depth (ADD) Program (Lindamood and Lindamood, 1997).

Gillon and Dodd (1997) studied reading-impaired children (ages 9–14). They found that strengthening their phonological processing skills dramatically improved not only their reading accuracy, but also their reading comprehension. Thus phonological awareness training is beneficial even in older students. This is why this chapter refers to the foundation skills rather than the early skills.

3.3. The Predictive Value of Phonological Awareness

A third group of studies looked at phonological competence as a possible predictor of later literacy success, and phonological difficulty as a possible predictor of literacy failure: Scarborough (1990), Muter (1995), Muter et al. (1997) cited in Hulme and Snowling (1997), and Lyytinen (1997).

Scarborough followed the development of children aged 30 months to eight years. Those at risk of dyslexia not only had poorer phonological skills at age five than their not-at-risk counterparts, but they also had poorer letter knowledge (Scarborough, 1990). Muter looked at a range of skills in four-year-old nonreaders, and tested the children again at the end of their first year in school. She found that segmentation (the ability to separate out the different sounds in a word) and letter knowledge, and in particular a combination of the two, were the skills which most influenced the degree of success in literacy in the first year of school. Rhyme was not an important factor, which was not in accord with the results of the Bryant and Bradley (1985) research. In a one year follow-up study (Muter, Snowling, & Taylor, 1994) they found competence in rhyme was a factor in spelling development.

The literature survey by Goswami and Bryant (1990) concludes that some phonological skills, in particular phonemic awareness, develop as a result of learning to read and not the other way round. They make the sensible observation that there are many different phonological skills, some of which develop before literacy and some which develop later. It seems that the answer to this "chicken and egg" conundrum lies in looking carefully at which phonological skills are being investigated.

3.4. Spoken Language and Memory: Other Important Factors?

Scarborough (1990) in her longitudinal study, found that in children who went on to have literacy difficulties, their early spoken language development was behind that of other children. In particular, their sentences were less complex and they were less able to accurately reproduce speech sounds. As these children got older (between three and five years), they exhibited poorer vocabulary comprehension and word-finding. A complex and wide-ranging study by Lyytinen is following the development of a large number of infants in Finland. So far, they have noted differences in auditory perception in six-months-old infants between the at-risk group and the controls (Lyytinen, 1997).

Muter (1995) used one visual and one auditory test to assess short-term memory in four-year-olds. She found auditory memory did not contribute to literacy development, and visual memory had a small influence on spelling. The latter is consistent with the findings of Goulandris and Snowling (1991), who also looked at the connection between visual memory and spelling. Muter's finding appears to be at odds with the work of Gathercole and Baddeley (1993), who found that early auditory memory skills are an important factor in predicting literacy success. As with phonological awareness, there are lots of different memory skills. Gathercole and Baddeley's data reveal that it is specifically phonological memory (in this case, repetition of nonwords) that is the reliable predictor.

3.5. Summary

- Early phonological skills, phonological memory, spoken language, and letter knowledge are the best predictors of literacy achievement.
- Some phonological skills develop after reading and appear to be, to an extent, dependent upon reading.
- Phonological skills are teachable, and direct instruction is effective, both as an end in itself and in the improvement of reading and spelling.

4. HOW DO THESE SKILLS RELATE TO LITERACY?

So far we have taken a top-down approach, considering the child as the subject of research. We should now consider the child in school. What are the main differences between the good reader and the struggler? It is reasonable to expect the child with better overall ability, which we may call intelligence or General Conceptual Ability (GCA), to do better than the less able child, and this is usually the case. The experienced teacher will probably have a low expectation of the child who enters school having a limited vocabulary or other spoken language difficulties, even if this child appears to be bright in other areas. Similarly, the child who finds it extremely difficult to pay selective attention to the spoken word may be expected to make slower progress than the good listener; there may also be implications for behavior here.

The development of good listening skills is dependent on environmental factors in the early years of life, provided that hearing and intellectual capacity are adequate. Teams of speech and language therapists have looked at the language environment of preschool children who had delayed spoken language development. They noticed how much background noise they had to contend with: radio, television, vacuum cleaner, and washing machine inside, and traffic and aircraft outside, for example. They asked the mothers to turn everything off for just one hour each day so that the children could hear language against a background of relative quiet, and measured their progress. This simple expedient turned out to be very effective and the children made impressive progress in spoken language.

It is worth considering the background noise levels in the average infant classroom, and the consequent problems this could be causing for children who already have poor listening skills. It is axiomatic among older teachers that children do not sit still and listen as well as they used to. Two recent studies go some way to supporting this. The first, by Evans and Maxwell (in press), found that children who live under the flight path of a New York airport do less well on tests of reading, phonological skills, and vocabulary comprehension. The other, the result of a questionnaire to teachers rather than a scientific study, was sponsored by one of the United Kingdom teaching unions. It suggests that the poor spoken language skills among five-year-olds are having an adverse effect upon their ability to learn to read. The proposed culprits are: shortage of talking time with parents; caretaking by non-English speaking au pairs or overstretched babysitters; exposure to too much television and too many computer games.

Phonological awareness is more important than general ability in the development of literacy. There is a built-in unfairness to the whole process, which Stanovich (1986) called the "Matthew effect." This is based on a biblical quotation from the book of Matthew (13:12), which says that "whoever has will be given more; whoever does not have, even that which he has will be taken away." This sums up the finding that children with the poorest skills do not just stay at the bottom, but fall further behind. Consider what has been said about the development of phonological awareness: some skills are in place before the child learns to read and others come later, partly as a result of reading. Now think about the child who enters school with well developed phonological skills and good spoken language. Everything is in place for this child to learn to read easily before developing the next level of phonological skills and moving forward without impediment. On the other hand, there is the child who arrives with poor phonological awareness and poor vocabulary. This child will struggle to learn to read, and will therefore lack the very reading skills which would promote the further development of phonological awareness. The playing field is definitely not level.

5. HOW DO THESE DIFFICULTIES RELATE TO DYSLEXIA?

The discrepancy model is frequently used to assess dyslexia. The idea behind it is that the dyslexic person has a discrepancy between his or her underlying ability and educational attainment. In other words, this person's reading, writing, spelling, and arithmetic skills are not as good as one would expect in someone of this ability. This person is underachieving. There may be many reasons for this. The skilled assessor will seek to rule out possibilities such as visual or hearing impairment, chronic illness, medication side effects, frequent change in school or environment, or emotional difficulties. In the absence of these the assessor will consider a specific learning disability, one of which is dyslexia, as a possible cause. Phonological skills play an important part in the diagnostic process, as a weakness in this area, combined with the sort of discrepancy described above, would be strongly suggestive of dyslexia.

Let us consider again the five-year-old child entering school. In the previous example, the child with good general ability sails through the literacy acquisition process. Suppose this child were dyslexic. Despite this child's promising start, his or her phonological skills, essential to learning to read, are not in place. She, or more often he, then begins to struggle. He has not enjoyed rhymes in the pre-school period, and he has never learned to play with sound or language. It may be that he will find it difficult to sit still and pay attention to the spoken word. Similarly, he may not yet have begun to recognize that letters symbolize sounds, and so he does not recognize many letters. We can see that the problems with which he entered school are likely to multiply in the school environment.

> Douglas was the eldest child of two college graduates, cultured people who had a love of literature, drama, and music. During his first term at infants' school Douglas' mother, herself a teacher, was summoned to the classroom to be asked by her son's teacher whether they had any books at home. It seemed that Douglas had no idea where to start looking at a book, even holding books upside-down. He did not know any nursery rhymes and could not attend well to stories. Far from being the environmentally deprived child that the teacher supposed, Douglas had enjoyed the almost undivided attention of his mother in his pre-school years. However, he struggled to master reading and writing. He was eventually diagnosed as dyslexic. Could it be that he was not very bright? It seems not; many years later he earned a degree from a highly regarded university.

As previously shown, the higher level phonological skills are acquired in the wake of reading development. It is widely recognized that much vocabulary development beyond the age of eight comes from experience of the written and not the spoken word. So, our dyslexic child's difficulties in learning to read stand in the way of progress in other areas, as well as making it difficult for him to keep up with the rest of the class.

The short-term auditory memory, sequencing, and handskill problems experienced by many dyslexic children will contribute further to their experience of failure. Teachers of dyslexic students often report multiple tasks as being a major problem for these students. Examples of multiple tasks include writing a story or solving a mathematical problem expressed in words. We have seen from the literature how dyslexic children process information slowly and inefficiently. It follows that a complex task, which requires information (especially verbal information) to be held in memory while it is being dealt with, is likely to be much more difficult than a series of simple tasks. Thus our dyslexic student may be able to produce fairly neat writing in a handwriting lesson, or spell single words in a test without too many mistakes, but may have poor handwriting and bad spelling when writing a piece of prose.

> Stephen was seven years old. He could read words on flashcards held up by his teacher if he had seen them often enough, and he could sound out some of the phonetically regular ones his special education teacher had taught him. However, he labored painfully over a page of the reading book. Afterwards he had no idea what he had been reading about. He could spell many one-syllable words by sounding them aloud. The handwriting in his four-line exercise book was exemplary, because his school taught cursive beginning with kindergarten. His "Monday morning news" consisted of a few messy, badly spelled words, despite his having talked his ideas through with the classroom assistant before starting to write.
>
> Although he was on the way to mastering some of the basic skills of literacy, he was not yet able to use them in the more complex tasks of real reading and writing.

6. THE RANGE OF SKILLS: THE RANGE OF DIFFICULTIES

6.1. Phonological Awareness

As this chapter initially stated, phonological awareness is the awareness of sounds within words. To appreciate the nature of the difficulties experienced by people with dyslexia, we must look at phonological awareness in more detail.

6.1.1. Some Useful Definitions

Phoneme is the smallest unit of speech capable of changing meaning; in other words, it is a single speech sound, e.g., /p/, /s/, /ch/, /l/, /a/. Two words which differ by a single phoneme are called a minimal pair; minimal pairs are very useful in auditory discrimination work.

Phonetics is the scientific study of speech sounds.

Phonology is part of phonetics; it is the study of speech sounds in context (in spoken language).

Grapheme is a letter or group of letters which represents a phoneme, such as s, -ss, -ce, ai, ay, p , m, sh, and so on. Sometimes it is useful to cluster phonemes and their graphemes, as in sp, str, cl, etc.

Phonics is the method of teaching reading by breaking words down into sounds, and building sounds up into words. It is important to remember that, in English, sounds and letters do not always have a 1:1 correspondence; sounds must be linked to their graphemes, rather than to single letters.

Rhyme is the identical sound of the end chunk of two or more words, irrespective of spelling, e.g., cow, now, bough.

Rime is the end chunk of a word, -ow or -ough, for example. Words have the same rime when they sound and look the same, e.g., *cow* and *now*, but not *bough* or *low*.

Onset is the initial sound or consonant blend (cluster) in a word, e.g., c / sh / dr / scr, as in cape / shape / drape / scrape. Words have the same onset when the spelling is the same, e.g., *cat* and *cot*, or *center* and *city*, but not *city* and *sun*.

Alliteration is the identical initial sound of two or more words, irrespective of spelling, e.g., shell, shop, champagne, sugar.

6.1.2. Levels of Phonological Processing

Words can be divided into *syllables* (wig / wam), into *onset and rime* (w-ig, w-am), which also takes account of *rhyming* (w-ig, p-ig, j-ig, or w-am, sh-am, scr-am, d-am), and into *phonemes* (sh-a-m, w-i-g-w-a-m, s-c-r-a-m). *Segmentation* is the splitting of a word into its component parts at any of these levels. This term is most often used to refer to splitting into phonemes.

6.1.3. Difficulties in Phonological Awareness

Counting the number of syllables in a word is a useful preliminary to reading and spelling. Mastery enables the child to read and spell unfamiliar words by breaking the word down into syllables. Dyslexic children, particularly those in the early grades, may experience difficulty with this exercise. At a more advanced stage, the perception of intonation patterns, including stressed and unstressed syllables, which does not develop until about ten years of age (Cruttenden, 1974), is important for the mastery of spelling rules.

When pre-school children play with sounds they experiment with the relationships between sounds, as in, for example, rhyme and alliteration. The dyslexic child in primary school may find it difficult to perceive these relationships and be unable to recognize rhyme or to produce a rhyming word. This is not only symptomatic of a wider problem in sound processing, but it has direct bearing on the child's ability to spell by analogy. "If I can spell *sing*, I can also spell *thing, king, bring* and so on," which is an important developmental stage in the acquisition of spelling skills.

The perception of the number and sequence of sounds in a word is a skill which develops once literacy acquisition has begun. It can be seen that this skill is essential to enable a child to access new words for reading and spelling. Word attack requires an understanding of the constancy of sound-symbol relationships and this understanding is a function of phonological awareness. This appreciation of sound-symbol constancy is particularly important when sounds are produced in context, and some of the auditory clues may be missing. For example, the skilled reader and speller will write *a n d* for *and*, whether it is pronounced "and," "an," or even "un," as in "fish un chips."

6.2. Phonological Awareness: The Domino Effect

The "*domino effect*" is the term used to describe the process when a communist regime in one country influences the political leanings of its neighbors. A deficit in phonological processing skills has a domino effect on other skill areas, which can in turn cause poor educational attainment.

6.2.1. Short-term Auditory Memory

As shown in the literature, phonological memory is linked to success in reading. The processing of incoming verbal information, by phonological storage and retrieval, is essential to other short-term verbal memory tasks (Snowling, 1996).

6.2.2. Listening and Attention

If a child struggles to process incoming information efficiently, then he or she will get left behind the rest of the class as the teacher talks. To understand what this feels like, imagine that you are listening to a talk in a foreign language of which you have some knowledge, but not total mastery. You may pick up most of what is going on, but you may slow down to grapple with a complex sentence or a tricky idiom. When you recover, the speaker has moved on and you must struggle to catch up. Two things may happen: 1) You will have an incomplete picture of the content of the lecture; or 2) if it is a long lecture, you will tire more easily and have more difficulty concentrating than if the lecture had been in your mother tongue. You may even decide that it is too hard for you and you become demotivated. From this analogy it is possible to appreciate the far-reaching consequences of a phonological processing deficit; the child misses some bits of the lesson or the string of instructions, the attention wanders and the motivation is reduced.

By a similar process, the child's difficulties in auditory processing may be compounded by weaknesses in vocabulary and syntax.

6.2.3. Sequencing

The importance of phonological processing in short-term verbal memory tasks has implications for the mastery of skills such as rote learning: multiplication tables; common sequences including the alphabet, days of the week, or months of the year. Mental arithmetic tasks are also likely to be affected. The dyslexic child may have some problem with grasping the language of time, sequence, and number. Vocabulary and other spoken language functions are dealt with in the text to follow and in Chapter 2. Evidence for language weakness in dyslexic children is consistent with the theory that dyslexia is a language and, particularly, a phonological problem.

6.2.4. Spoken Language

Chapter 2 covers this subject in detail. In this section only those aspects of spoken language linked to phonological processing skills will be considered. Word-finding (also known as word retrieval or verbal naming) problems are often reported in dyslexic students. We all experience, from time to time, the feeling that a word we need is just beyond our mental grasp. The dyslexic student "knows" the word; he or she has heard it and learned its meaning, but when the student needs it to use in a sentence, either spoken or written, it is inaccessible. This word retrieval system depends on a reliable phonological storage system.

More advanced vocabulary development, after the age at which literacy skills are acquired, depends to some extent on learning new words from the written medium rather than the spoken. For the poor reader, this is likely to be an impoverished source of new learning. Similarly, the poor speller and writer will select words which are easy to spell, thus bypassing an important means of vocabulary extension—trying out new, long, or difficult words. The effects of having a limited vocabulary have been explained in sections 6.2.2. and 6.2.3.

6.3. Summary

As demonstrated, the consequences of a dysfunction in phonological processing are far reaching. Listening and attention, short-term verbal memory, many aspects of sequencing, and some aspects of spoken language can all be subsumed under the heading of phonological awareness as a core deficit in dyslexia.

... the status of children's underlying phonological representations determines the ease with which they can learn to read. Performance on a range of phonological tasks including tests of phonological awareness, verbal short-term memory or verbal naming also requires access to phonological representations. It is probably for this reason that performance on such tasks tends to be highly correlated with reading performance. (Snowling, 1996)

6.4. Fine Motor Skills

Disabilities in fine motor skills are more often associated with dyspraxia, than with dyslexia. *Dyspraxia* is a neurologic problem that affects planning and execution of motor activity. The two conditions may co-exist in some children. Dyslexic people who have not been diagnosed with dyspraxia, may also have non-neurologic problems with fine motor skills. Hand–eye coordination is what we use to control a pen, knife and fork, or a pair of scissors. Some dyslexic children find these skills hard to master. The implications for learning to write are obvious, particularly in light of the observation that dyslexic children struggle with multiple tasks. Writing a story is a highly complex multiple task. Spatial skill is less associated with reading and writing; it involves the perception of space and distance. Impairment in this area may lead to clumsiness and poor ball skills. It can also cause the child to have trouble processing visually presented information, such as maps and charts.

7. EARLY IDENTIFICATION OF DYSLEXIA

In recent years, a number of techniques and assessment procedures have been developed to identify children at risk of dyslexia or who show dyslexia-like tendencies. Remedial help is available at an earlier stage than was possible in the past. It is not universally acknowledged that this is a good thing. Let us examine some of the issues.

7.1. What Are the Advantages of Early Identification?

Robert, at the age of eight, was acknowledged to be bright. He made excellent verbal contributions in class and had interesting ideas. In spelling and multiplication tables tests he did fairly well, because he worked hard at home. His written work was brief, messy, and limited in vocabulary and sentence structure. It used poor spelling and had no punctuation at all. Everyone at school agreed that he must be lazy. His class teacher spoke severely to him. He was kept in at playtimes to finish his work. His parents and teachers met to try to think what to do with him. He described himself as "not good at anything" and explained that there was no point in getting worked up about exams because he knew what the results would be before he took them—a disaster. It took four years for Robert's problem to be identified as dyslexia, and four more years before Robert began to benefit from specialist teaching and achieve his potential. Years later, Robert was awarded a first-class honors degree.

This brief case history illustrates clearly the disadvantages to a child's academic progress and self-esteem when the diagnosis of dyslexia is left until the child has experienced some years of failure. In this case, the story had a happy ending.

In the beginning of the chapter, we showed how the child with poor skills not only lags behind, but slips further and further behind the peer group. Early diagnosis can provide help before the child has slipped too far. Remedial help will be more effective if the child is only a little way behind; if several years have elapsed, there is likely to be a huge chasm that has to be bridged. One has to question not only the ethics but also the common sense of a policy which requires a huge difference between ability and attainment before help is made available. Early intervention leads to shorter intervention time, and therefore more efficient use of scarce resources. Would any doctor wait until an illness became severe, with complications, before treating it?

Let us consider what else may happen to a child whose difficulties are undiagnosed and not addressed. First, he or she fails, or at least experiences difficulties in learning to read, write, and spell. The other children appear to find it quite easy; so what does this child think about his or her own ability? The child may have a poor self-image. His or her motivation may suffer, and this will result in even less progress. It is a vicious circle. If the child is believed by parents or teachers to be lazy, naughty, or not trying hard enough, then the child's fragile

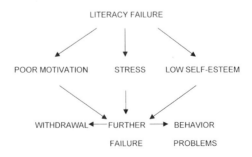

Figure 1. The Vicious Circle

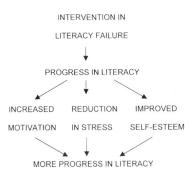

Figure 2. The Virtuous Circle

self-esteem may be further reduced. Equally, when a child is erroneously regarded to be of low overall ability, and given remedial help or differentiated work appropriate to such a child, or if praise is given for trivial achievement, the child's sights will be set very low (see Figure 1).

When a child receives the appropriate remedial teaching and support in the classroom, this downward spiral can be reversed. The vicious circle can become a virtuous circle (see Figure 2).

7.2. The Disadvantages of Early Identification

One oft-quoted disadvantage of early (mis-) identification of dyslexic-type disabilities is that it yields a number of false positives. This means some children who are identified as having a disability go on to develop literacy normally. It may be suggested that early intervention could be a waste of resources, and we should wait to see if there is really a problem (e.g., failure to read) before intervening. If the child becomes very anxious about the assessment process, then the distress caused to the child outweighs any possible benefit. There is a school of thought that labeling children is somehow unfair, because it may lead to lower expectations at school. A label such as dyslexia is considered to be damaging to the self-image. It is questionable whether it is of any use to identify a problem early if the means of dealing with that problem is not available.

Should a child be unduly distressed by the assessment process, then we may need to question the appropriateness of the assessment session. A skilled educational psychologist who is experienced in dealing with young children is usually able to make the assessment session be a positive experience. Such psychologists are understandably reluctant to label a young child; the reader will notice the term *dyslexic tendencies* used in the context of children below the age of seven. This, too, should be a positive statement; it is saying that there is a recognized pattern of difficulties and that there is a recognized way to deal with those difficulties before they turn into a more complex problem.

Is early identification appropriate in the absence of early intervention? Consider these two points. First, intervention is not necessarily something special; it may be that there are things the parents can do to help at home, and the choice of school may be informed by the child's needs. Second, if it is known that the child has, or is at risk of a learning disability, then the adults involved can take steps to ensure that the child's strengths and talents are nurtured and developed. In this way the problems of low self-esteem may be mitigated.

The fear of wasting resources by teaching children who turn out not to have a problem is easy to counter. It is well recognized that what helps the dyslexic pupil benefits the whole class, so good classroom practice may be all that is needed to prevent real problems in those who are not severely affected. Good practice is never wasted. In summary, the purpose of early assessment is to inform a program of intervention, but it must be the right intervention.

7.3. Early Identification by Assessment

There are many good assessment resources available to help teachers assess young children. Literacy attainment tests are unlikely to be appropriate, and the teacher will need to look at those skills which are predictive of literacy development. Such assessment will identify underlying difficulties in a child of whom it might otherwise be said that he or she is "not ready for reading" or "will catch up in time." It will also help to identify or to eliminate other causes for the apparent difficulties, such as a visual or hearing impairment, and to point toward areas which may need further investigation.

7.3.1. Screening Tests

The Dyslexia Early Screening Test (DEST) by Fawcett and Nicolson (1996) is a useful battery for identifying dyslexic tendencies in young children. The Cognitive Profiling System (CoPS) by Singleton, Thomas, and Leedale (1996) is a computer-based assessment which claims not only to identify dyslexia, but to provide a range of information about a child's cognitive strengths and weaknesses on school entry.

7.3.2. Tests of Phonological Awareness

Another way of assessing risk factors is to examine phonological awareness skills. The Sound Linkage Test, by Hatcher (1994, 1996), is a wide-ranging battery of tests of phonological processing skills, including sound blending, rhyme, phoneme deletion, and transposition. It is standardized to the end of Year 3 (end of the academic year in which the child becomes eight and has completed between 10 and 12 terms in school). It has value as a criterion referenced test for older students. The Phonological Assessment Battery (PhAB) tests a wider age-group, but is available only to those with an appropriate qualification (qualified Special Educational Needs Coordinator, or a recognized dyslexia qualification, for example).

7.3.3. Tests of Spoken Language

Competence in spoken language is a valid indicator of later literacy achievement, and it may therefore be helpful to test this in the young child. Spoken language assessment is specialized work, but some resources are available to teachers. The British Picture Vocabulary Scale (BPVS) tests vocabulary comprehension, and the latest edition has a facility for assessing children who have English as an additional language. A straightforward test of word-finding, the Word-Finding Vocabulary Scale, by Renfrew, may be used with the BPVS. The AFASIC Checklists is a useful classroom resource. It allows a teacher to observe a range of spoken language and related skills in an individual child, over a period of time, and identify areas of difficulty. Teacher assessment is not used to label the child but to identify any learning problems the child may have so that he may receive appropriate help as early as possible.

7.4. Early Intervention

The nature of early intervention depends on the child's age and the nature and severity of his or her disabilities. This is dealt with in some detail later in the chapter. Here we will consider the statutory provision that is available and examine whether it is likely to help the young child with dyslexic tendencies.

The Literacy Hour, introduced into schools in England and Wales in September 1998, and the California Reading Initiative, both seek to link the teaching of literacy in schools to recent research and to spread and encourage best practice. The emphasis is on using a sound phonics base for work at word level and to teach decoding. From there, it stresses developing higher literacy skills in sentence level and text level work. This initiative is very much to be welcomed, but to what extent will it help the struggler? For the child with minimal difficulties, or the "at risk" child whose phonological skills are a bit insecure, it may be just what is needed: structured, cumulative, and predictable. However, it quickly moves from point to point, with little time for the consolidation which is so essential to the dyslexic student. It may be safe to assume that the child with no problems in literacy will be able to transfer the skills learned in the Literacy Hour to the rest of the curriculum. For the dyslexic child, these links need to be made explicit. Someone will need to find time to do that.

8. HOW DO THE PRINCIPLES OF SPECIALIST TEACHING RELATE TO THESE SKILLS?

Chapter 5 discusses the principles of teaching the dyslexic child. Those which are particularly relevant to the teaching of these foundation skills include a structured, multisensory approach to the teaching of specific skills, with a logical progression and adequate opportunity for reinforcement and the promotion of metacognition. We will examine these in more detail.

8.1. Structure

A structured approach breaks written language into its component parts and presents it in small steps, each building on what has gone before. The progression must be logical and the links between steps need to be made explicit. The National Literacy Strategy word-level work is an example of a structured program. At the earliest stages of literacy development, this logical progression may take the form of moving from splitting a compound word (flowerbed, sunshine) into its components, to splitting into syllables and then to splitting into onset and rime, before segmenting a word into phonemes. Many complex tasks may be divided into simpler tasks: Learning to proofread could begin with tracking activities, for example. Similarly, sound–symbol relationships provide a secure foundation upon which to build word attack for reading and sound blending for spelling.

8.2. Multisensory

A multisensory approach uses as many sensory channels as possible to input information. While it is considered to be an essential element in the teaching of dyslexic people of all ages, it is particularly appropriate to the teaching of young children. Multisensory learning is active and interactive, which makes it memorable and encourages good attention to stimuli. The child's auditory and visual perceptual skills are developed through practice and through linking one modality to another. This is most important in literacy, where multisensory learning of how a phoneme sounds, how it feels in the mouth, how the grapheme looks, the name of the letter or letters and how it feels to write it, all contribute to secure learning of the association between sound and symbol. The stronger, more developed sensory channels will support and inform the weaker ones. Closely linked to multisensory teaching is the important principle of Directed Discovery. This technique enables the pupil to discover the new information or skill, but not in a random way; the teacher must structure the lesson carefully so that the child is led directly and without confusion to the point. If the material has been discovered, in an active, interactive, multisensory exchange between teacher and pupil, it is much more likely to be retained than if it had simply been imparted.

8.3. Reinforcement

Children with dyslexia need many opportunities to practice the skills they have learned and to preserve them in long-term memory. Practice work must be presented in a variety of ways to maintain interest; this has the additional benefits of encouraging a flexible approach to tasks and promoting transfer of the skill to a range of applications. It is also necessary to introduce an element of rote learning; phoneme–grapheme correspondence, for example, is so fundamental to mastery of written language that it needs to become automatic. Automatic access to this information is the only way for a child to become independent in attempting to read and spell new words.

8.4. The Teaching of Skills

Useful and transferable skills, rather than facts and information, should be taught. This relieves the burden on a fragile short-term memory and lays the foundations for later learning. Examples of this are phonological awareness as a foundation for reading and spelling, and cursive writing as a foundation for all later written work.

8.5. Metacognition

Metacognition is not an independent unit; it is the thread running throughout this section. Metacognition is the awareness of the learning process and includes transfer. Transfer (or bridging) is the ability to apply knowledge or skills learned in one context to another. The highest levels of cognitive self-examination are not available to the young child; indeed Piaget (1928) stated that "second order thoughts" (thinking about thinking), develop in the early teenage years. However, even a young child is able to consider "Shall I do it like this or like this?" and to see which strategy works better. The use of analogy in spelling, which may be considered to be a form of skill transfer, is a normal developmental stage in early literacy (Goswami, 1994). It is also amenable to teaching. Dyslexic children do not readily transfer skills or develop a wide range of alternative strategies for tackling literacy work, and these links need to be made explicit by the teacher. However, once they have been mastered the child is on the way to becoming an independent learner.

8.6. The Advantages of Early Intervention

It is widely believed that the "neural and cognitive plasticity" (Locke et al., 1997) of young children means that their difficulties are more amenable to remediation than would be the case when they are older. Increased effectiveness is a powerful argument in favor of early intervention. It would give earlier access to the whole curriculum, and mitigate the damaging effects to their self-esteem which follows failure.

Many techniques and materials necessary to teach the foundation skills, such as simple vocabulary, large print, and short, multisensory activities, will be quite acceptable to the young child. It is a sensitive and delicate matter to introduce such material into a lesson for either an older child, teenager, or adult. The availability of appropriate resources is important when the efficient use of time and money is an issue.

As already stated, what is good for the dyslexic child is good for the whole class. Sound teaching of the foundation skills underpins later literacy skills, such as essay writing. The establishment of good learning habits early in the educational process will set any child on the path to achieving his or her potential.

9. TEACHING THE FOUNDATION SKILLS

Here are some practical ways to teach these foundation skills.

9.1. Phonological Awareness

9.1.1. A Few Golden Rules

In phonetics, we can represent sounds clearly by an internationally recognized set of symbols called the International Phonetic Alphabet. This enables the phonetician to write down any speech sound, which means we can show, in written form, the difference in pronunciation between the same word in different parts of the country. We cannot do that with spelling.

This symbol /ə/ is called the schwa. It represents the unstressed vowel sound in standard English, as in the second syllable of "sister," the first syllable of "again," and the first and third syllables of "collector." In American or Scottish English, the final r is pronounced, and better examples for them would be the second syllable of "henna" or the first and third syllables of "manila." There are at least 17 ways of spelling this sound in English!

When isolating sounds, make the sounds pure: The sound /s/ is a phoneme and is one sound. If you say "suh," that is two phonemes, two sounds, /s/ and /ə/.

The sound /m/ is one phoneme, but "muh" is /m/ and /ə/, two sounds. If you use the two-sound pronunciation, you mainly hear the vowel sound. This masks the real differences between the consonant sounds. The volume of speech is carried largely by the vowels, while much of the contrast between words is carried by the consonants. Try it yourself: say "suh, muh, puh," then say the pure sounds (not the letter names) "ss, mm, p-"; can you hear the difference? When teaching children with poor phonological awareness, you must be careful to make sounds in isolation as closely as possible to the way they would sound in a word. This is crucial to sound blending: For example, the word cat has three sounds, /c/ /a/ /t/, not five (cuh (2) ă (1) tuh (2)).

Pictures or the spoken word are the usual medium of presentation throughout these activities. If we present, for example, lists of words to be sorted into rhyming groups, then the student will likely look for the pattern on the page. This becomes a visual matching task and not a task of phonological processing. In work on onset and rime, teachers may find it helps their students if they link the auditory with the visual, to illustrate the usefulness of onset–rime segmentation in reading or spelling by analogy. If you cannot draw, buy packs of small adhesive-backed pictures from a good educational supply store. Once you have made them, you will use the exercises and games many times.

When making exercises using written language (onset–rime dominoes, for example), ensure that the onsets are placed against the right edge of the card, and the rimes against the left edge of the other card, at the same level and use print of the same size. When the pieces are put together, they will form a real word.

Always make students repeat words or sounds and have them listen and feel how the sounds are made. We learn most effectively from the sound of our own voice, and the centrality of this multisensory approach has already been established.

Be phonologically aware yourself. I once heard a teacher trying to explain to a child that he should be able to hear the short vowel /ă/ sound in "chair," while the child was insisting that he could hear the short vowel /ĕ/. In fact, the sound /air/ is much closer, phonetically, to /ĕ/ than to /ă/. One has to ask who was more phonologically aware in that case. It is a very easy mistake for a literate person to make, for there is the letter in black and white. We all need to *listen*. Words which look alike do not always sound alike; say them out loud and listen to yourself to check. What about boot and foot, or bear and near, or cow and low? But sometimes . . . shoe, glue, do, boo!

9.1.2. Rhythm

Practice rhythm by clapping patterns. Clap in time to simple tunes, using castanets, drums, or other bought or homemade percussion instruments. Reciting nursery rhymes or chanting the alphabet are good for memory too.

9.1.3. Syllables

You could begin with splitting or building compound words by using pictures: butter + fly, snow + man, sand + pit. This is an easy and superficial introduction to segmentation. Move on to sorting activities: two-syllable words in one line, three-syllable in the next and so on (there are long words you can use, such as helicopter and hippopotamus, but the lines do tend to get shorter). One popular game can be created from any game board and a pile of small pictures: each child picks up a card and moves one square for each syllable in the name of the picture. The longer the name, the more spaces moved; for example, "train" would allow one space, "engine" would allow two, but "locomotive" would allow you to move four spaces. This, then, is not only good for syllable counting, but also for encouraging vocabulary extension at the same time.

9.1.4. Rhyme

Rhyme is an important skill to teach if it is not present in the early stages of literacy acquisition. Sorting and matching activities for pictures of things that rhyme, and games such as "Go Fish," "Rummy," "Old Maid," "Concentration," and "Dominoes" lend themselves well to practice in rhyme for individual children and small groups. Activities for a larger group or a class could include: picking out two rhyming words from a list of three or four, or from a short sentence presented orally by the teacher; picking out the word that does not rhyme from a short list read by the teacher; generating as many words as possible to rhyme with a word supplied by the teacher. When the rhyming words are put on the board, this leads neatly into onset and rime, and the visual patterns of many rhyming words.

Other activities with a visual component include picking out matching "chunks" such as "–ist" or "–amp" in a passage, or in a book from the class reading scheme. A group investigation of the result could lead to interesting discoveries being made about word families, which leads into analogy "Which parts of the word are the same? Can we think of some more words in that family? Can we spell them? Can we read them all tomorrow? Can we use some of them in sentences?"

9.1.5. Onset–Rime

Activities involving parts of words, such as cards, spinners, or word ladders are useful for onset–rime practice. For example, if a rime, such as "–in" is displayed, a range of onsets (p-, t-, sp-, ch-, m-) can be tried to see how many real words can be made. This activity will inevitably result in the reading of some nonwords to see if they work; this is itself a valuable exercise in word attack skills. It can be done on a board or overhead projector, or by getting children to hold up cards with an onset or a rime written in large print. Young children would enjoy finding a partner to make a real word. "Dominoes," in which onset has to be matched to rime, is a popular tabletop activity.

An oral activity for a class or a group is to select an onset (single consonant sound, digraph, or blend) and have the students think of as many words as possible with that onset. This practices alliteration. When teaching children on any kind of structured program, including the National Literacy Strategy, it would be sensible to choose the sound or sounds currently being worked on as the onset. A more difficult exercise, and more sophisticated than thinking of words that rhyme with a given word, is to supply just a rime for the children to generate real words. They should also be encouraged to say what they have added to make this word. If the rime is "–in," the student may say "I can add /ch/ to make chin." Once students have mastered the skill of splitting words orally into onset and rime, then they can begin to make links with the written word.

9.1.6. Phoneme Segmentation

Phoneme segmentation is a relatively advanced phonological skill. It involves being aware of all the sounds in a word. Activities could include: orally identifying the initial or final sound, the initial or final consonant blend (cluster), the medial consonant sound or blend, or the vowel sound in a word or group of words. Sorting activities to put together the pictures of the words that have a feature in common, such as the same vowel sound, may also be used. The teacher could ask, for example, "What are the sounds in the word pig?" For younger children I would use either a picture, model, or toy robot and say "This robot speaks in a funny way: He says cup like this: /c/ /u/ /p/. How do you think the robot would say pig?" This is the beginning of learning how to tackle the spelling of a phonically regular word.

Sound blending is a complementary skill that leads effectively into phonic attack of unfamiliar, but phonically regular, words. The child is asked to listen to a string of sounds and put them together to make a word. Again an alternative strategy would be to say "The robot is saying /m/ /a/ /n/; what word do you think he is trying to say?" The teacher can help the child who has severe problems in segmentation and blending at the phonemic level by taking a small card and using it to cover the word and expose a syllable at a time or a phoneme at a time, or an onset and then a rime. Alternatively, the word could be written out, spread across the page in suitable segments for the child to read, or each segment could be put on a different small card.

9.1.7. More Advanced Phonemic Segmentation Work

Sound sequencing activities, such as determining which sound comes before /p/ in staple, or before /i/ in rabbit, is a relatively difficult task. It needs to be mastered because it leads on to accurate segmentation of consonant clusters ("What are the *two* sounds at the end of *jump*, or the *three* sounds at the beginning of *string*?"). Similarly, phoneme deletion ("Say bend . . . now say it again without /b/; say meant . . . now say it again without /t/."), is demanding of good phonological skills. It may be introduced by first learning to delete half of a compound word, (e.g., cowboy, sandpit, toothpaste) or one syllable of a two-syllable word (e.g., before without *be*, or without *fore*).

Finally, it is important to remember that phonological awareness is a means to an end, namely literacy, and not an end in itself. Therefore, as the skills are taught, their relevance to literacy must be clearly made. Remember that a dyslexic student is unlikely to make such links without guidance. For example, letter recognition is an important skill, and one which may be taught as part of phoneme–grapheme correspondence. It is possible to acquire good phonological skills but still be unable to read and write. Students make the best progress in literacy when they are exposed to a program that includes training and practice in reading *and* phonological awareness.

9.2. Promoting Attention and Listening

For details of programs for listening skills, see Borwick and Townend (1993). Tasks to develop attention to verbal stimuli must at first be very brief, and immediately followed with a reward. One possibility, when working with young children, would be to make a hand puppet appear when an instruction is accurately carried out. Impulsiveness may be a problem; encourage children to wait for the whole instruction before beginning to act upon it. For small group, tabletop activities, use highly motivating games which require attention either to the teacher or helper, or to each other. "Go Fish" is an obvious example.

Large group activities in which students take turns offering a contribution combine listening with output skills. In the absence of any reading and writing, these tend to be perceived as play. For example, the teacher supplies a short word, and students take turns to change the word by one sound: cat > hat >hot > pot > spot > spit > spill > kill > chill and so on. You could make up a class sentence in which each member adds a word or phrase at the beginning, middle, or end, or even do a class story and have each member of the class add a sentence. Alternatively, the teacher could read a story. Each child, supplied with beads or counters and a pot, must put a bead in the pot each time a certain word is mentioned in the story. A count at the end will reveal who was listening carefully (and an eye kept on known nonattenders will show if they were loading in their beads at random, or when everyone else did. This may be overcome by having teams listen for different words.)

There is a wealth of commercially available material, much of it designed to be read by the child, with instructions to follow leading to interesting activities. However, many of these activities lend themselves very well to being done orally, either in person or with a tape recorder. An excellent resource for this is *Headwork*, a series of eight books spanning Key Stages 2 and 3, (age 7–14) by Culshaw and Waters (published by Oxford University Press). Also look at materials produced by specialist publishers for SEN materials, such as Learning Development Aids (LDA) and Learning Materials Ltd.

9.3. Developing Spoken Language

Chapter 2 covers spoken language in detail, so I will mention here only a few group activities for generating vocabulary, particularly to lead into writing. Any of these could equally well be used with a child or a pair of children in a teaching support or withdrawal situation.

Nouns can be produced under collective headings, such as furniture or utensils, or grouped according to what they are made of. Sadly, it is no longer relevant to group according to which store sells each item, because children are often unaware of the origin of even the most familiar items. Verbs may also be collected in groups: transport words, movement words, what might you do if you felt . . . words. Similarly, you could elicit adjectives linked to a theme, such as feelings, the weather, or animals. A thesaurus is an invaluable tool once a child can read, and there are many junior versions on the market. The two color version is better for the dyslexic child to use. Even without a thesaurus, students can find oral work on synonyms or near-synonyms fun and be introduced to the richness of the English lexicon. People remark upon the number of words the Inuit people have for snow, but how many words and phrases do we have in English for rain?

9.4. Fine Motor Skills and Handwriting

For a discussion of cursive handwriting, see Chapter 5. There is a wealth of published material, attractively presented and ready to use, for prewriting and other early handskill exercises. My only warning about using any published material, especially if it has not been designed with special needs in mind, but even if it has, is that it may go too quickly through the stages with inadequate reinforcement. The dyslexic child needs an individual program designed with his or her needs in mind, even if this program is going on as part of the curriculum. We have already considered the need for plenty of repetition; one way to reconcile this with a published activity is to construct extra exercises at each level, or to devise intermediate activities if the leap from one page to the next is too great. For example, instead of following a maze once, why not follow it several times, using different colored pencils, trying to get the line steadier each time. An excellent source of motor skill activities is *Take Time* by Nash-Wortham and Hunt, (Robinswood Press, 1994). Training in letter recognition could usefully be linked to the teaching of handwriting, particularly the variety of print forms that can represent one letter.

9.5. Sequencing and Directionality

Some direction activities are closely linked to handskill exercises: Lines and patterns should go from left to right, not from right to left. Tracking exercises, first for shapes, then for letters, then words, both individual and in a sequence to form a sentence, are excellent for reinforcing the left to right direction of print. It is also the first stage in learning to proofread. For prereaders, picture books in which the pictures make a story, have a similar function and are also good for listening and spoken language.

Other sequencing activities include work with the alphabet, first using wooden or plastic letters and finally moving on to a dictionary. Months of the year and days of the week need to be taught. Many dyslexic children do not have any idea that the seasons are linked to the months. One ten-year-old boy complained to me that it was not fair that his sister had her birthday party in the garden and he was never allowed to: his birthday was in February and hers in May, but he remained hopeful. Linked to sequencing is the concept and vocabulary of time. Again, this needs to be taught to many dyslexic children. The overriding principles are: all this material must be presented in an interactive and multisensory way; there must be opportunities for discovery; and there needs to be a great deal of reinforcement. The progression must be at the right pace for the child, and the steps must be as small as necessary.

9.6. Improving Short-term Verbal Memory

Many of the activities suggested for attention and listening, spoken language and sequencing have, or could be made to have, an element of practice in memory skills. Some of the segmentation activities in phonological processing have a short-term verbal memory component. There are many techniques for training the memory, and those which are most suitable for older students are covered in Chapter 9. For the young child, all the techniques we have mentioned so far are relevant: attention and listening; repetition of the stimulus by the child; multisensory, interactive learning; practice and reinforcement. The development of memory skills may be better considered as an integral part of the learning rather than a separate part of the lesson. However, this does not mean that it can be neglected; instead, for each thing you teach, ask yourself how you are going to help your student to remember it.

9.7. Task Analysis and Multiple Tasks

Finally, it is the teacher's responsibility to ensure that each student is presented with work that he or she can tackle with some expectation of success. It is often very difficult, as we have established, for dyslexic students to cope with complex tasks. For those at the stage of emerging literacy, analyzing the task may be beyond them. Therefore it will be necessary for the teacher to split the task into manageable pieces, which can then be done, one by one, and put together. For example, if a child is required to write a story, he or she should first be presented with a framework, such as a series of six boxes with a question in each: Who? Where? When?

What happened first? What happened next? How did it end? Alternatively, the child could set down the main ideas as single words or as pictures, or use a tape recorder. Then the work could be done in draft form and then corrected. At the same time, it is necessary to encourage these students to develop their own task analysis skills; this is part of metacognition, which was mentioned earlier.

10. CONCLUSION

A broad range of skills support and accompany literacy development. These are all teachable skills. For the child who exhibits dyslexia or dyslexic tendencies, certain techniques (including structured, multisensory teaching) have been shown to be successful. Phonological awareness is the skill area most closely associated with success in literacy. This may be taught from a very early stage, even before reading and writing have begun to be acquired. For those who have experienced failure in literacy learning, a program of phonological awareness training, with reading experience, is the most likely path to success in literacy. As with all teaching, the aim of any such program should be to enable the students to reach their potential.

REFERENCES

Borwick, C., & Townend, J. (1993). *Developing Spoken Language Skills*. Staines, Middlesex: The Dyslexia Institute.

Bryant, P., & Bradley, L. (1985). *Children's Reading Problems*. Oxford: Blackwell.

Cruttenden, A. (1974). An experiment involving comprehension of intonation in children from 7 to 10. *Journal of Child Language, 1*, 221–231.

Department for Education and Employment. (1998). *National Literacy Strategy*. London: HMSO.

Evans, B. (1997). Coloured filters and dyslexia: what's in a name? *Dyslexia Review, 9*(2), 18.

Evans, M., & Maxwell, L. (in press). The effects of noise on pre-school children's skills. *Journal of Environmental Psychology*.

Frith, U. (1997). Brain, mind and behaviour in dyslexia. In C. Hulme and M. Snowling (eds.), *Dyslexia: Biology, Cognition and Intervention*. London: Whurr.

Gathercole, S., & Baddeley, A. (1993). *Working Memory and Language*. Hove, Sussex: Lawrence Erlbaum Associates.

Gillon, G., & Dodd, B. (1997). Enhancing the phonological processing skills of children with specific reading disability. *European Journal of Disorders of Communication, 32*(2), 67.

Goswami, U., & Bryant, P. (1990). *Phonological Skills and Learning to Read*. Hove, Sussex: Lawrence Erlbaum Associates.

Goswami, U. (1994). A special link between rhyming skills and the use of orthographic analogies by beginning readers. *Journal of Child Psychology and Psychiatry, 31*, 301–311.

Goulandris, N., & Snowling, M. (1991). Visual memory deficits: A plausible cause of developmental dyslexia? Evidence from a single case study. *Cognitive Neuropsychology, 8*, 127–154

Hatcher, P., Hulme, C., & Ellis, A. (1994). Ameliorating early reading failure by integrating the teaching of reading and phonological skills: The phonological linkage hypothesis. *Child Development, 65*, 41–57.

Hulme, C., & Snowling, M., eds. (1997). *Dyslexia: Biology, Cognition and Intervention*. London: Whurr.

Jager Adams, M. (1990). *Beginning to read*. Oxford: Heinneman.

Lindamood, P. (1985). Cognitively developed phonemic awareness as a base for literacy. Paper presented at National Reading Conference, *San Diego, California*.

Lindamood, C., & Lindamood, P. (1997). *Auditory Discrimination in Depth*. Austin, Texas: Pro-Ed.

Locke, J.L., Hodgson, J., Macaruso, P., Roberts, J., Lambrecht-Smith, S., & Guttentag, C. (1997). The development of developmental dyslexia. In C. Hulme & M. Snowling (eds.), *Dyslexia: Biology, Cognition and Intervention*. London: Whurr.

Lyytinen, H. (1997). In search of the precursors of dyslexia: A prospective study of children at risk for reading problems. In C. Hulme & M. Snowling (eds.), *Dyslexia: Biology, Cognition and Intervention*. London: Whurr.

Muter, V. (1995). Predictors of beginning reading: Their role in early identification. *Dyslexia Review, 6*(3), 4.

Muter, V., Hulme, C., Snowling, M., & Taylor, S. (1997). Segmentation, not rhyming, predicts early progress in learning to read. *Journal of Experimental Child Psychology, 65*, 370–396.

Muter, V., Snowling, M., & Taylor, S. (1994). Orthographic analogies and phonological awareness: Their role and significance in early reading development. *Journal of Child Psychology and Psychiatry, 35*, 293–310.

Piaget, J. (1928). *Judgment and Reasoning in the Child*. New York: Harcourt Brace.

Scarborough, H.S. (1990). Very early language deficits in dyslexic children. *Child Development, 61*, 1728–1743.

Snowling, M. (1995). Phonological processing and developmental dyslexia. *Journal of Research in Reading, 18*, 132–138.

Snowling, M. (1996). Developmental dyslexia: An introduction and theoretical overview. In M. Snowling & J. Stackhouse (eds.), *Dyslexia, Speech and Language: A Practitioner's Handbook*. London: Whurr.

Snowling, M.J., & Nation, K.A. (1997). Language, phonology and learning to read. In C. Hulme & M. Snowling (eds.), *Dyslexia: Biology, Cognition and Intervention*. London: Whurr.

Stackhouse, J., & Wells, B. (1997). *Children's Speech and Literacy Difficulties*. London: Whurr.

Stanovich, K.E. (1986). Matthew effects in reading: Some consequences of individual differences in the acquisition of literacy. *Reading Research Quarterly, 21*, 360–406.

Vellutino, F. (1979). *Dyslexia: Research and Theory*. Cambridge, Massachusetts: MIT Press.

Wise, B.W., Olsen, R.K., & Ring, J. (1997). Teaching phonological awareness with and without the computer. In C. Hulme & M. Snowling (eds.), *Dyslexia: Biology, Cognition and Intervention*. London: Whurr.

TESTS

AFASIC Checklists. (LDA).1991.

British Picture Vocabulary Scale (BPVS) 3rd Edition. Windsor: NFER Nelson.

C.H. Singleton, K.V. Thomas, and R.C. Leedale. (1996). CoPS Cognitive Profiling System by Chris Singleton. (Hull University). Beverley, East Yorkshire: Lucid Research Ltd.

Dyslexia Early Screening Test (DEST) by Angela Fawcett and Rod Nicholson. (1996). London: Psychological Corporation.

Phonological Assessment Battery (PhAB). (1997). Limited availability. Windsor: NFER Nelson.

Sound Linkage Test by Peter Hatcher. (1994). In *Sound Linkage* (London: Whurr) and *Dyslexia Review, 8*(1).

Word-Finding Vocabulary Scale by Catherine Renfrew. (1976). Winslow Press.

RESOURCES

Take Time by Mary Nash-Wortham and Jean Hunt. (Robinswood Press, 1994).
Headwork Books 1–8 by Chris Culshaw and Deborah Waters. (Oxford University Press).
Also look at material published by:
Learning Development Aids (LDA), Duke Street, Wisbech, Cambs.
Learning Materials Ltd., Dixon Street, Wolverhampton.
Philip and Tacey (small pictures) Andover, Hants.

2

Spoken Language

Caroline N. Borwick

1. INTRODUCTION

Spoken language is the normal means of human communication. The progressive development of language skills characterizes the effective level of communication between people. Competence with speech and language precedes and has a direct effect on literacy development. The relationship between early speech and language difficulties and ensuing literacy difficulties is well documented in the literature (Stackhouse and Wells, 1997; Catts, et al., 1994). The *verbal deficit hypothesis* proposed by Vellutino (1979) has become progressively accepted as fundamental when diagnosing and working with dyslexic children.

2. SPOKEN LANGUAGE DEVELOPMENT

To detect and understand the implications of a *verbal deficit* one must be aware of the normal development of speech and language in children and the factors which affect this. As an infant develops into a preschool child, he progresses from merely expressing his basic needs of hunger, anger, pleasure, and discomfort to being able to articulate complex ideas and emotions. Children have to learn to "crack the code" of spoken language and develop a "speech processing system" (Pring and Snowling, 1986), which will enable them to become progressively competent with spoken language and later literacy development.

Caroline Borwick, The Dyslexia Institute, 133 Gresham Road, Staines, Middlesex, TW18 2AJ, United Kingdom

Language development must be considered in the context of the whole child, his environment, his relationships, and his general development. A child's development depends on the interrelationship between a number of factors to ensure normal language acquisition. Some factors to consider when examining language development are:

1. The language used interactively with the child within his environment and the relationship bonding this child is able to establish in his early years.
2. The child's general physical and mental development: A child who is generally slower with his developmental skills will probably be slower with his language development.
3. The child's expanding experiences: Language is used to help make sense of the world around him. As he becomes exposed to more situations he will endeavor to make sense of his evolving world by using language to interpret and identify significant things, people, and emotions.
4. Interpersonal and emotional development: Language is an interactive function. The child must communicate and interact with others to reinforce language development.
5. The general home environment: Security and consistency are vital ingredients in effective early language development. Many children who feel insecure fail to develop adequate language skills.
6. Play: A young child learns a great deal about his world through constructive play. Play is an essential precursor to language. The child who shows impairment in his ability to play almost always has difficulty in learning to talk.
7. The child's attention levels: As a child's ability to direct and maintain his auditory and visual attention selectively to sounds and objects develops, so does the child's ability to focus on relevant features in spoken language.
8. Neurological and audiological competence: A child will develop normal speech and language if he has competent neuromuscular development and adequate consistent hearing levels. Many young children suffer from repeated bouts of otitis media (middle ear infections) which causes intermittent hearing loss. It is becoming increasingly apparent that children who suffer from dyslexia may be particularly susceptible to upper respiratory tract disorders.

The child's progress, from babbling to understanding and using complex sentences, has been documented by a number of authorities. A summary of these stages can be found in *Developing Spoken Language Skills* (Borwick and Townend,

1993.) Stackhouse and Wells (1997) relate spoken language difficulties to literacy development in their identification of five distinct stages that children progress through in the process of developing spoken language. These are as follows.

2.1. The Prelexical Stage

This stage is characterized by babbling, speech-like sounds, intonation, emergent turn-taking, and a progression toward word-like and consistent verbalized patterns. Progressive recognition of some familiar words and intonation patterns also emerge.

2.2. The Whole Word Phase

In this stage, the first real words emerge. These are largely the names of significant people, things, and needs that dominate the first words of the one-year-old child. Many of these words are used flexibly within the context of the child's environment, and their articulatory accuracy is determined by the child's neuromuscular development. We see many simplifications and child-specific names at this stage; often these patterns are only understood by those in the child's immediate circle.

2.3. The Systematic Simplification Stage

This stage demonstrates the progressive emergence of the child's awareness of sound patterns in words. His use of contrastive sound patterns begins to map on to a systematic system. Although the patterns may be simplified from the adult form, they begin to follow a predictable pattern. The child begins to use his inherent knowledge of language to distinguish between words within his vocabulary and to form some basic rules which allow him to distinguish between similar sounding words such as "bag" and "back." Progressive practice and exposure to speech results in the child developing increasing accuracy in his speech. He also learns the distinctive features of sounds and their contrastive usage in words. Stackhouse and Wells (1997) propose that children who progress without difficulty through the whole word and systematic simplification phases create a foundation for the development of segmentation skills which can later be applied to literacy acquisition.

2.4. The Assembly Phase

At this stage the child has to integrate complex speech patterns such as blends as in "strand," multisyllable words such as "ketchup," morphological indicators such as *s* to indicate more than one in "boys." He is attempting to absorb and progressively use more complex clauses and sentence structures. This stage is often characterized by simplification and over-application of the rules of grammar, e.g., "The mens slept in the beds." As the child attempts longer and more complex sentences this stage is often accompanied by dysfluency and repetitions. The child is also learning the metalinguistic aspects of language, such as intonation and appropriate use of pitch and volume.

2.5. The Metaphonological Phase

This phase emerges as the child enters school and is characterized by his progressive ability to reflect on language. He becomes able to segment words and syllables into their constituent parts. He can not only detect rhyme or the common onset of words in games such as "I Spy" but can also progressively analyze words into increasingly more discrete segments. Competence at this stage of language development is essential for the development of reading and spelling. This links with the Alphabetic stage of learning to read following the work of Frith (1985). Stackhouse and Wells (1997) related the phases of development in language to the stages of literacy development and demonstrated the linkage of breakdown at the different levels (see Figure 1). The interrelationship of Bloom and Lahey's triad of Form, Content, and Use must be remembered throughout the consideration of all aspects of speech and language, both in the developmental phases and in evaluating the efficacy of communication (see Figure 2).

3. THE STRUCTURE OF LANGUAGE

Speech and language are the means by which we communicate with one another. To do this effectively, we have to achieve a balance in all aspects of our message. There can be breakdown of effective communication if any of the aspects covered under the general headings of form, content, and use are inadequately developed.

3.1. Form

3.1.1. Sounds

Phonology is the study of speech sounds. We use 46 contrastive sounds, or phonemes, in English. The accurate use of the sound system both in terms of production of the sounds and of their order within words is critical for producing intelligible speech. By the time the child is six or seven, he should have acquired the complete range of contrastive phonemes used in English. His use of the sound system can be context dependent. Certain sounds are seldom used in some dialects. This can result in the child having considerable difficulties with accurate spelling patterns. For example, if the use of /f/ for /th/ is acceptable for spoken communication, the child will have problems in learning to hear and use the /th/ pattern in his written language.

Phonological competence is considered to be the root of building literacy skills. (See Chapter 1 for a detailed discussion of phonological skills.) Current research on the close relationship between language skills and dyslexia with a particular focus on phonological competence is summarized by Thomson (Thomson, 1997) in his review of the 4th BDA International Conference at York.

3.1.2.

Grammar encompasses a number of aspects including word order, sentence structure, and morphology.

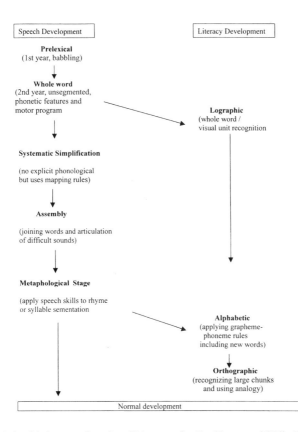

Figure 1. Relationship between Speech and Literacy, after Stackhouse and Wells. Reproduced with permission from Michael Thomson (1997) and Joy Stackhouse and Bill Wells (1997). Figure adapted by Thomson from Stackhouse and Wells (1997), p. 331.

Word order is a critical factor in determining the case of words within a sentence.

The   dog   chased   the   cat.

(*subject*) (*verb*)   (*object*)

but

The   cat   chased   the   dog.

(*subject*) (*verb*)   (*object*)

The case, and therefore the function of the words within the sentence, is determined by the word order.

Sentence structure is the shape or pattern of an utterance. Progressive competence in managing complex sentence forms develops with increasing awareness of, and exposure to, language.

Simple SVO (subject–verb–object) sentences can be represented in the passive form:

The cat was chased by the dog.

as a question:

Did the dog chase the cat?

denial:

The dog did not chase the cat.

determiners added:

The farmer's dog suddenly chased the big black cat.

subordinate clauses:

The dog, which is lame, chased the cat.

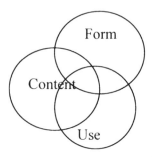

Figure 2. The interrelationship between different aspects of language.

phrase addition:

> The dog chased the cat around the farmyard.

embedded clause:

> The dog, which chased the cat, was brown.

By the time the child is in his second year of school, he should be able to interpret the complex sentence structure of embedded clauses and tell who, in the last sentence, was brown.

3.1.3.

Morphology is the structure of words. A morpheme is a unit of meaning. Understanding word structure and how morphemes can combine to alter the meanings of words is a critical factor in developing competence and flexibility in language. For example:

help	is a morpheme. It is also a word which can stand on its own. We know it can be a verb or a noun.
un-	is a morpheme indicating negation.
-ful	is a morpheme meaning "has the quality or characteristic of."
-ness	is a morpheme denoting state.

Thus   un   +   help   +   ful   +   ness   = unhelpfulness.
    (prefix)   (root word)   (suffix)   (suffix)

We have built one word, an abstract noun, which consists of four morphemes or separate meaningful units. (Example from Borwick and Townend, 1993)

Children in the process of developing language form hypotheses as to how words are structured, so we have emergent forms such as *"bringed," "two sheeps," "the mans camed."*

3.1.4.

Rhythm, *stress*, and *intonation* are all important aspects which influence how spoken language is used effectively. The rhythm or tune of a language is detected early in development, even at the babbling stage it is possible to determine the native language of the infant. Stress is often used to change the meaning of a sentence.

> *He* lent me some money.

> He *lent* me some money.

> He lent *me* some money.

> He lent me *some* money.

> He lent me some *money*.

3.2. Content

3.2.1.

Vocabulary use and *comprehension* are important aspects to consider. The child will generally understand more words than he uses in his spoken language. However, it is important to remember that the progressive understanding of words depends on the child's language exposure and his awareness of language in context. Many dyslexic children have restricted meanings for the words in their lexicon. Interpreting a sentence which contains words which have a variety of meanings could be problematic. For example, the word "mole" has a number of meanings depending on the context: a small burrowing animal; a growth on the skin; a tool for digging drains; a subversive person. Reading offers the child a wider experience of language, although his vocabulary will expand only if he understands the words and their meanings in context.

A word is only useful if it is readily accessible. The ability to easily retrieve a word is an essential aspect of competent language. We all have experienced the frustration of having a word on the tip of our tongue. Poor *word finding ability* is a frequent characteristic of the language of the dyslexic person.

3.2.2

Semantics, or the study of meaning in language, is crucial both to the interpretation and appropriate use of language. While a sentence may be structurally and grammatically correct, it may not necessarily be meaningful, for example:

> *The lampshade wound the idea.*

A classically structured SVO sentence with no meaning.

Children who have difficulties with semantics do not understand idiom, simile, and metaphor. Jokes and implied meaning are frequently misunderstood and this can result in significant difficulties in relationships both in the home and at school. The child who does not appropriately interpret the hidden imperative in a request such as:

> *"Would you like to straighten your desk, please?"*

will find himself being regarded as disobedient and uncooperative. The ability to interpret successfully the *intent* of what is said is critical for being able to function in both the home and school environment.

3.2.3.

The primary purpose of language is to convey *Information*. To do this effectively we need to be able to use concise appropriate language. The understanding and use of collective nouns, kinship labels, appropriate labels and descriptive terms all aid the effective transfer of information. Too many fillers such as "you know" interfere with the message.

3.3. Language Use

The pragmatics of language is the way in which we use language appropriately in a social setting. It is the subtle ability to use the nonverbal cues of communication, which are critical for developing effective relationships. Some aspects of the pragmatics of language include the comprehension of: turn-taking, different intonation patterns, context appropriate vocabulary and terminology, and styles of address. "The ability to utilize nonverbal language effectively is the very basis of solid and satisfying social and vocational success throughout life; the absence of this ability is an identifiable and correctable cause of social difficulties" (Duke, Nowicki, & Martin,1996).

4. SPOKEN LANGUAGE DIFFICULTIES OF THE DYSLEXIC STUDENT

As already described, spoken language is the precursor to written language, and dyslexia is acknowledged to be a language-based disorder. Breakdown can occur at any stage of the language acquisition process. Particular aspects of language which are frequently found to be areas of difficulty include:

- Lack of phonological awareness
- Verbal memory deficit
- Organizational difficulties
- Storytelling problems
- Working memory deficit
- Auditory processing difficulties
- Naming and word-finding difficulties
- Sequencing of ideas
- Concepts of past and future
- Poor memory strategies

5. ASSESSMENT

It is important to assess a child's spoken language skills objectively using both standardized assessments and structured observation. A detailed history gathering information from parents, teachers, and other professionals contribute to compiling a profile of the language strengths and weaknesses of the child. Sometimes a family history of speech and language difficulties will be found as well as a history of otitis media.

5.1. Standardized Tests

5.1.1.

The *British Picture Vocabulary Scales* (Dunn, et al., 1982) measures receptive vocabulary. The single words are graded in difficulty. The child receives four pictures from which he has to make a choice. Children who score more than two years behind their chronological age will have great difficulty in understanding the language of the classroom.

5.1.2.

The *Test of Word Finding* (German, 1989) was standardized in America for children aged 6–12. This test measures accuracy in naming and is divided into five sections: picture naming for nouns; sentence completion naming; description naming; picture naming for verbs; and category naming.

5.1.3.

The *Test of Word Knowledge* (Wiig and Semel, 1992) is designed to assess a student's skill in the reception and expression of an important component of language—semantics, or the meaning system . . . students who evidence difficulty with semantic development will be severely hampered in both communication and learning. (Wiig and Semel,1992)

5.1.4.

The *Renfrew Language Tests* (Renfrew, 1991). This battery of readily accessible tests comprise a test of continuous speech *The Bus Story*, a test of word finding, the *Word Finding Vocabulary Scale*, and the *Action Picture Test*, which is a test of information and grammatical structure. These tests are all suitable for children aged three to six.

5.1.5.

The *Afasic Language Checklists* (LDA) are designed to help mainstream teachers identify children, aged four through ten, who have speech and language problems. Checklist 4–5 focuses on what children aged four through five can be expected to do and contains three main sections: Language and Structure; Language Content; and Ability to Communicate. Checklist 6–10 is a "problems" checklist focusing on behavior that may indicate impaired speech and language development. This list includes an assessment of (1) Response to sound; (2) Movement and motor skills; (3) Cognitive processes; (4) Errors in sound; (5) Communication; (6) Play and recreation; (7) Vocabulary; and (8) Grammar. This is a useful teachers' tool.

5.2. Nonstandardized Language Sampling Procedures

5.2.1. Observation

Observation in the classroom, both in formal and informal situations, gives the teacher an indication of the child's levels of receptive and expressive language. It is helpful in some situations to keep a detailed record of the child's interactions. Have an adult record a short sample of the child's speech as well as what the child is doing at ten-minute intervals throughout the day. When later analyzed this may reveal some interesting patterns of the child's behavior and language skills. Note whether the child responds to questions or waits to follow the responses of other children, and observe his or her vocabulary and the use of gesture. It is important that the child not feel "observed" in an informal information-gathering session.

5.2.2. Taking Language Samples

This can follow a more formal pattern. The teacher and the child need some quiet time in a place on their own without too many distractions. Use a good quality tape recorder that has a free-standing microphone. Be sure the tape recorder is set up prior to the session with the *pause* button activated. Use some appropriate material which will require a response indicating comprehension or expressive language. LDA produce many suitable materials. Record the conversation and also write down any gestures, symptoms of distress, or other behavioral patterns. Transcribe the material later for analysis, because it is easier to detect language patterns when they are written down. See *Developing Spoken Language Skills* (Borwick and Townend, 1993) for a number of sampling procedures.

5.2.3. Story Sequence

Provide the child with a series of pictures which tell a story, and ask the child to arrange these in order and tell you the story. This can be made more interesting by having the child describe the story to another child who cannot see the pictures. The other child then has to rearrange the pictures according to his understanding of the story as related to him. This game will extend from an assessment to a language teaching tool whereby the children monitor themselves for the efficacy of their language.

5.2.4. Syntactic Comprehension

Syntactic comprehension may be sampled informally using the nonstandardized procedure for the Comprehension of Syntax in Appendix 5D of *Developing Spoken Language Skills* (Borwick and Townend, 1993). This utilizes everyday toys. The teacher asks the child to act out the instructions with the toys.

5.2.5. Sentence Construction

Teachers can discover if a child has a certain grammatical feature by having him produce it himself after presenting a model. For example:

> *Teacher:*   "I like pears."
>
> *Pupil:*   "I like pears."
>
> *Teacher:*   (Presents picture of strawberries)
>   "See if you can make a similar sentence about the picture."
>
> *Pupil:*   (We hope!) "I like strawberries."

The constructions increase in complexity and can investigate any aspects which are causing concern. It is important to remember that children will not use a construction in written language that they are not able to use in spoken language (Borwick and Townend, 1993).

5.2.6. Following Multiple Instructions

Multiple instructions are often given in the classroom situation. The child who is having difficulty following these will be at a disadvantage. He may have problems because of a number of different factors: poor short-term memory, poor verbal comprehension, poor sequencing ability, short attention span, auditory figure–ground difficulties, slow verbal processing, or inadequate vocabulary. These problems can be tested by giving instructions of increasing length and complexity. This has the added benefit of making the teacher aware of the structure and level of the language she is using to instruct the class! For example:

Single instructions:

- Hop to the white line.
- Bring me the big book.
- Go and touch the window.

Double instructions:

- Touch the door and bring me a pencil.

- Put away the yellow blocks and the red bricks.
- Go to the blackboard and draw a cat on it.
- Go to the office and give Mrs Black this note.

Instruction sequence:

- Show me a crayon, then a book, and then a brick.
- Give me a big, square, red, thin shape.

Addition of a distracter:

- Don't go to the computer, but get me a book.
- Instead of putting away the blocks, put away the balls.

Adverse order of mention:

- Turn on the computer after you have put away the books.
- Before you go to the playground, put this note in the pigeon hole.

Students with poor short-term verbal memory or with language comprehension difficulties will have to slow down and work harder to follow instructions as the sentences increase in length and complexity. It is important to ensure that the child understands the vocabulary used so that the teacher does not confuse sentence structure problems with immature receptive vocabulary.

5.2.7. Auditory Discrimination

Auditory discrimination can be tested by an informal sampling procedure readily assembled by the teacher. This will gauge whether auditory discrimination is an area which needs further investigation. The teacher can create a set of minimal pair cards, or use materials found in the LDA catalogue which have the same function. Minimal pairs are words where there is only one sound difference between the words, for example:

pin / bin	fin / thin	sip / ship	Kate / gate	sheet / sheep
win / wing	back / bag	ran / ram	boat / beat	bin / Ben

A collection of cards of minimal pairs which focus on consonants in initial position; consonants in final position; and medial vowel contrasts are a useful resource for the teacher, both for assessment procedures and for working on auditory discrimination.

5.2.8. Sound Production

A set of cards, which illustrate consonant sounds can investigate a student's ability to say these sounds. *Developing Spoken Language Skills* (Borwick and Townend, 1993) in Appendix 5G has a set which may be photocopied, mounted on cardboard, and colored. *Launch into Reading Success, through Phonological Awareness Training* (Ottley and Bennett, 1998) contains a good selection of simple pictures and instructions on how to help five- and six-year-olds with sound development.

5.2.9. Storytelling Ability

It is important for older children to be able to organize, sequence, and develop an idea into a coherent account. Many dyslexic children have enormous difficulties in telling stories (Westby, 1984). This skill can be evaluated by using a tape recorder and picking a subject the child is familiar and comfortable with. The younger child might like a familiar story, such as "Goldilocks and the Three Bears." The older child could be asked to discuss an incident or activity he is interested in as though he were talking to a friend. Another good exercise would be to have the child give instructions to a Martian on how to boil an egg. *Headwork* (Culshaw and Waters) books has a number of useful ideas which may be used orally.

Assessment and language sampling can gain a full picture of all aspects of the child's language functioning in any number of situations. The teacher needs to observe the child's social relationships and his metalinguistics skills: How aware is he of the language about him? Is he gaining information from different situations? For some children, the language they need to learn and use has to be made explicit. Once the teacher has a child's profile, she can then plan a program which addresses specific weak areas, both in the context of special needs sessions and in the classroom.

6. PRACTICAL SUGGESTIONS FOR ADDRESSING SPOKEN LANGUAGE DEFICITS

There are three areas to consider when planning a program that focuses on helping a child develop his speech and language: home, special education lessons, and the classroom. The special education teacher should include parents and classroom teachers when implementing activities that help a child develop his language skills.

The following outlined suggestions fall into the main groups of form, content, and use of language. More extensive suggestions can be found in *Developing Spoken Language Skills* (Borwick and Townend). There are many useful articles on language in *Special Children* (Questions Publishing Company). Also, many aspects of the curriculum can be adapted appropriately if the student's specific needs are kept in mind.

6.1. Working on Language Form

This section we will consider Articulation (the sounds the child uses in speech), and some aspects of Grammar.

6.1.1. Card Games

Create card games for playing "Snap," "Concentration," "Picture Lotto," "Go Fish." Collect cards with pictures that all start with the same sound, e.g., pen, paint, pony, pod, peel, post, pin. There can be a number of sets, which can be integrated. Avoid blends or clusters (prank, play) to begin with, and increase the complexity of the selection as the child's ability increases. Card games are useful for many activities including discrimination, for example a set of minimal pair cards (bin/pin; bat/pat) is a helpful resource. *Launch into Reading Success* (Ottley and Bennett, 1997) has some excellent early exercises and photocopyable material. *Expressive Language Skills* (Wood, 1998) suggests using *"monster" words:* phonetically regular words used as names for monsters such as "spish," "plong," "frip." These can be incorporated into a story, a naming game, or an activity such as the one suggested by Rosie Wood in which students collect the sounds off the "leaves" in a "lily pond." The game "Twister" can be used here. Sound blocks can be attached to each color and the children can collect their own blocks and create their own names. This can be extended into expressive creative language by encouraging them to create a character for their name. Have them draw it, create characteristics, and activities. One language activity can be expanded into a number of areas which involve sequencing of ideas, vocabulary expansion, story development, and concepts of past and future.

6.1.3. Word Chains

Try going around the class and having the children alter words one sound at a time, e.g., bat > bad > band > brand > bran > brat.

6.1.4. Shopping Game

Each item in the basket has to begin with the target sound. "I went to the store and I bought a **p**en, a **p**ostcard, a **p**enny whistle, a **p**aper doll . . . etc.

6.1.5. Rhyming and Alliteration

Play word games which focus on rhyming, such as "Ben has a hen and a pen in a den and ten wrens for Len, " or tell nonsense stories which have alliteration: Penny and Posie painted pretty pictures of ponies and peonies. Parents can play games such as these with their child in the car on their way to school. This is an excellent way to make use of dead time.

6.1.6. Syllabic Awareness

Write the syllables of words on separate cards and play "Concentration" with the pieces to create the whole word. Play "Go Fish" with the syllables and the whole target word in sets, e.g., picture of an umbrella, um brel la, helicopter, hel i cop ter. Expand this activity to the appropriate conceptual and language development level of the child. Even advanced adult students gain from activities where complex and technical words are broken up into syllables. This will help with spelling as well as pronunciation. For older students, there is a helpful explanation of word roots in *Developing Literacy for Study and Work* (Bramley, 1993).

6.1.7. Word Order

Read a short sentence or story to the children. Write out all the words on to separate cards. Invite each child to pick up a card and arrange them into the order of what they have heard. Build up the complexity, for example:

The dog ate his dinner.
The dirty dog ate his dinner.
The fat, dirty dog ate his dinner.
The fat, dirty dog ate his dinner hungrily.
The fat, dirty dog ate his delicious dinner hungrily.

Progressively introducing more complex and descriptive language in a situation such as this generates auditory reinforcement, repetition, and a concrete framework, which will ensure comprehension.

6.1.8. Question Games

Experiment with the use of intonation and ask the children to detect the difference between a statement and question. Try, for example: We are going tomorrow. He likes me. Teach intonation patterns by putting simple sentences on a card that they pull out of a bag followed either by a period or a question mark. Many dyslexic children have great difficulties in detecting and using intonation patterns appropriately.

6.1.9. Plurals

Plurality needs to be marked both for nouns and for verbs. Take simple cards which have a single object such as a cup and a card with 2 cups; ask the child to give you the cup or the cups, then extend this with a number of common objects. See the Appendix for other useful material.

Games like "Concentration" can be played with single items and multiple items. Include irregular plurals such as "sheep" and "men."

Mark plurality in verbs, using concrete examples, such as "I am eating my lunch and they . . . eating their lunch."

6.1.10. Negatives

Flexibility in using negative structures and contracted negatives contributes to effective language.

Practice using negative sentences by having each child pick a card from a pile of cards, which have an activity given on them. Have the other children guess what the activity is. The child with the card is only allowed to reply in complete sentences: "He is not cleaning his teeth." To shorten the game, give a clue, like "this is an activity you would do outside, maybe on a school field" for an activity such as football.

Grammar books have exercises which involve shortening a sentence to the contracted negative. These can be adapted to verbal work.

A concentration game can be made where the matching pairs are:

Is not	isn't
Do not	don't
Does not	doesn't
Have not	haven't
Can not	can't
Would not	wouldn't
Will not	won't

6.1.11. Morphology

Morphological awareness can be built up with domino-style games where prefixes and suffixes are written on cards and attached to base words. Children get points for words they build from the component parts. Some useful morphemes would be:

PREFIXES	BASE WORDS	SUFFIXES
un	help	ful
in	do	less
pre	dress	ment
re	cede	ing

6.2. Working on Language Content

This section looks at the vocabulary the child or adult uses and the information he imparts.

6.2.2. Overview

A language learner gains his vocabulary from a wide range of sources. Home, school, books, friends, relationships, caregivers, teachers, video, television, activities, hobbies, the Internet, peers, and older children are all sources. To learn and make constructive use of new language the speaker must experience it in a multisensory way, find it useful and relevant. We all have a larger receptive vocabulary than we have expressive vocabulary. Words can be understood in both written and spoken contexts which are not available to be used in either.

A vocabulary extension program needs to use language that is relevant, consistent, repeated in a number of contexts, useful, and built on existing knowledge.

Also, bear in mind the person's age, language level (and this involves evaluating the social context), and interests and needs. For example, many adults require help with technical language and vocabulary when filling out employment applications.

Language extension can be tackled in a general manner but it is more effective to focus on some specific categories. The grammatical functioning of words and the need to develop the ability to express oneself effectively in a variety of situations provide a structure on which to base a language development program.

6.2.2. Word Categories

Word categories include the parts of speech, such as nouns, verbs, adjectives, prepositions, adverbs, pronouns, and conjunctions. It also includes words that express emotions and feelings or technical terms and subject specific vocabulary.

Whole class activities are valuable when devising activities to aid vocabulary development.

6.2.3. Whole Class Activities

Suggested ideas can be adapted and extended to involve the whole class. Project work focused on a central theme is useful here. The children could all collect vegetables, furniture, clothing, types of trees, pets or items of transport; the list is endless. Use categories which encourage the children to share experiences. Topic collection activities can generate a family's focus on language by steering parents to the encyclopedia, as dads search for different herbivores! The level and the concepts can be adapted to the needs and levels of the children.

6.2.4. Small Group Work

In small group work, the more anxious children will learn to be comfortable enough to contribute if there are only a few children in a secure group. Working in a small language group where the children learn to take turns and feel that their contribution is valued is a crucial part of gaining confidence in language. Many learning disabled children do not feel confident enough to contribute verbally in a large class situation. Their confidence with using language only comes when they actually use it. Many notable speakers were reluctant contributors in school because they felt stupid or inadequate. They overcame their fear and built their self-esteem by developing skills about which they then felt able to talk. Small group work is a good situation to explore children's individual skills. Children can be encouraged to share their interests and strategies. This situation also presents an opportunity to develop metacognition in learning as children share their strategies and insights.

6.2.5. One-on-One Teaching

Some children will also attend structured multisensory literacy lessons. It is important to include vocabulary development in these sessions. As with all aspects of the teaching of dyslexic pupils, the vocabulary development program needs to focus on hearing, seeing, saying, doing, generalizing, feeling and understanding. The aim is for the student to be able to *use* and *recall* what he has learned.

6.2.6. Games

Games and activities are very useful ways to reinforce vocabulary and many of the areas covered in the lessons. Activities such as "Simon Says" can be adapted to reinforce the knowledge of body parts, positional terms, prepositions, adverbs, and action verbs.

6.2.7. Semantic Links

This idea is a useful tool which can be adapted to a number of areas such as Nouns, Verbs, Adjectives, Adverbs. The idea is to start with a central theme and encourage brainstorming to extend conceptual development.

6.2.7.1. Noun semantic links. For example, if working on nouns, choose the central position of "cat" and have children suggest: other domestic animals, characteristics of a cat, what the cat likes to eat, who he likes to associate with, what colors he could be. This will generate a great deal of language. Children can discuss whether the contributions fit into the category of a noun. This gives the opportunity to discuss the grammatical function of words (see Figure 3).

6.2.7.2. Verb semantic links. When working with verbs, brainstorm for different verbs to describe an activity. Encourage children to think where and why we undertake the activity and how we undertake the activity. Children could be di-

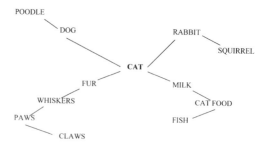

Figure 3. Noun semantic links.

rected toward thinking of the conditions required to enable an activity to take place. For example, a football game needs a ball, goal posts, flat ground, safe area, referee, an even number of players, a whistle, some drink, a clock, etc. (see Figure 4).

6.2.8. Adjectives

Adjective work is a great way to encourage children to use *all* their senses. When you go to the seaside what do you *see*? What color is the sky, sea, sand, beachballs, etc.? What do you *hear*? How do the children sound, are they happy? What do the sand, sea, or wind *feel* like? How does the ice cream *taste*? What can you *smell*?

Take the children outside and encourage them to use all their senses to experience a market with all the stalls, feel the materials, rattle the buttons in the little containers, smell the spices and the fresh bread, listen to the chatter and the stall-holders' patter, discuss how his language is special and what effect it has on the people listening.

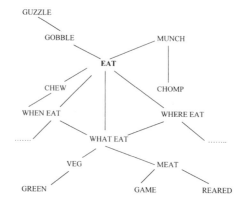

Figure 4. Verb semantic links.

6.2.9. Vocabulary Building

A thesaurus is essential to every classroom and children should be encouraged to use it. There are some very useful activities for older children in the *Vocabulary Module* (English Skills; Burgess, 1986).

6.2.10. Prepositions

Prepositions need to be experienced in a multisensory way. Physical education activities are useful. *Developing Spoken Language Skills* (Borwick and Townend) has a 100-square grid which requires following instructions for filling it in. Draw a castle by using prepositions, such as up, along, beside, between, under, over, left, right, down. Develop a design tailored to the children's language levels.

Encourage the awareness of synonyms for different prepositions, such as: under; beneath; below. "Hide and seek" games can be fun and help the children integrate the language they may have acquired for receptive vocabulary into their expressive language.

6.2.11. Adverbs

An adverb game can be played by taking turns in a circle. Start with a simple sentence qualified by an adverb. Have each child use the sentence with a different qualifying adverb:

- I eat my dinner slowly.
- I eat my dinner hungrily.
- I eat my dinner greedily.
- I eat my dinner ravenously.

Get the children to mime the feeling of the adverb at the same time so they convey the sense of the word to the other children.

For adverb grab, put a number of adverbs onto cards, mime something in the manner of the word (for example, "run quickly") and have the children find the right adverb. Extend and vary this activity using two piles of cards with verbs in one pile and adverbs in another. Get the children to select one from each and have them mime the activity in the manner of the adverb while the other children guess the activity and the adverb.

Books such as *Round the World* (Picture Word Book) (Watson, 1980) have plenty of activity in the pictures, which can be used usefully for vocabulary extension work.

6.2.12. Pronouns

Fill in the blank sentences are useful for helping children to develop appropriate pronoun use.

Fred and Jane went to the cinema and ____ had a great time.

Johnny wanted to play football but he had lost ____ football.

Semantic links for pronouns can also be fun. Put up a picture of a boy and a girl and attach all the relevant pronouns to each (see Figure 5).

6.2.13. Answers and Questions

Give a list of interrogative pronouns. Provide answers such as "I went to the cinema" and get the students to provide the question which might have been asked to elicit that answer. At a higher level, provide open answers such as "Three." Get the children to think of a question which would be relevant.

Highlighters can be a good tool. Use different colors, pink for female and blue for male, and get the children to go through their text highlighting the relevant pronouns according to whether they indicate male or female. This will engender the discussion of terms like "their" where it is not specific or may refer to a male and a female.

6.2.14. Emotions and Feelings

Many children need help building the language of emotion into their vocabulary. Use pictures of people and describe how they are feeling. LDA has some good material which can be used for this. Get children to describe how they would *feel* if their cat was run over: Sad, miserable, unhappy, desperate, lonely, tearful, etc. Try using a number of incidents.

Read an article from the newspaper about something topical, for example a football hooligan incident and get the children to think about all the participants, the mugged granny, the storekeeper whose store was vandalized, the policeman, the gang members, the football manager. Discuss how they all felt, why they acted as they did, and what will be the consequences.

6.3. Use

The effective use of language is critical to good communication and a number of aspects need to be considered. Extensive research and a great number of

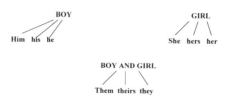

Figure 5. Pronoun semantic links.

practical suggestions are in *Teaching Your Child the Language of Social Success* (Duke, Nowicki, & Martin, 1996). The nonverbal features of language contribute significantly to the interrelationships among people. Some subskills which can help children work with both the perception and use of the nonverbal aspects of language are rhythm, stress, intonation, gesture, and facial expression.

6.3.1. Rhythm

Listen to the rhythm in a nursery rhyme and clap to it. See if the children can identify a familiar rhyme by the rhythm you are clapping out. Beat out simple rhythms with percussion instruments. Listen to the "tune" of different dialects and encourage children to echo the tunes; there is wealth of different cultural "tunes" surrounding us all. A task for children may be to listen to a television program selected by the teacher and identify where the people involved originate from.

6.3.2. Stress

Identify the stress within the word. Use a beat with the hand or a visual clue such as a highlight on the stressed syllable. Point out the difference in meaning indicated by stress in such words as **con**tract versus con**tract**. Stress can change the meaning of the sentence: "Where are we going?" versus "*Where* are we going?" Give the children sentences and have them change the meaning of the sentences by altering the stress. This is a high level activity suitable for children aged ten and up.

6.3.3. Intonation

Intonation is important for children to understand and detect. Practice changing a statement into a question by changing the intonation pattern.

"*The duck is here*" with a falling intonation pattern is a statement. "*The duck is here?*" with a rising intonation pattern is a question.

Urgency and control are often exercised through intonation. Acting out different roles are excellent activities to help children experiment with using their voices effectively.

6.3.4. Gesture and Facial Expression

Collect pictures of people looking happy, sad, angry, or pleased. Discuss what features indicate the feelings being expressed. Act out short sequences of emotions (happy, sad, angry, or pleased) and have the other children guess the emotion being expressed. Watch a video with the sound turned down and have the children discuss how the people were feeling. Ask them to identify what helped them detect these emotions. Discuss how it feels when someone comforts you, rejects you, is angry with you and is pleased with you. Ask what gestures indicate this.

7. CONCLUSION

Language difficulties are fundamental and a continuing challenge to the dyslexic student. Ginny Stacey observes:

> Sometimes I am fluent, sometimes I can apply concentration to get me through and sometimes I have to wait several hours until the dyslexic mode of operation dies down and normal, effective functioning can resume. (Stacey, 1997)

The observation that there are different ways of thinking and processing language and ideas is critical to understanding and teaching dyslexic children and adults. Facilitation and encouragement along with acknowledgement of individual differences will help children build their self-esteem and their skills in communication. Give students tools to be effective in life by finding out what helps them learn best and by encouraging them to learn in a safe environment where language can be experimented with and reinforced. Language learning never stops; it grows and develops, nurtured in the evolving environment of a person's experiences.

REFERENCES

Bloom, L., & Lahey, M. (1978). *Language Development and Language Disorders*. New York: John Wiley.

Borwick, C., & Townend, J. (1993). *Developing Spoken Language Skills*. The Dyslexia Institute Skills Development Programme. Cambridge, England: LDA Publishers.

Bramley, W. (1993). *Developing Literacy for Study and Work*. Cambridge, England: LDA Publishers.

Burgess, C. (1986). *English Skills* (six books). Huddersfield, England: Scholfield and Sims.

Catts, H.W., Hu, C-F., Larrivee, L., & Swank, L. (1994). Early identification of reading disabilities. In Watkins, R.V. and Rice, M. (Eds), *Specific Language Impairments in Children. Communication and Language Intervention Series 4*. London: Paul H. Brookes.

Culshaw, C., & Waters, D. (1984). *Headwork Series*. Oxford, England: Oxford University Press.

Duke, M.P., Nowicki, S., & Martin, E.A. (1996). *Teaching Your Child the Language of Social Success*. Atlanta, USA: Peachtree Publishers Ltd.

Dunn, L.M., Dunn, L., Whetton, C., & Pintillie, D. (1982). *British Picture Vocabulary Scales*. Windsor, England: NFER-Nelson.

Frith, U. (1985). Beneath the surface of developmental dyslexia. In K.E. Patterson, J.C. Marshall, & M. Coltheart (Eds), *Surface Dyslexia* (pp. 301–330). London: Routledge and Kegan Paul.

German, D. (1989). *Test of Word Finding*. Leicester, England: Taskmaster.

Ottley, P., & Bennett, L. (1997). *Launch into Reading Success Through Phonological Awareness Training*. London: The Psychological Corporation.

Pring, L., & Snowling, M. (1986). Developmental changes in word recognition: An information processing account. *Quarterly Journal of Experimental Psychology, 38A*, 395–418.

Renfrew, C.E. (1991). *Renfrew Language Tests*. Revised. Available from C.E. Renfrew, 2a North Place, Headington, Oxford, England.

Stacey, G. (1997). A dyslexic mind a-thinking. *Dyslexia*, 3: 2, 111–119.

Stackhouse, J., & Wells, B. (1997). *Children's Speech and Literacy Difficulties*. A Psycholinguistic Framework. London: Whurr Publishers.

Thomson, M. (1997). An overview of papers on speech and language. *Dyslexia CONTACT, 16*(2), 12–14.

Vellutino, F. (1979). *Dyslexia: Theory and Research*. Cambridge, MA: MIT Press.

Watson, C. (1980). *Round the World* (Picture Word Book). London: Usborne Publishing.

Wood, R. (1998). *Expressive Language Skills*. The Dyslexia Handbook. Pub. BDA. Reading, England.

Wiig, E.H., & Semel, E. (1992). *Test of Word Knowledge*. London: The Psychological Corporation.

3

The Bilingual Dyslexic Child

An Overview of Some of the Difficulties Encountered

Christine Firman

1. INTRODUCTION

Dyslexic children have difficulty with acquiring literacy skills in one language. It becomes more problematic when they are obliged to develop competence in two languages. This chapter attempts to discuss some of the problems of dyslexia in bilingualism and will relate it to dyslexic children in Malta.

2. GLOBAL CONCERNS

Appropriate literacy development for all has become a global concern as countries attempt to reduce their level of illiteracy. Political developments and improved means of communication have necessitated the development of literacy in more than one language. Bilingualism has become a necessary way of life in many countries because monolinguism has been found to be restricting, unprofitable, and culturally excluding. Although some children adequately cope with the development of two languages, there are others who face significant difficulty in just one language. Concerted efforts have been made to investigate limited literacy development. Dyslexia is given considerable attention.

Christine Firman, SpLD Service, Education Division, The Mall, Floriana, Malta

3. WHAT IS BILINGUALISM?

Many studies evaluate the manifestations of dyslexia in one language but few studies actually *compare* the performance of bilingual dyslexics in two languages. There are various reasons for this but it is possible that the magnitude of the term "bilingualism" could be one of the factors.

Disputes have continued over the precise implications and boundaries of the term. To the lay person "bilingualism" means one who is *equally skilled* in two languages. Equal competence in reading, writing, speaking, and listening is therefore expected. The exact level of attainment in the different skills is hard to determine because it necessitates comparisons which also consider the child's educational, cultural, social, and geographical positions. Thus, studies on bilingualism are fraught with complexities: Who is the bilingual individual? Which factors are most likely to contribute to the development of the bilingual individual who has "equal competence in terms of production and reception of oral language" (Baker, 1988)?

Research on the performance of bilingual people must therefore include a wide variety of individuals. "If the sample is restricted or possibly includes a particular type of bilingual the results may have little validity and applicability" (Baker, 1988).

4. BILINGUALISM IN MALTA

The bilingual individual in Malta can be considered to be "a communicator of a different sort" (Grosjean, 1992). This section will outline Malta's language policy and consider the difficulties experienced in relation to bilingualism and dyslexia before covering some of the problems teachers and students encounter.

Malta has two official languages: English and Maltese. Maltese is a Semitic language with a Romance script and shallow orthography. Children are exposed to English and Maltese in greater or lesser degrees. Because of the direct mappings between sounds and symbols, Maltese words can be accessed by both direct and indirect routes. Once formal education begins, Maltese children are necessarily expected to develop written and verbal competence in both languages. The dyslexic child has much to struggle with when faced with the burden of bilingual literacy development.

5. BILINGUALISM AND DYSLEXIA

Much research work has been carried out on the manifestations of dyslexia in the English language among them subtypes, error classifications, case studies, and manifestations (Seymour, 1994; Stanovich, Siegel, & Gottardo, 1997; Boder, 1973; Snowling, Hulme, & Goulandris, 1989; Miles, 1983). In the course of my work with Maltese children, it has been suggested that lack of transparency of the orthography of the English language may lead to further difficulties. Given that neurological differences (Frith, 1997) contribute to the manifestations of dyslexia, such a view is untenable. Furthermore, there is a worldwide awareness of the problem (Salter and Smythe, 1997). Studies undertaken for example in the Dravidian, Kannada (Ramaa, Miles, & Lalithamma, 1993), and the Chinese languages (Leong, 1997) indicate dyslexia is not restricted to one orthography.

Yet most studies tend to investigate difficulties manifested only in a single language. There are few studies of the difficulties encountered by bilingual dyslexics. Furthermore, literacy development tends to be discussed in relation to English. It is thus necessary to exercise caution in discussing difficulties encountered in languages other than English because the differences in language structure together with the methods employed for teaching reading and writing could give rise to the use of different channels for the purposes of reading.

Wimmer and Goswami (1994), in their comparative study of word recognition in English and German children, suggested that a universal model of reading development is not possible. They believe German children may not necessarily pass through the three stages of reading development (logographic, alphabetic, and orthographic) proposed by Uta Frith (1985). Languages which have a close grapheme–phoneme correspondence might lead to the omission of the "logographic" stage of reading development. The Wimmer and Goswami (1994) study indicates that German children were able to decode nonsense words, but English children attempted to force nonwords into real word patterns thereby showing their reliance on visual routes even to decode unknown words. This again serves to accentuate that bilingual children exposed to languages of *different* orthographies encounter different difficulties.

The nature of the orthography also contributes to the diversity of difficulties encountered in the development of literacy. For example, Wimmer (1993) indicates that though German-speaking children might encounter initial decoding difficulties, unlike English children, they overcome them within a short period of time. The rapid progress is attributed to the consistency of the orthography. Such differences clearly illustrate the importance of indepth assessment of the languages the child is exposed to. As Karranth (1992) appropriately proposes, an understanding of the teaching of reading in different scripts will "contribute to the management of developmental dyslexics and rehabilitation procedure for acquired dyslexics." This also has much relevance for the Maltese bilingual child.

Goswami (1997) explored the literacy development of dyslexic children exposed to languages of different orthographies. She cited studies illustrating how children growing up in different linguistic environments appear to go through the same sequence of phonological development—the ability to identify onsets precedes awareness of phonemes. However, difficulties encountered by the dyslexic child appear to depend on the phonology and orthography of the language. This may contribute to our understanding of the development of reading and writing in languages of different orthographies. Such studies could facilitate our comprehension of the problems the bilingual dyslexic child encounters and enable us to create more appropriate teaching strategies.

It is necessary to refer briefly to spelling strategies and to highlight some differences that can be detected through different teaching systems and orthographies. In Firman, 1994, I analyzed the error pattern of five monolingual dyslexic students educated in England and five bilingual dyslexic students educated in Malta. Both groups had attained the same level on a standardized English spelling test. When the test of words of increased syllable length (Snowling, 1985) was administered, I found some obvious differences. The Maltese bilingual children were able to attain a larger proportion of phonically correct polysyllabic words though they lacked orthographic correctness. The English group tended to omit syllabic clusters and displayed greater weakness in coping with polysyllabic words. Also, while Maltese children experienced difficulties with monosyllabic words because of confusions (Maltese–English) caused by two distinct orthographic systems, English children experienced no such difficulties. Again, this illustrates the necessity of taking into consideration the orthography of the language and teaching methods when discussing and analyzing literacy difficulties.

6. LEARNING DISABILITY OR LIMITED EXPOSURE TO THE ENGLISH LANGUAGE?

It can be problematic to identify a child's learning disability in countries where majority and minority languages are spoken. This is because a child's limited development can be erroneously attributed to insufficient exposure to the English language. Grosjean (1992) does not consider the possibility of a "language deficit" in any child who has not been offered every opportunity to learn. Such general judgments can prove to be extremely detrimental to a child's well being because he might be allowed to continue in his pattern of failure without being offered the necessary intervention. Bilingual children can therefore be wrongly classified (Hall, 1995). Edbury and Rack (1998) note this in their paper on literacy difficulties in second language learners.

In countries, such as Malta, where it is necessary for every child to have knowledge of two languages, the delayed identification of a learning disorder can also cause parents considerable apprehension. Much depends on the teacher's awareness of the usual manifestations of dyslexia, the difficulties experienced by the average bilingual child, and the aggravated difficulties the child is experiencing because of compulsory exposure to two languages.

It is hard to investigate a bilingual child's literacy difficulty. There is a concern over the tendency to use English as a standard of measurement and the "varieties of the reading disorders seen in English as the norm" (Karanth, 1992). As we have established, the concise measurement of the bilingual individual's skills can be enigmatic; understandably, investigating difficulties in relation to both bilingualism and dyslexia is complex.

Baker (1988) suggests bilingual research tends to generalize too freely across countries and continents. Children are often tested with culturally loaded tests. A low result does not necessarily reflect the child's ability, rather it reflects the test's inappropriateness. Similar problems occur when a bilingual dyslexic child is assessed. Tests that measure deviancy from the norm or establish patterns of functioning in the different languages are not easily available in countries where the study of dyslexia is relatively new and much is "borrowed" from the English language. For example, verbal tests, such as The British Picture Vocabulary Scale (Dunn, Dunn, and Whetton, 1982), are inappropriate for the assessment of Maltese bilingual subjects, because scores tend to be significantly lower than expected. The 1996 edition, however, has an additional scale of scores for children who have English as an additional language.

The digit span test, of short-term auditory memory is one clear illustration of the danger of simply translating tests into another language. Following Ellis and Hennelly (1980) I asked 14 Maltese dyslexic children, ages 8–14, attending a Special Centre for dyslexic children, to repeat a series of digits in both English and Maltese (Firman, 1995). Maltese digits are generally polysyllabic (as opposed to the preponderance of monosyllables in English digits), thus the children were able to recall a larger number of digits in English than Maltese. Such minor differences in word length must also be kept in mind when using tests in different languages.

7. ASSESSMENT MEASURES

It is necessary to begin by determining, even informally, whether the child has a dominant language by asking routine questions such as:

1. What languages are spoken at home?
2. What television programs are watched?
3. What opportunities does the child have to hear and learn two languages?
4. How often does the child have to communicate in the two languages or is one language used predominantly?

The answers to these will help the teacher develop an overall picture of the child's verbal ability and to determine which tests could be administered.

After working for some time in the field of literacy difficulties and having considered various language tests and techniques which adequately highlight areas of difficulty in monolingual speakers, I feel the following areas should be investigated. This ideally should be done in the two languages the child is exposed to, before a teacher embarks on a program of specialist intervention.

7.1. Phoneme Discrimination

It is of primary importance to establish whether the child is aware that the languages to which he is exposed might employ different phoneme to grapheme correspondences.

7.2. Blending Skills

The child's ability to blend sounds together to produce words must be investigated in both languages. Any problems with this skill could reveal an area of difficulty which is not necessarily restricted to one language.

7.3. Segmentation Skills

Segmentation of words into syllables, in both languages, can also highlight a child's area of weakness. Such a skill is not usually restricted to one language. Yet a larger proportion of errors in one language than in the other can be significant.

7.4. Reading Strategies

A qualitative assessment is required to comprehend the nature of the child's difficulties (Snowling, 1985; Miles, 1983). Boder's categories of error classification (dysphonetic, dyseidetic, and mixed) may be worthwhile to implement for the purposes of "transcultural studies" (Boder, 1973). An analysis of the skills of bilingual dyslexics should extend to the established categories to consider more particularly the possible language interference or overlap.

In my assessment of Maltese bilingual children, I found some children would attempt to access words on a Maltese Word Reading Test (Bartolo Word Reading Test, 1988) via the semantics of the word rather than by using phonological strategies. For example, the Maltese word *ballun* (ball) was read as "ball," the Maltese word *kelb* (dog) was read as "dog." It is also necessary to investigate the level or extent of phoneme–grapheme interference. For example the English word "cat" read as "chat" (/ch/ in English is the equivalent of /č/ in Maltese) or "box" as "bosh" (/sh/ in English is the equivalent of /x/ in Maltese) reveals the child's inability to draw a distinction between the two languages.

7.5. Spelling

Spelling strategies can reveal the nature of the child's difficulties. It is important to investigate whether there is any obvious interference between one language and the other. Some children experience much language confusion at the level of the phonemes ("politician" written as "politixin," "ship" written as "xip"). It is not possible to claim this phenomenon is unique to dyslexic students, but it is more commonly found among language-impaired children, including those with dyslexia.

Having briefly discussed some of the areas of difficulty teachers and therapists might be faced with when working with bilingual children, I shall present two case studies to illustrate further some of the difficulties children encounter in bilingual environments.

8. CASE STUDIES

Tommy and Peter are both being brought up in similar educational systems yet both have underlying deficits which have caused them to develop different language preferences.

8.1. Tommy

Tommy (9 years, 2 months) is a Maltese male of low average ability who is experiencing severe difficulties in the development of his literacy skills. Maltese is the dominant language at home, but he is exposed to both English and Maltese at school. Tommy has short term memory deficits, and sequencing and naming difficulties. His ability to segment words and identify the constituent phonemes is limited in both languages.

An analysis of his Maltese spelling errors shows that he is unable to write sounds in sequential order. He writes *suf* as "futri," *tacci as "c̈arta," and *moda* as "mutr." It was expected that because Tommy is having such difficulty in coping with sounds in the language he is most familiar with, he would also have even greater difficulty in English—a language in which he has limited verbal competence. However, Tommy managed to spell a total of four words correctly and some were close to target. It appears that Tommy could not cope with encoding his dominant language because he could not adequately access his phonological system.

Tommy uses the direct or visual strategy to read English words. His Maltese reading patterns point to a significant language interference. He reads the Maltese word *ballun* (ball) as English "balloon," *papra* (duck) as "up," and *zewg* (two) as "zoo." However, the rest of his errors clearly show Tommy lacks phonic skills. He attempts to read by making use of minimal visual cues or by trying to bypass his phonological strategies to supposedly access the semantics of the word. Like the Swedish subjects discussed by Miller-Guron and Lundberg (1997), Tommy considers English to be the easier language.

8.2. Peter

Peter, a child whose mother is English and father is Maltese, spent only limited periods of time in Malta during his early infancy. His dominant language is English: He speaks fluently and has a wide vocabulary. His verbal Maltese is satisfactory. Peter demonstrates an unstable pattern of difficulties; he is able to generate more rhyming words in English than Maltese, but able to segment more words in Maltese than English.

An analysis of his English error patterns shows Peter relies heavily on his phonic recall of words and has not yet reached the orthographic stage of development. He considers Maltese spelling to be easier and says he experiences limited difficulties. Yet, Peter considers English to be the easier language to read.

These two children show partially contrasting preferences. Tommy, exposed mainly to Maltese, considers English reading and spelling to be easier, while Peter, whose first language is English, considers Maltese spelling and English reading to be easier. Tommy has phonological weakness while Peter has phonic strengths. This limited evidence points to the possibility that phonic strengths and weaknesses could determine literacy development in the different languages.

9. CONCLUSION

This study illustrates that the identification and assessment of dyslexia in bilingual students calls for understanding of the structure of both languages. It is not possible to state categorically that one language poses greater hurdles than another. Assessment must attempt to investigate a child's underlying strengths and weaknesses in relation to the languages of different orthography. Thus, language preference is not necessarily determined by social and family conventions but can be unconsciously determined by a child's individual learning pattern.

Individual differences have to be considered before embarking on a program of remediation. An indepth literacy assessment is required to help a child in a bilingual teaching environment maximize his full learning potential rather than have any complex language issues further undermine his ability.

REFERENCES

Baker, C. (1988). *Key Issues in Bilingualism and Bilingual Education*. Avon: Multilingual Matters.

Bartolo, P.A. (1988). Maltese Word Reading Test. Test Construction Unit, Education Department, Malta.

Boder, E. (1973). Developmental dyslexia: A diagnostic approach based on three atypical reading-spelling patterns. *Develop. Med. Child Neurol., 15*, 663–687.

Dunn, Ll.M., Dunn, L.M., Whetton, C., & Pintilie, D. (1982). *British Picture Vocabulary Scale*. Windsor: NFER-Nelson.

Edbury, J., & Rack, J. (1998). Tackling literacy difficulties in second language learners. *Special Children, 108*, pp. 14–19.

Ellis, N.C., & Hennelly R.A. (1980). A bilingual word-length effect: Implications for intelligence testing and the relative ease of mental calculation in Welsh and English. *British Journal of Psychology, 71*, 43–45.

Firman, C. (1994). Phonological Deficits in Bilingual Dyslexic Learners. Paper presented at the 3rd International Conference of the British Dyslexia Association. Manchester, U.K. April 7, 1994.

Firman, C. (1995). Word Length Effect on Bilingual Dyslexic Learners. Paper presented at the 22nd Annual Conference of The New York Branch of The Orton Dyslexia Society, March 23, 1995.

Frith, U. (1985). Beneath the surface of developmental dyslexia. In K.E. Patterson, J.C. Marshall, & M. Coltheart (eds.), *Surface Dyslexia*. London: Erlbaum.

Frith, U. (1997). Brain, mind and behaviour in dyslexia. In C. Hulme & M. Snowling (eds)., *Dyslexia: Biology, Cognition and Intervention*. London: Whurr.

Goswami, U. (1997). Learning to read in different orthographies, phonological awareness, orthographic representations and dyslexia. In C. Hulme & M. Snowling (eds.), *Dyslexia: Biology, Cognition and Intervention*. London: Whurr.

Grosjean, F. (1992). Another view of bilingualism. In R.J. Harris (ed.), *Advances in Psychology—Cognitive Processing in Bilinguals*. Amsterdam: Elsevier Science Publishers.

Hall, D. (1995). *Assessing the Need of Bilingual Pupils Living in Two Languages*. London: David Fulton Publishers.

Karanth, P. (1992). Developmental dyslexia in bilingual-biliterates. *Reading and Writing: An Interdisciplinary Journal, 4*, 297–306.

Leong, C.K. (1997). What Can we Learn From Dyslexia in Chinese? Paper presented at the International Conference on Dyslexia: Advances in Theory and Practice. Norway, Stavanger, November 22, 1997.

Miller-Guron, L., & Lundberg, I. (1997). Dyslexia and second language reading—A second bite at the apple? Paper presented at the 4th International Conference of the British Dyslexia Association. York, U.K., April 4, 1997.

Miles, T.R. (1983). *Dyslexia: The Pattern of Difficulties*. London: Granada.

Ramaa, S., Miles, T.R., & Lalithamma, M.S. (1993). Dyslexia: Symbol processing difficulty in the Kannada language. *Reading and Writing: An Interdisciplinary Journal, 5*, 29–42.

Salter, R., & Smythe, I. (1997). (eds.). *The International Book of Dyslexia*. London: World Dyslexia Foundation.

Seymour, P. (1994). Variability in dyslexia. In C. Hulme & M. Snowling (eds.), *Reading Development and Dyslexia*. London: Whurr.

Snowling, M. (1985). The assessment of reading and spelling skills. In M. Snowling (ed.), *Children's Written Language Difficulties*. Windsor: NFER-Nelson.

Snowling, M., Hulme, C., & Goulandris, N. (1989). Phonological coding deficits in dyslexia. In G. Hales (ed.), *Meeting Points in Dyslexia: Proceedings of the First International Conference of the British Dyslexia Association*. Reading: British Dyslexia Association.

Stanovich, K.E., Siegel L.S., & Gottardo A. (1997). Progress in the search for dyslexia subtypes. In C. Hulme & M. Snowling (eds.), *Dyslexia: Biology, Cognition and Intervention*. London: Whurr.

Wimmer, H. (1993). Characteristics of developmental dyslexia in a regular writing system. *Applied Psycholinguistics, 14*, 1–33.

Wimmer, H., & Goswami, U. (1994). The influence of orthographic consistency on reading development: Word recognition in English and German children. *Cognition, 51*, 91–103.

4

From Assessment to Teaching

Building a Teaching Program from a Psychological Assessment

Martin Turner and Angie Nicholas

1. INTRODUCTION

Teachers often say a student should not be received into a special education program without first being psychologically assessed. Such a touching faith in the efficacy of such assessments might come as a surprise to some educational psychologists. What are the reasons for this faith? Is it justified? Who can deliver such an assessment?

This chapter will first consider if a special education teacher may acquire the skills necessary to perform an individual psychological assessment. It will next look at the place and structure of such an assessment. From there it will review the assessment features that have particular implications for the teacher who will deliver the education program. We identify some kinds of further information needed. Finally, this chapter examines some external aspects of the management of the teaching, such as liaison and planning of time.

Martin Turner, The Dyslexia Institute, 133 Gresham Road, Staines, Middlesex, TW18 2AJ, United Kingdom   Angie Nicholas, The Dyslexia Institute, 133 Gersham Road, Staines, Middlesex, TW18 2AJ, United Kingdom

2. CAN A SPECIAL EDUCATION TEACHER PERFORM A PSYCHOLOGICAL ASSESSMENT?

An experienced special education teacher, without access to restricted tests,[1] can be trained to produce a serviceable psychological assessment, using psychological tests.

There are, to be sure, some provisos.

A teacher assessor will not be able to make authoritative clinical judgments even though she or he may be experienced in recognizing dyslexia. Such decisions frequently concern the *differential diagnosis* between dyslexia and other developmental disorders with which dyslexia may be confused, or with which it may co-occur. A practitioner needs much training and clinical experience before she or he can formulate these opinions.

Similarly, the opinion of a special education teacher, who has received additional training in psychometric[2] methods, is not usually acceptable as the sole clinical judgment of an individual who may need special arrangements in timed, written, public examinations or who may have special educational needs (SEN). Their opinion is, however, a valuable contribution to a multiprofessional assessment.

A teacher may use tests of ability, and these may furnish some estimate of *general intelligence*. However, the measurement of an IQ implies the use of a restricted or closed test by a qualified psychologist to survey several distinct domains of ability and produce, based on six to 12 such individual test results, a reliable composite score. Because of the long-term predictive significance, justified and unjustified, associated with such measurement, any shorter procedure, using less powerful tests, is best described, not as IQ, but as an *estimate* of general ability.

Dyslexia is a *cognitive deficit*, that is, a specific difficulty with the management of certain kinds of (mainly verbal) information. Psychological tests are therefore indicated to help diagnose this disability. Many other developmental problems are diagnosed by using a range of assessment methods that do not center around testing.

Conversely, the special education teacher has strengths unparalleled in other professions, notably in his or her ability to design and implement a specialized learning program. Here the teacher has a wealth of specific knowledge and experience on which to draw. Moreover the special education teacher's knowledge of tests and testing may already be greater than that of many other professionals.

---

[1] A *restricted* test is one not supplied freely by publishers and distributors to all would-be purchasers. Most test publishers require customers to complete a questionnaire giving details of their professional qualifications. Tests of various levels of restriction are supplied in accordance with these levels of qualification. Codes are assigned to customers as a form of *security clearance*.

[2] *Psychometric psychology* is the term usually applied to the development, construction, use and interpretation of psychological tests.

These factors, together with the teacher's experience with dyslexic individuals, especially if offered as provisional, with caution and respect for evidence, make the findings and recommendations of a teacher's assessment uniquely valuable.

3. THE PLACE OF ASSESSMENT IN GUIDING TEACHING

Any form of assessment will play a fundamental part in determining a student's educational needs. Upon realizing a dyslexic student's specific needs and how this affects his or her classroom performance, the teacher should adopt appropriate methods and strategies.

In almost all cases, the student is being assessed because he has already experienced failure in some aspect of his school career. It is important to be aware of what has gone wrong. This may involve evaluating the student's early background and even considering the family's own history of learning difficulties. Adults are often prompted to seek an educational assessment either because of experiencing difficulty with work aspects, or because they're embarking on a course of further education and need an explanation for the learning barriers which stem from their school career. In all situations it is vital to gather as much background information as possible, as this often provides a useful insight into the provision currently available to the individual and can help determine which recommendations will be effective.

An educational psychologist's assessment will serve to determine the nature of the individual's difficulties. The psychologist is statistically evaluating discrepancies between the individual's ability, information skills, and attainment. The individual's strengths and weaknesses will become evident. The assessment will have provided a unique picture of how these difficulties manifest themselves in all the areas of literacy; reading, spelling, writing, comprehension. Finally, any assessment should provide practical and comprehensible recommendations to those professionals involved with the individual.

A psychologist's report will allow the teacher to identify and clarify a student's disabilities. The inclusion of recommendations for educational support in the classroom, individualized instruction, or test preparation will be valuable. Of equal importance, the report helps the individual understand the nature of his or her difficulties. It is necessary, therefore to include an explanation of how these problems will affect class performance and how the student can be helped to overcome them.

4. THE PLACE OF INTELLIGENCE QUOTIENT TESTS

The place in psychological assessment of tests of general intellectual ability continues to be controversial, perhaps because "such tests tap the most important general way in which people differ psychologically" (Brand, 1996, pp. 1–2).

Accordingly people object to them because they feel these tests objectify human inequalities, and this offends their political sensibilities. But in special education, ability tests are recognized as valuable simply because intellectual ability affects learning ability.

> The relationship between [intelligence] test scores and school performance seems to be ubiquitous. Wherever it has been studied, children with high scores on tests of intelligence tend to learn more of what is taught in school than their lower-scoring peers...intelligence tests...are never the only influence on outcomes, though in the case of school performance they may well be the strongest (Neisser et al., 1996, pp. 77–101, 82–83).

Their use in assessment follows the logic of science and of the controlled experiment. What do we need to know about any individual to predict the likely level of their achievement in learning? *Their age*, would be most people's first answer to this question. If we know a child is ten years old, then we can narrow down somewhat their likely range of achievement. However, ten-year-olds vary widely in their achievement. Therefore the next biggest single contributor to this variance is IQ. This is the single summary statistic that, based on between six and ten subtests, has greater reliability than any of its components.

After we know a person's age and level of general intellectual ability, we can closely predict their level of *expected* scholastic achievement. Other variables may be important, such as their first language (if not English), their absence from school or lack of exposure to adequate teaching, but age and IQ are the most important. If we establish, through administering other tests for reading or spelling that the individual's performance is below expected levels, then this *discrepancy* may be evaluated statistically by two criteria:

1. Is the discrepancy large enough to be distinguished from mere chance variation? Is it statistically significant?
2. If the difference is a real one, and so interpretable, how common or uncommon is this size of gap? How prevalent or acute is this level of underachievement?

The latter can be done most easily in the form of a table (see Table 1).

This estimation of the frequency or *exceptionality* of the individual's problem is the end point of the assessment, furnishing a watertight argument for identification and provision that may be found convincing by all parties.

How do we evaluate, then, and report on the *degree of exceptionality*? This is obviously a matter of personal discretion, but the convention in Table 2 has proved a useful guide. Note that these percentages are not the percentile equivalents of standard scores, but are estimates of the prevalence (or frequency of occurrence)

Table 1. Attainment Scores Expected at Age 8 Years 5 Months on the Basis of an IQ Score of 95

	Expected standard score	Observed standard score	Difference	Statistical Significance	Frequency
Basic Reading	97	74	23	0.01	1%
Spelling	97	72	25	0.01	1%
Reading Comprehension	97	84	13	0.05	10%
Numerical Operations	97	82	15	0.05	10%

of observed levels of statistically significant underachievement. Note, too, that *age equivalent scores* (or reading, spelling, and "mental" ages) are quite inadequate for serious measurement purposes: they simply have no constant meaning (see Table 2).

The assessment of an individual's conceptual ability is integral to any diagnosis of a specific learning disability. A test of an individual's inherent ability provides a crucial baseline from which to measure attainment levels in areas of literacy and numeracy. If we know what an individual is capable of, then we can clearly identify any areas of failure. It is the evidence of a discrepancy between an individual's underlying ability and their levels of achievement in reading, writing, and arithmetic that begins to suggest a picture of specific learning difficulty.

Table 3 illustrates the classification of IQ scores that are obtained from the Wechsler Intelligence Scale For Children 3rd edition (WISC-III[UK], Wechsler, 1992) and the British Ability Scales 2nd edition (Elliott, et al., 1996).

An IQ is commonly given either as a standard score or its direct equivalent, a percentile. Both express performance in relation to an individual's age-peers. For example, someone with a percentile score of 50 in relation to his IQ is performing above 50 percent of the population of others of his own age. The

Table 2. Qualitative Evaluations of Observed Underachievement

Above 25%	An acceptable level of achievement
15–25%	On the low side but not exceptional
10–14%	Unexpected but not extreme
5–9%	Unexpected
Below 5%	Highly unexpected

Table 3. Conventional Classification of IQ Scores by
the Two Main Batteries in Use in the United Kingdom

Full scale IQ or GCA score	% of population in category	Description (WISC-III)	Description (BAS-II)
130 and above	2.2	Very Superior	Very High
120–129	6.7	Superior	High
110–119	16.1	High Average	Above Average
90–109	50.0	Average	Average
80–89	16.1	Low Average	Below Average
70–79	6.7	Low Extreme	Low
69 and below	2.2	Mentally Retarded	Very Low

This table illustrates the classification of IQ scores that are obtained from the Wechsler Intelligence Scale for Children 3rd Edition (WISC-III[UK], Wechsler, 1992) and the British Ability Scales 2nd edition (BAS-II: Elliott et al., 1996).[3]

standard score has an average value by convention of 100 and a standard deviation of 15; that is, two-thirds of the population fall between 100 + 15 and 100 − 15 (or between 85 and 115). This has a constant meaning at every age and is subject only to the technical qualifications of the test used. Table 4 shows the relation of standard scores and percentile equivalents at selected intervals throughout the normal distribution.

Although standard scores describe equal intervals, with equal numbers of possible scores between them, percentile equivalents reveal that most people are actually bunched in the middle or average range, with progressively fewer individuals toward the extremes.

5. DEVELOPMENT AND THE PROFILE OF STRENGTHS AND WEAKNESSES

Learning difficulties may arise from many sources:

- Impairment of vision or hearing, either at an early age or still present; glue ear,[4] for instance, may have caused problems with listening comprehension or short-term auditory memory
- Motor problems, sometimes called dyspraxia or developmental coordination disorder (DCD)
- Problems with spoken language, which may be delayed or deviant

---

[3]The summary score provided by BAS-II is called the GCA or index of General Conceptual Ability.

Table 4. Percentile Equivalents for
Selected Standardized Quotients

Standard score	Percentile equivalent
60	0.4
70	2
80	9
90	25
100	50
110	75
120	91
130	98
140	99.6

- Inherited difficulty in the phonological processing[5] that is central to the learning of print skills
- Health problems resulting in long absences from school
- Frequent changes in schools or a lack of early schooling
- Behavioral and emotional problems, such as poor self-esteem or lack of motivation
- Family difficulties arising from divorce, imprisonment, remarriage, financial problems
- Cultural differences, including the position of English as the learner's second language

One or more of these factors may operate together to create or aggravate a specific learning difficulty.

All such possibilities need to be considered throughout the assessment process and used in the drawing of conclusions, because they may be key to an individual's poor academic performance. The individual may display learning problems despite having satisfactory general intellectual ability. Moreover, repeated school failure may have led to learning failure, frustration, and lack of motivation. However, these may be effects rather than primary causes, and the emotionally disturbed or socially or environmentally disadvantaged individual may well also have dyslexia.

[4]Otitis media.

[5]The ability to hear, store, reproduce, and manipulate the *sounds* of speech, such as the sequence of syllables in *car park* or *barbecue* (rather than *par cark* and *cubeybar*).

Diagnostic testing establishes an individual's proficiency in the processing of information. It is important to emphasize that dyslexia comes from within and is not simply the result of external factors, such as poor teaching or a lack of opportunity.[6] An objective psychometric assessment aims to secure information that reflects an individual's development at the biological or cognitive-developmental level. The dyslexic pupil is likely to have weaknesses in one or more of the following areas:

1. Short-term memory
2. Phonological awareness
3. Speed of information processing

It is worth enumerating some of the many features of learning difficulty that appear in assessment and create obstacles to teaching.

Weak phonological skills make it difficult to segment syllables, distinguish between similar sounding letters, and blend and sequence sounds.

Poor speech and language skills cause difficulties such as word-finding, mishearing, labeling difficulty (right–left, up–down), the use of convoluted explanations, the need to play for time before answering so that information can be successfully processed.

Literacy difficulties are apparent where the pupil exhibits the problems of erratic spelling, avoidance spelling (restriction of vocabulary to words he knows he can spell), poor syntax and punctuation. An individual may be able to read a word on one line but unable to read the same word further down the page. There may be a weakness in comprehension caused by a slowed decoding, which interferes with retention.

Numeracy difficulties often accompany reading disabilities in the younger dyslexic child, because the early stages of mathematics are predominantly verbal. The dyslexic may take longer than expected to perform simple calculations. There may be difficulty in counting backwards or adding long columns of figures. Multiplication tables may be read or written in the wrong order or numbers reversed. The student may need to rely on the use of concrete aids for simple calculations. The language of mathematics may tax poor comprehension skills. Memorizing the order in which to carry out procedures, copying accurately, and confusing mathematical symbols are other problems the dyslexic student may encounter.

Sequencing time, dates, days of the week, and months of the year can be difficult. Remembering the sequence of the alphabet and multiplication tables may cause similar problems. The sequencing of words, sentences, and ideas in continuous prose is often a weakness. The students may also find that he has problems

---

[6]It is assumed that good teaching will lessen and poor teaching aggravate, but these factors may be hard to disentangle when dealing with the effects of dyslexia. For an extreme view that quality of teaching alone explains cases of dyslexia, see McGuinness (1998).

following instructions, completing homework by the date required, and revising previous work.

Motor skills difficulties tend to affect the planning or execution of movement skills, and range from difficulty with dressing, tying shoe laces, using buttons, throwing and catching to the fine motor skills of handwriting, and layout and presentation of work.

Memory difficulties affect the dyslexic student's ability to remember instructions, messages, facts, and formulas and, again, to copy from the blackboard or from books.

Poor organization of work, projects, and belongings can be a feature. Dyslexic individuals often have difficulty with producing the correct equipment at the right time, completing homework on time, or having the books needed for a particular lesson.

Behavior difficulties, even minor ones, can affect concentration, memory, listening skills, and general attentiveness. Students may have difficulty putting thoughts together coherently for writing, coupled with a belief that the less they write, the less they will have to have corrected.

6. THE SURVEY OF ATTAINMENTS

To complete the survey of skills in the psychological or educational assessment, we look for evidence of achievement in the areas of basic academic processes: reading, spelling, writing, and arithmetic. Once again, we need to be able to compare a child with his or her contemporaries and choose, therefore, sensitive, informative and technically modern tests of attainment in these areas.

Unless progress remains rudimentary, reading should always be tested in more than one way. Word recognition is the engine that drives reading. Unless individuals can recognize words out of context fast and accurately, they cannot do complex integrated reading. Comprehension, for instance, depends critically upon the achievement of reasonable fluency. A traditional test of word reading is essential. However, a child's *decoding* skills may be determined by using a *nonword reading* test in which there is no story, no sentence structure, no pictures, and no words. The typical dyslexic person finds this kind of an investigation of his alphabetic coding skills to be difficult. Then there is, for the more advanced reader, integrated passage reading, not necessarily aloud, in which the student is asked purely about the meaning of what is read. A profile can emerge on these three levels of reading, that is characteristic of dyslexics, whose comprehension typically is better than their word recognition, and whose recognition of words is better than their decoding of nonwords (Turner, 1995).

Spelling is easily tested, and all tests of spelling tend to correlate together at high levels. Words are dictated, supplied with sentence context, and repeated: The child writes just the one word. Here the technical consideration is to choose a modern test that reflects current national standards in spelling, because these seem to have declined. An older test, therefore, may exaggerate a student's level of difficulty. Spelling ability, however, may be better on an actual test of spelling than it is in free writing, when the pupil has to integrate creative composition, planning, punctuation, and other writing skills together with spelling.

Of course number skills come to encompass much more than the written arithmetic skills. Nevertheless the latter are affected in dyslexia. In the long term, number skills seem to be less affected than reading skills in dyslexia. It is important not to omit number skills from an assessment. The tendency is to accord them a lesser priority, in spite of their constant utility in daily life, with the result that reading improvements often occur while dereliction in number skills worsens.

7. INTERPRETING THE PSYCHOLOGIST'S REPORT

The special education teacher needs to be able to understand the implications of the skill deficits identified in a psychologist's report. Sometimes the terms used are unfamiliar. Table 5 summarizes several commonly used expressions and explains their meanings.

8. THE VALUE OF EARLY INTERVENTION

Dyslexia cannot be prevented or cured, but the symptoms can be alleviated to some extent. Early identification may lessen the long-term effects if it is supported by effective remediation; this in turn may diminish the effects of the difficulties upon the individual's self-esteem (see also Chapter 1).

The Code of Practice (Department for Education, 1994) states:

> Because early identification should lead to a more timely assessment and intervention which in turn should avoid the escalation of a difficulty into a significant special need, it is important that any concern about a child's development and progress should be shared at the earliest possible moment. (Code of Practice, para 5:16)

There are many helpful checklists for parents and professionals that give developmental indicators of characteristics of specific learning difficulties. However, many signposts can apply at any stage of learning for any child and not specifically the dyslexic child. These performance indicators can only be helpful insofar as they trigger further evaluation to pinpoint areas of weakness in learning development.

It is possible to achieve an accurate learning profile of the young child. There is often concern about the consequences of applying a *label* to any difficulties. Some believe that labeling a child may lead professionals to have negative expectations of that child. There is also the question as to whether or not any weaknesses are because the young child has not yet developed the relevant skills. However, any detailed assessment that labels an individual's problems is really seeking to apply a widely accepted term that will go some way to explaining the nature of the difficulties and prompt the healthy understanding of these difficulties. The child, his parents, and the professionals involved can take some comfort in knowing that the child's problems are due to internal factors beyond their control. This relieves a great deal of pressure on the child himself and all those involved with him educationally because the pathway to effective teaching through understanding has been revealed.

It is important to emphasize that a detailed assessment at an early age is not a panacea for identifying dyslexia. Some students' problems do not become evident until they start high school or even before they take their college entrance examinations. Dyslexia that was previously coped with shows up under pressure at all stages of people's careers, including just before a managerial promotion in middle life. In contrast there are preschool children who exhibit signs of specific learning difficulties.

9. BUILDING A SUCCESSFUL TEACHING PROGRAM

Each dyslexic individual has a unique profile of strengths and weaknesses in learning. The special education teacher must skillfully design a teaching program tailored to each student. The dyslexic student will have specific needs, and each of these needs will have a different priority at any one time. The special education teacher, therefore, must integrate different resources that will successfully enhance the individual's learning. The student may have had programs of remediation in the past but *ad hoc* programs that do not follow a structured, progressive and cumulative design often produce disappointing progress.

When compiling a teaching program for any dyslexic student, the special education teacher must take into consideration the following elements:

1. *Age and ability* of the student
2. A *cumulative, multisensory, structured teaching program* of reading or spelling
3. *Teaching materials and approaches* that support and complement an individualized teaching program
4. A *balance* between the individual's long-term needs and more immediate needs by understanding their learning disabilities and the stage they have reached in their educational career

Table 5. Understanding the Psychologist's Report: Explanations of Some Common Terms

Skill	Means	May cause difficulties in
Short-term auditory memory	Cannot hold information while processing it	Mental arithmetic, multiplication tables, learning by heart, following instructions, spelling, remembering what he or she has heard, attentive listening
Visual memory	Remembering shapes or patterns	Checking spelling, look-and-say reading, copying shapes
Auditory sequencing	Managing sequential order in material heard	Oral spelling or tables, alphabet and reference skills, following sequence of instructions
Visual sequencing	Organizing symbols or shapes in order	Spelling (especially irregular words), copying, arithmetical routines, some aspects of CDT
Visuomotor skill (or hand–eye coordination)	Coordination of vision with movement	Handwriting, ball skills, PE; clumsiness—may spill food, paint
Visuospatial ability	Perception of objects in space, position, distance, speed, abstract form	Page layout, aspects of handwriting, relative size, map work, shape work in mathematics
Listening or auditory comprehension	Understanding the spoken word	Following instructions, attending to any verbal material, including stories; distractible, low attention span, easily confused, slow to learn, especially literacy. May depend on following others, looking at gesture, pointing.

Auditory discrimination	Hearing fine differences between sounds	Even when this is said to be satisfactory there may still be difficulties with sounds of *speech*—rhyme, sounds within words (segmentation)—that are essential for literacy.
Phonological awareness	Perception of sounds within words	Sequence of sounds in words; beginnings and endings of syllables; rhyme; alliteration; identification of individual sounds or blends
Speed of information processing	Mental or clerical speed	Inefficiency with the management of streams of information, especially written symbols, as in copying

Table 6. Selected Literacy Teaching Resources

Literacy Program	Description	Age Application	Strengths
Alpha to Omega (Hornsby and Shear, 1980) Published: Heinemann, 1980	A structured, cumulative program based upon a phonetic hierarchy. It is divided into three sections and gives regular opportunities to test knowledge, understanding, and consolidation	KS 1 and KS 2 Ages 5–11	Emphasis on the sounds of spoken language
Letterland (Wendon, 1987, 1989) Published: Cambridge: Letterland Ltd	Letterland characters reinforce the relationship between letters and sounds. Instructional stories centre around the Letterland characters. Specific spelling rules as such are not taught. The holistic approach incorporates reading for meaning, word recognition and creative writing skills.	KS 1 Ages 5–7	Visual emphasis
The Bangor Dyslexia Teaching System (Miles, 1992) Published: Whurr, 1992	A structured program where the central feature is the teaching of phonetic structures formulated by the Dyslexia Unit at the University of Bangor. Contains both a primary and secondary application and provides age appropriate secondary material.	All ages	Written from the practical experiences of practicing teachers of dyslexic students
Teaching Reading Through Spelling (Prince, et al., 1992) Published: Frondeg Hall Technical Publishing, 1992	A structured, cumulative phonics program based on the original Orton-Gillingham Program.	All ages	A clear and detailed structure that can also be accessed by the class teacher

Program	Description	Ages	Comment
DISTAR (e.g., Engelmann, et al., 1983, 1988; Dixon and Engelmann, 1979, 1990) Published: SRA, 1998	Direct Instruction System of Teaching Arithmetic and Reading: The reading programs include both decoding and reading comprehension; spelling programs use morphology.	All ages	Independent comparative research strongly favors direct instruction programs
Active Literacy Kit (Walter Bramley) Published: LDA, 1998	A program designed to develop the skills of basic literacy through structured activities so that they develop accuracy, fluency, and automaticity.	All ages	Suitable for all literacy difficulties and applicable to individual or group teaching
The Dyslexia Institute Literacy Programme (DILP: Walker and Brooks, 1993)	Currently the fullest development of the Hickey structured cumulative phonic and multisensory literacy teaching programme. Published only as courseware for the Dyslexia Institute Postgraduate Diploma with the University of York.	All ages	A highly structured and detailed programme for both reading and spelling
Units of Sound (Bramley, 1994, 1998) Published: LDA	An audiovisual program of reading, spelling, and comprehension.	Ages 9 and above.	Structured and cumulative program
Developing Literacy for Study and Work (Bramley, 1993) Published: LDA	Teaching programs for spelling, writing, and study.	KS 3 and above Ages 11 and up	Versatile literacy resource for older individuals
Spelling Made Easy: MultiSensory Structured Spelling (Brand, 1989) Published: Egon Press	A comprehensive spelling program focusing on developing and applying spelling skills.	Primary and secondary Ages 5–16	A resource for whole school policy and classroom work

5. Inclusion of the principle of *overlearning* at every stage
6. Elevation of *self-esteem* and self-belief

A student's age and ability directly influence the teaching approaches adopted. For any teaching to be successful, all elements must challenge and motivate the individual student and must take into account his or her intellectual ability. A high school student may have skill deficits similar to an elementary school student but may need a different pace and presentation of concepts.

A special education teacher usually includes reading and spelling in any structured teaching program. Inevitably the choice of teaching program will to some extent be determined by availability and teacher familiarity but this must not be at the expense of a consideration of its individual suitability and effectiveness for the student. Table 6 is an overview of the many highly structured and individualized teaching programs available and designed for use by the special education teacher.

Dyslexic students typically have poor short-term memories. Therefore, continued revision and reinforcement of previous work taught are necessary to ensure that the work is stored for maximum effective retrieval. This need not mean that a lesson's content becomes repetitive and tedious. On the contrary, previous knowledge is incorporated into the progressive teaching program and this, in turn, serves as a constant review of progress. It also serves to indicate through a continual diagnostic process whether weaknesses are being addressed.

Students can be motivated and their self-esteem raised by continuously encouraging their strengths and talents throughout the teaching process. Learning disabilities should only be highlighted in the context of deriving alternative strategies, which should be broken down into small, achievable targets. Many dyslexic students, feeling that they have failed totally, blame themselves and it is the responsibility of all who work with the individual to create opportunities for realistic and genuine success so that self-belief is restored, albeit through a gradual process. At the same time, there will be dyslexic students who fall back upon their dyslexia as an excuse for weak performance rather than work to overcome their personal difficulties.

A core literacy program often relies upon additional support materials or resources. These cater to the student's specific needs and provide a method of bridging skill areas into their specific studies. For example, a student who has weak study skills will require specifically targeted work.

Although integral to the teaching of the dyslexic individual, each of the previously listed schemes will not in isolation be a sufficient course of remediation. There are many other skill areas that would need, if they were areas of weakness, to be addressed. The teacher must clarify what vital skills need to be built up at any one time. Given the constraints of timetables and the amount of time available for special education, the teacher should prioritize issues despite everyone's desire to alleviate all problems simultaneously. The teacher must consider whether the following skills areas should be included in a teaching program in light of any assessment.

1. Organization
2. Information processing
3. Improving speed
4. Study skills
5. Information technology, including keyboard skills
6. Written work as a whole
7. Oral communication
8. Motor skills
9. Social skills

For the special education teacher, the psychological assessment is a starting point for teaching. An assessment may provide a profile of the individual's learning strengths and weaknesses, however, it may not be deep enough to help the special education teacher design a successful, individual teaching program. If the assessment does not give enough information about the individual's behavior and attitude to learning, then the teacher should collect additional information from both school and home.

10. THE INDIVIDUAL'S ATTITUDE TO HIS OR HER LEARNING DIFFICULTY

Each individual will have unique problems. Therefore, any teaching program must be specific and allow students to work from their strengths while special education teachers work to strengthen their weaknesses. It is important equally to weigh strengths and weaknesses. This enables the teacher to design a teaching program that provides a balanced but specific learning regime tailored to the student. A successful and effective teaching program will use the individual's strengths in learning to support and develop that individual's weaknesses in learning. By considering the individual's strengths, the teacher can accurately determine his or her learning style.

Students must be closely in tune with their own learning styles, and it is the role of the teacher to encourage experimentation with learning styles. No modality is reliable because it may change according to the subject or task in question. The individual may need to use all senses to ensure the effective transfer of information to long-term memory.

11. LIAISON WITH THE STUDENT'S SCHOOL

Here there are both advantages and disadvantages. Such liaison may:

- Increase awareness of student's specific difficulties
- Gain consistency of approach and attitude toward student
- Enable more effective planning of short-term objectives
- Enable a more effective system of review and monitoring

Equally, however, such liaison may:

- Be time-consuming
- Be interpreted as threatening, while
- Methods of communication often rely on the student remembering to circulate pieces of paper!

Liaison with the student's school is a fundamental aspect of any teaching program, though it must always be approached with diplomacy and tact. It is important to raise awareness of the individual's difficulties in as many of his or her teachers as possible. Teachers need to feel that they can help effectively, using their own expertise. A teacher may feel threatened or vulnerable, or feel their skills as a teacher are being scrutinized, or that the student's dyslexia is a result of their poor teaching.

Provision and recommendations for teaching should take into account how the classroom environment can be adapted so that the dyslexic student can have access to the daily curriculum just as much as his nondyslexic peers. Ongoing communication is crucial for schools that are working to the best of their abilities to help the dyslexic student. Still more advantageous is the special education teacher working regularly within the school. Where the special education teacher is independent of the student's school, a large responsibility for lines of communication falls upon the student's parents.

12. THE USE OF SCARCE TIME

Time provision is an important consideration when creating a teaching program or writing recommendations after an assessment. There are no reliable predictions for how long an individual may require special provision. It is rare for an individual to receive individual attention throughout their whole school career. Effective teaching must therefore effectively target the individual's current needs. Identification, too, must be effective and early; if remediation begins during a child's first two years at school then there is likely to be less need for prolonged periods of individual support. If the child progresses through school without his difficulties being recognized, then the gap between his performance and that of his peers widens to such an extent that the amount of time needed for special education may be greater than special education resources or financial constraints will allow.

A seven-year-old child who has mild specific learning difficulties can often be helped within the mainstream classroom by the class teacher, who has some assistance. Effective improvement can be achieved through weekly tutoring sessions lasting no more than an hour.

As mildly affected individuals progress through their school careers, they begin to specialize in curriculum subjects, perhaps shedding some that cause them especial difficulty and lessening the amount of time needed for individualized support. If these individuals continue to receive support in English, they may be expected to perform satisfactorily without support in other curriculum areas.

Nevertheless other curriculum areas may present a continuing need. Work may need to be differentiated in respect of difficulties in written output rather than intellectual presentation. For example, the language of course textbooks should be accessible to the student, if possible including both those with sophisticated vocabulary skills and those with spoken language difficulties. The special education teacher working within the school may be effective in this context. However, the special education teacher working outside the school can only suggest and recommend.

The special education teacher, whether working within or outside the student's school, will need advance knowledge of the curriculum content for the term or academic year. In this way preparation can be made, foundations laid and consolidated, and weak short-term memory difficulties aided. Subject-specific vocabulary can be focused upon, study skills relevant to course assignments targeted and practiced. Students can benefit when greater time is given to literature to be studied. New mathematical concepts can be tackled and, when later encountered by the dyslexic student in a classroom situation, met with familiarity and confidence.

The depth of effective teaching and support may be dependent upon:

- The local education authority's policies and resources
- Teacher knowledge and training
- Faculty or department attitudes at the school

There are great differences in the provision available from state to state and area to area as these factors all have a direct influence upon the resources available. The purchase, allocation, and application of appropriate resources depend also, however, on the expertise and awareness of those involved with the education of the dyslexic student.

With the introduction and implementation in Britain of the National Literacy Strategy and in particular with the Literacy Hour, it is now even more vital that the dyslexic student be supported effectively within the classroom and his specific needs addressed, since there is now still less time for special education within the timetable. Any time allowed for specialist provision has to be incorporated in all English lessons where possible, making the implementation of individual training programs far more of a challenge.

13. TWO CASE STUDIES

When building an individual teaching program the teacher must analyze in great detail a wide range of skill areas. The aim is to compile as complete a picture as possible of the individual's strengths and needs. However, the skill of the teacher lies in the ability to combine and even prioritize the areas that require attention. The correct balance will determine the student's future success and improved self-esteem.

The following two cases show how assessment findings were used to create an individual special education program.

Sarah
9 years, 11 months

Summary of Attainments

Verbal IQ	116	86th percentile	above average
Nonverbal IQ	101	53rd percentile	average
Full Scale IQ	109	73rd percentile	high average
Word Recognition	95	38th percentile	9 years, 4 months
Decoding Skills	89	24th percentile	8 years, 1 month
Word Comprehension	97	42nd percentile	9 years, 5 months
Passage Comprehension	95	36th percentile	9 years, 2 months
Global Reading	94	36th percentile	9 years, 2 months
Comprehension	96	40th percentile	9 years, 4 months
Spelling	95	36th percentile	average
Arithmetic	91	27th percentile	average

Pattern of Strengths and Weaknesses
Strengths in Learning:
- Verbal intelligence
- Phonological awareness

Weaknesses in Learning
- Short-tem working memory
- Visual memory
- Spelling
- Numeracy

General Intellectual Ability
The Kaufmann Brief Intelligence Test (K-BIT), which measures verbal and nonverbal skills, was used for this assessment. Sarah's general conceptual ability places her at percentile rank 73 (above that of 73 percent of pupils at her chronological age).This would be described as being high average, so it should naturally follow that Sarah achieves a similar ability level with respect to her literacy and numeracy skills.

There was quite a marked difference between Sarah's verbal and nonverbal skills.

Conclusions
Sarah is a delightful girl who is clearly not functioning at a similar level to her peers. She is performing consistently at slightly below her chronological age. However, her general conceptual ability suggests this is still further below her potential. At her current level of functioning, she is undoubtedly experiencing a great deal of frustration with her literacy skills.

Sarah shows some evidence of having specific learning difficulties (dyslexia).

Recommendations
Sarah's current specific needs can be best addressed through a structured, cumulative multisensory program of reading and spelling. This will improve automation in reading and spelling and bring these to a more functional level so that she can access the National Curriculum. All teaching must allow for regular opportunities for the consolidation and revision of skills acquired. Auditory and visual memory skills can also be developed through multisensory teaching. As well as raising the level of spelling and reading it is also vital that Sarah is helped to improve her reading comprehension and the standard and speed of both her handwriting and written work.

Above all, Sarah needs to have her self confidence raised within the classroom by experiencing success. Classwork and homework that is sensitively differentiated to allow her to demonstrate her understanding rather than highlight her difficulties with basic educational attainments could achieve this. Tasks need to be broken down into small manageable chunks.

The following aims and resources could be identified as being those appropriate to dealing effectively with Sarah's individual needs:

To Improve Reading Accuracy and Spelling
Units of Sound (published LDA, Duke Street, Wisbech, Cambridgeshire PE13 2AE). This is a structured program, developed by The Dyslexia Institute over twenty years, which encourages independent and active learning. It is available on audio cassette and CD-ROM.

The following structured spelling programs would be suitable for equipping Sarah with effective reading and spelling skills:

> *Spelling Made Easy* by Violet Brand
> *Alpha to Omega* by Bévé Hornsby

To Improve Sight Vocabulary
Sarah must be helped to build her sight word vocabulary by targeting the reading and spelling of high frequency words such as those listed in the Murray and McNally Word List.

To Develop a Joined, Legible, Cursive Style of Handwriting
Sarah must be taught correct letter formation initially leading on to cursive script which can be taught simultaneously with spelling patterns.

To Improve Speed and Fluency of Writing
Create opportunities for speed writing whereby Sarah is given a list of ten nouns and has ten minutes in which to write a short passage, or initially form ten sentences. Also it is important to explore ways in which she can plan and organize her work.

To Improve and Develop Effective Study Skills
Sarah will need tutoring in study skills which should include strategies for organizing thoughts and planning writing, memory training.

To Improve Sequencing Skills
Sarah must be given strategies for sequencing the months of the year.

Sarah would benefit from at least two sessions of additional support a week (totaling 2 hours), where the methodology is based on cumulative multisensory techniques.

Colin
26 years, 11 months

Summary of Attainments

Verbal IQ	90	25th percentile	average
Nonverbal IQ	96	39th percentile	average
General IQ	92	30th percentile	average
Word Recognition	85	16th percentile	14 years, 0 months
Decoding Skills	105	63rd percentile	18 years, 6 months
Word Comprehension	88	20th percentile	15 years, 9 months
Passage Comprehension	87	19th percentile	13 years, 10 months
Global Reading Score	91	27th percentile	14 years, 0 months
Spelling	59	0.7th percentile	low extreme

Pattern of Strengths and Weaknesses
Strengths in Learning
• Nonverbal reasoning
• Decoding skills

Weaknesses in Learning
• Short-term auditory memory
• Phonological processing
• Sight vocabulary
• Reading comprehension

Background
Colin is currently attending college where he is studying for a National Vocational Qualification in Landscapes and Ecosystems. There is a background of learning difficulties from Colin's school career when no remediation was available. Consequently Colin may not have achieved

his true potential at school. He wishes to pursue a career in conservation management, and so it is necessary that he is able to reach his potential to gain access from his current studies.

General Intellectual Ability
The Kaufmann Brief Intelligence Test (K-BIT), which measures verbal and nonverbal skills, was used for this assessment. Colin's general conceptual ability places him at percentile rank 30 (above that of 30 percent of individual's of his chronological age). This would be described as average and so Colin should achieve a similar level of achievement in literacy and numeracy skills.

Conclusions
Colin shows some evidence of having specific learning difficulties (dyslexia). This can be seen in the differences between his general ability and relative attainment levels in reading and spelling, which are below his expected potential. Diagnostic tests relevant to specific learning difficulties highlight weaknesses of phonological processing and auditory short-term memory.

At this current level of functioning, Colin undoubtedly experiences a great sense of frustration as he is unable to use the written word to express himself. He may also find that he has an increasing difficulty in deriving accurate meaning from text, as his studies become more sophisticated and demanding.

Recommendations
Colin would benefit from additional support based upon cumulative multi-sensory techniques in order to alleviate his under-functioning in reading and particularly in spelling. This will raise automaticity in spelling and reading and bring them to a more functional level. All teaching must allow for the regular consolidation and revision of skills acquired.

This additional support should also aim to improve Colin's reading comprehension and accuracy of reading by developing an understanding of reading strategies. There should be regular opportunities to improve his ability to gather accurate detail and respond to viewpoints from exposure to a variety of styles of literature.

As well as Colin's level of spelling and reading comprehension, it is vital that Colin is helped to improve the standard, speed and presentation of his written work. A structured program of study skills that will help him to approach his studies with greater efficiency with respect to time would be of extreme importance.

14. SUMMARY

Special education teachers, through both their knowledge of tests and testing and their knowledge of effective teaching methods, play a vital assessment role. They have strengths that cannot be easily replicated by other professions, most notably in their ability to design and implement a teaching program.

Although the measurement of IQ remains the domain of the psychologist, the special education teacher is able to apply an estimated measure of general intelligence by using shorter and less powerful tests. Although the judgment of a special education teacher, who has received additional training in psychometric testing, is not usually accepted as sole judgment in the case of an individual who may need special arrangements, it is a valuable contribution to a multiprofessional assessment.

Early identification of a specific learning difficulty may lessen the long term effects if supported by effective remediation. Early intervention relieves the negative emotions of guilt and shame and the emotional stresses relating to failure. It also makes financial sense through the ability to provide remediation and support for a far shorter length of time.

When compiling a successful teaching program, the special education teacher will take into consideration the dyslexic student's specific needs and the varying priority of these needs. The teacher must also consider these factors when designing a teaching program: age and ability of the student; the use of structured teaching programs; teaching materials that complement and motivate; appropriate balance and pace; the inclusion of overlearning opportunities and the constant but credible raising of self-belief on the part of the student.

Liaison with a student's school can have as many advantages as disadvantages but must be seen as fundamental to any teaching program. Always to be approached with diplomacy and tact, it should not be a form of liaison which is left solely to student and parents. Special education teachers have an obligation to the student to help to raise awareness of their specific and individual learning needs amongst the teachers who are doing their best to guide them through their educational journey.

REFERENCES

Bramley, W. (1993). *Developing Literacy for Study and Work*. Staines, Middlesex: The Dyslexia Institute.

Bramley, W. (1994). *Units Of Sound*, second edition. Staines, Middlesex: The Dyslexia Institute.

Bramley, W. (1998). *Units of Sound*, CD-rom third edition. Wisbech, Cambridgeshire: The Dyslexia Institute.

Brand, C. (1996). *The g Factor*. Chichester, West Sussex: Wiley.

Brand, V. (1989). *Spelling Made Easy*. London: Egon.

Department for Education. (1994). *Code of Practice on the Identification and Assessment of Special Educational Needs*. London: HMSO, May 1994.

Elliott, C.D., Smith, P., & McCulloch, K. (1996). *British Ability Scales Second Edition* (BAS II). Windsor, Berks: NFER-Nelson.

Engelmann, S., Carnine, L., & Johnson, G. (1988). *Corrective Reading Programs*. Chicago: Science Research Associates.

Engelmann, S., Haddox, P., & Bruner, E. (1983). *Teach Your Child to Read in 100 Easy Lessons*. London: Simon and Schuster.

Hornsby, B., & Shear, F. (1980). *Alpha to Omega: The A–Z of Teaching Reading, Writing and Spelling*, third edition. London: Heinemann.

McGuinness, D. (1998). *Why Children Can't Read—And What We Can Do About It*. Harmondsworth, Middlesex: Penguin Books.

Miles, E. (1992). *The Bangor Dyslexia Teaching System*, second edition. London: Whurr.

Neisser, U., Boodoo, G., Bouchard, T.J., Boykin, A.W., Brody, N., Ceci, S.J., Halpern, D.F., Loehlin, J.C., Perloff, R., Sternberg, R.J., & Urbina, S. (1996). Intelligence: Knowns and unknowns. *American Psychologist, 51,* 77–101 and 82–83.

Prince, M., Cowdery, L., Morse, P., & Low, S. (1992). *Teaching Reading through Spelling: The Kingston Programme (8 books).* Wrexham, Clwyd: Frondeg Hall Technical Publishing.

Turner, M. (1995). Assessing reading: Layers and levels. *Dyslexia Review, 7*(1), 15–19.

Walker, J., & Brooks, L. 1993. *Dyslexia Institute Literacy Programme.* London: James and James.

Wechsler, D. (1992). *Wechsler Intelligence Scale for Children,* third edition UK (WISC-III[UK]). New York: Harcourt Brace Jovanovich.

Wendon, L. (1989). *First Steps in Letterland.* Barton, Cambridge: Letterland Ltd.

Wendon, L. (1987). *Big Strides in Letterland.* Barton, Cambridge: Letterland Ltd.

5

Teaching Basic Reading and Spelling

Jean Walker

1. INTRODUCTION

The dyslexic student fails to read and spell at the level of his intellectual and social group, and this failure is unexpected in view of his ability. He does not pick up literacy skills "naturally," that is, by the teaching methods which are adequate for the majority of his peers. He is taxed by the synchronization of skills required for reading and spelling. He is, by definition, hard to teach. It is important to his self-esteem and for his survival in school and the working world that he learn the skills of literacy. His struggles with the written word attract growing numbers of interested parties, researchers, and theorists who try to understand what is going wrong as well as teachers and helpers who produce toolkits to fix the problem. It is the special education teacher who combines theory and practice to bring a coherent understanding and rationale to the teaching. There are four areas in which she needs to be knowledgeable and in which she will constantly augment and deepen her understanding.

1. Normal acquisition of literacy for the competent reader and speller
2. Particular difficulties of her dyslexic learner
3. Principles of multisensory teaching
4. Structure of words, and the organization of written English

Jean Walker, The Dyslexia Institute, 53 Queen Street, Sheffield, S1 1UG, United Kingdom

I will deal briefly with each of these topics in turn, before discussing practical teaching within a structured language program, some problems which a student may encounter; and suggestions for dealing with them.

For the sake of clarity, I will refer to the dyslexic student as "he" and the teacher as "she," which incidentally reflects the gender distribution of the majority of dyslexic learners and special education teachers.

2. THE NORMAL ACQUISITION OF LITERACY

The researchers and theorists produce models of reading and spelling which can illuminate how the normal reader acquires literacy.

Uta Frith (1985) presents a model of reading development, positing that the normal child progresses through three stages: logographic, alphabetic, and finally orthographic. She points out the importance of acquiring accurate grapheme–phoneme links in the alphabetic stage, and the crucial role of kinesthetic learning when the beginner reader shapes his letters and says their sounds. Thus the young reader becomes aware of the details of the shapes and sound of each letter and begins to feel familiarity and ownership with those vital 26 letters.

The Seidenberg and McClelland (1989) (Figure 1) model shows the interconnecting processes involved in reading. It reminds us that the skilled reader

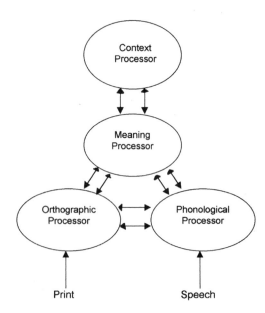

Figure 1. Model of word reading. Adapted from Seidenberg and McClelland, 1989 (in Firth, 1990).

processes print at several levels simultaneously. It is the complexity of this task, particularly the very accurate timing and sequencing of the skills that is so amazingly synchronized in the competent learner–reader. Thus begins the virtuous upward spiral of the child who has cracked the code, and is acquiring the synchronized skills of phonology, along with knowledge of the orthography and morphology of words. For these processes to work smoothly other attributes are also needed. The successful reader and speller also has the following skills:

- Attention and listening. He can attend to the target written word or to the relevant sounds or speaker (Borwick and Townend, 1993).
- Adequate phonological awareness. He is aware of the patterns of sounds in words, such as rhyming, and alliteration and he can segment speech sounds (Bryant and Bradley, 1985; Snowling, 1987).
- The use of analogy to appreciate orthographic patterns. Good readers use existing knowledge to generalize and read new words (by knowing "peak," he can read "beak") (Goswami & Bryant, 1990).
- Accurate awareness of letters. The young child who knows the alphabet on school entry is at a reading advantage (Adams, 1990).
- Adequate fine motor control to learn to write letters, linked to their sounds and names. Automaticity in such motor responses is needed for fluency in literacy skills (Fawcett and Nicolson, 1994).
- Adequate visual memory for words to check if a spelled word "looks wrong" (Peters and Smith, 1993).

As children begin to read what interests them, they practice all these skills concurrently and so constantly improve their processing of the written word.

3. THE DYSLEXIC LEARNER

The dyslexic learner fails to adequately acquire many of the previously described skills. His teacher must be aware of where his weaknesses may lie:

- *Attention and listening.* He has trouble understanding an array of symbols and has difficulty in linking sounds to those symbols correctly. His attention may wander because he receives little reward from his efforts to concentrate.
- *Phonological awareness.* He is particularly vulnerable to difficulties in phonological processing and short-term memory. He is used to fuzzy representations of words in his own lexicon so that words which are similar in sound may become confused. ("Specific" and "pacific" sound the same, and he may hear "bet" and "bed" as the same word.) Phonemic awareness is needed not only in initial reading, but also

when acquiring new, more complex vocabulary ("metamorphosis" in biology and "reformation" in history).

- *Use of analogy.* With poor phonological awareness, the dyslexic learner has very little appreciation of patterns in words and, therefore, does not use analogy as a reading or spelling strategy. He may learn a single word well, such as "bend," but be unable to use the information about that word to decode other words such as "mend," "send," and "spend" and fail to perceive it as the base word in "bending."
- *Letter awareness.* His memory for sequences is poor. He cannot remember the order of the alphabet or the match between the name and shape of individual letters.
- *Automaticity.* He has difficulty linking the handwritten shape of the letter to its sound. This is not an automatic response for him. If phoneme–grapheme links are laborious, then higher level skills, such as planning the story and sequencing the words, will be accordingly slowed down. For the dyslexic learner, such multitasking leads to overload, confusion, and panic.
- *Visual memory.* His visual memory for words is poor, so reading is difficult. He may not distinguish visually between "felt" and "left" or "difficult" and "different." Correct spelling is very difficult because he cannot tell if a word "looks right."

As these weaknesses have a direct impact on his learning, the dyslexic student often cannot make progress when taught by teaching methods which work well for other students. He may have failed at understanding reading and spelling, because of the teaching methods used, before arriving to the special education teacher for help.

3.1. Reading Instruction

3.1.1. Using His Strengths

Teachers are often told to teach to the child's strongest channels. If the student has a good visual memory, then he should learn to read using a visual approach, such as a whole word method. However, a single sensory channel is insufficient. Both visual and phonological processing is needed for reading.

3.1.2. Look-and-Say, or Whole Word Method

The whole word method is mainly a visual approach. It encourages the student to look at the outline shapes of words and guess from the context. However, we know that good readers notice the fine details of letters in words. (Adams,

1990). The dyslexic student, therefore, needs to have his attention directed to the letters and structure of each word, not just its outline shape.

3.1.3. Phonics

Phonics teaching directs the student's attention to grapheme–phoneme links, but is often introduced as /b/ "buh is for bat." Further digraphs and letter strings are often not taught systematically enough to allow him to decode words which are presented to him. So for example, having learned some single letter sounds, including the letter **b**, he may be asked to read bun, bat, brick, bake, beak. But he is unable to cope with the consonant blend /br/, the /a-e/, or the /ea/ digraph as these patterns have not been taught. Phonics teaching is rarely sufficiently detailed, thorough or cumulative for the dyslexic student. A purely phonic approach cannot help much with irregular words such as "said," "through" and "laugh."

3.1.4. Real Books

The Real Books practice is based on the philosophy that children learn to read by reading; that, given stimulating materials, and a skilled reader to model the process for them, the failing readers will be motivated to learn. This tends to ignore the complexities of subskills which make up the reading process. The patient parents of many a dyslexic child will attest that this is just too much to expect. Such overload leads to confusion and panic, and very little learning, apart from wild guessing.

3.2. Spelling Instruction

Often children have had next to no formal instruction in spelling but may have spelling words to learn at home. Some methods of teaching and practicing spelling, such as visually based schemes or rote learning of lists, do not work for the dyslexic learner:.

3.2.1. A Spelling Word List

A spelling word list may have one or two spelling patterns, for example:

- beat
- stream
- bread
- deaf
- sigh
- right
- fright

The dyslexic child may not notice the patterns "ea" and "igh," nor realize that the "ea" has two sounds here /ē/ and / /ĕ/ and that the "igh" represents the sound /ī/, and is usually followed by **t**. A great deal of explicit teaching and practice would be needed for the dyslexic student to establish each of these patterns in memory, individually, before being presented together.

3.2.2. Spelling Rules

Spelling rules include rules such as "**i** before **e** except after **c**" or doubling the consonant before a vowel suffix in words like "shopping" or "bidder." These rules appeal to teachers, because their bright dyslexic students often understand the rule well. However, spelling is not an intellectual exercise like a crossword puzzle, and teachers are often disappointed that such students fail to remember and apply the rules in their own writing.

3.2.3. Look, Cover, Write, Check

The Look, Cover, Write, Check method, introduced by Charles Cripps, (Cripps, 1988) is widely and successfully used with many children. Its premise is spelling is learned by visual inspection and by the motor memory of handwriting patterns. For dyslexic children, this method omits the grapheme–phoneme links and letter naming, thus excluding the important part of the alphabetic principle which underlines the English spelling system.

3.2.4. Dealing with Spelling Mistakes

Children will inevitably misspell words. Some spelling instruction focuses only on correcting a child's mistakes. Spelling mistakes are dealt with in several ways by teachers:

3.2.4.1. Uncorrected. Uncorrected errors may be ignored by a teacher who wants to encourage freeflow creative writing and does not want to discourage a student by covering the work in corrections. This can lead to well-practiced misspellings. A teenager will continue to write "befor" if the error is never corrected.

3.2.4.2. Writing out. The student must write out several times the corrected spelling of a word. Unless the teacher's writing is very clear, this can misfire with the student copying incorrectly. Mere copying does not help the student see word structure or remember it.

3.2.5. Topic Spellings

For children writing about a class topic, spelling of new words appropriate to the topic are given (e.g., pharaoh, pyramid, mummy). Such words have a semantic theme but lack spelling patterns or word structure consistency. This just reinforces the dyslexic child's belief that spelling is a mystery with neither rhyme nor reason to it. He cannot learn much about the spelling regularities of his own language in this way.

So how does the dyslexic learner need to learn?

4. PRINCIPLES OF MULTISENSORY TEACHING

Generations of teachers have been puzzled by the problem of the average or bright child who is difficult to teach when he tries to read and spell. Special education teachers, increasingly strongly backed by research, continue to use and refine structured, multisensory methods for dyslexic children. These methods have long been established as necessary for dyslexic students. Gillingham and Stillman (1958), in collaboration with the neurologist Samuel Orton (1967), first trialled and promulgated methods which were structured, cumulative and multisensory. In Britain, Kathleen Hickey (1977) and Beve Hornsby (1975) used the same principles, adapted to the sounds and spelling of British English. According to these principles, teaching should be:

- Multisensory
- Phonic
- Structured
- Cumulative
- Sequential

4.1. Multisensory

The multisensory approach relates most directly to the need to change the dyslexic person's neural pathways so his fuzzy representations of oral and written language become clear, direct, automatic. Just as physiotherapy aims to reestablish responses in the muscles, multisensory teaching aims to establish

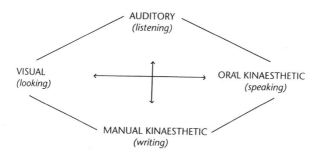

Figure 2. The four modalities of the multisensory approach. (From Walker & Brooks, 1996.)

automatic responses to phonemes and graphemes, leaving more working memory available for higher thinking and writing skills.

The multisensory approach is based on the knowledge that we use four sensory modalities for reading and spelling: visual, auditory, oral kinesthetic, and manual kinesthetic (see Figure 2).

In terms of literacy, we learn through the channels of looking, listening, speaking, and writing. When the normal learner reads a new word, he looks at the letters in the word, links each to the remembered sound, and pronounces the word—thus using three modalities.

When spelling, he hears the sounds in the word, repeats them to himself, produces the hand movement to give the correct shape for each letter, then checks it visually against the remembered spelling of the word. Thus he uses all four modalities.

However one or more of these modalities is likely to be weak in a dyslexic student. By learning in a multisensory way, he will learn to use them in synchrony. This will make full use of his strengths while awakening and integrating his weak areas in the process.

Initial multisensory learning ensures grapheme–phoneme correspondence at a basic behaviorist, connectionist level. The speed, strength, and timing of these connections then need to be increased (Adams, 1990). This gives a firm basis for the important higher order skills.

4.2. Phonic

A phonic approach is necessary to decode a writing system, such as English, which is based on an alphabetic–phonetic system. Because it works with an alphabet of 26 letters and a language which is conveyed in about 44 phonemes, phonics need to be taught as more than a 1:1 correspondence. So not only does the student need to know single letter sounds: that the letter **b** makes the sound /b/, but also the sound associated with groups of letters such as "igh" /ī/ and "tion" /shun/. Once the regularities of a phonic system are established and the student has cracked the code, then irregular words can be dealt with.

4.3. Structured

The structure chosen should follow the structure of the English language. The segmentation skills required should be taught within the structure and include phoneme segmentation and blending, syllable segmentation, and analysis and synthesis of affixes.

A particular program may include a structured letter order, governing the sequence in which the graphemes are introduced to the student (Hickey, 1977; Dyslexia Institute Literacy Programme, 1996).

4.4. Cumulative and Sequential

Cumulative and sequential aspects can hardly be separated in any well thought-out language program. The structure of the English language should be presented in a clear sequence so that simple responses and concepts are taught before more complex ones. Each new concept is taught thoroughly and the practice tasks incorporate only those points which have been previously learned, in a gradually accumulating set of skills.

Table 1 summarizes the reason for each principle in relation to the requirements of written English and to the needs of the dyslexic learner.

4.5. Memory

Memory plays an important role in any teaching program for dyslexic students. Strategies for remembering are incorporated into the routines of structured multisensory programs, especially when establishing the links between letters and sounds. Some structured programs have reminders, such as reading and spelling cards, built into their system. These are to be practiced to provide the necessary overlearning. Memory strategies are used, such as the grouping and classifying of words, spelling choices, and suffixing rules, to help the dyslexic student remember some language patterns. For important irregular words, mnemonics may be devised. Audio feedback through self-voice recording may help extend auditory memory when students are reading or spelling.

Overlearning is a necessary means of improving memory. Language tasks and concepts need to be revisited several times, perhaps using the same vocabulary in a different context. It is important to revisit the original word list or prose to see if the student can read it again more quickly and fluently. The stop watch will give measurable evidence of improvement.

5. LEARNING THE STRUCTURE OF ENGLISH SPELLING

Special education teachers must be aware of the structure of English orthography. English is a synonym-rich, luxurious language which has derived from many other languages. English spelling appears to be illogical and inconsistent. In its orthography we have preferred to maintain the history of the language as in the Old English "knight," the French word "station," and in Greek spellings such as "psychology," instead of a more phonetic representation which is often demanded by spelling reform groups.

So English readers and spellers have to learn not only a one-to-one correspondence of letters to sounds which would be found in a transparent language such as Italian and Swahili, but also the more colorful irregular spellings which

Table 1. Why Use Multi-Sensory Teaching?

Principle	Description	Written English	Relevant skills to Dyslexic Student
MULTI-SENSORY	Links four sensory modalities: visual, auditory, oral and manual.	Words need to be seen and read: heard and spelled.	The student must use all four sensory channels in synchrony to reinforce strong modalities, imrpove the weak ones and ensure automaticity.
PHONIC	Links graphemes to phonemes.	English is basically an alphabetic-phonetic system.	Student with poor phonologial awareness must improve phonic skills.
STRUC-TURED	An imposed order of presentation of graphemes, ortho-graphic patterns and concepts.	The language can largely be ordered and classified into a coherent system of patterns and regularities.	The dyslexic student may show good understanding of rules and classification. By applying this skill to language he can use analogy and reduce the burden of learning.
CUMULA-TIVE	Built up in small steps, to ensure mastery of each, before progressing to the next.	Simple letters build into morphemes and thence into longer words.	The dyslexic student is slow to establish automatic responses. They ensure he can consolidate single responses before more complex skills.
SEQUEN-TIAL	Simple responses and concepts are taught before more complex ones. Easy before hard. High frequency before more esoteric.		

English has inherited. These do, however, have patterns and consistency, and as such, they can be taught and learned. The teacher must be thoroughly familiar with the patterns, regularities, and structures of English words. The tree diagram (Figure 3) presents a skeleton overview of the main information about words which the teachers should know and understand.

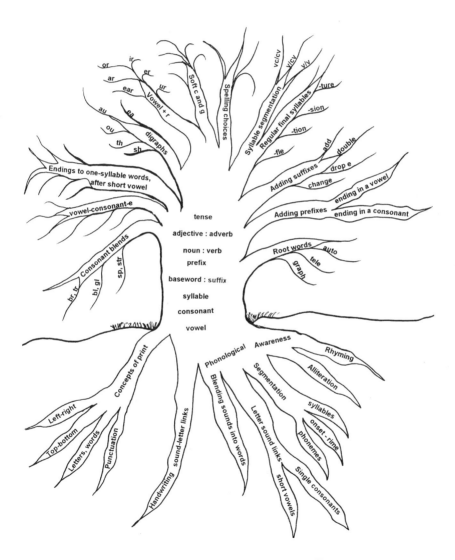

Figure 3. Learning the structures of English spelling.

The roots of the tree represent the basic knowledge which is needed by the beginning or struggling reader or speller in the early stages of reading and spelling.

5.1. Concepts of Print

Would-be readers when faced with a book need to understand the concepts of print: how the symbols are spaced, and how they are arranged on the page to represent spoken words. They need to know we read from left to right, across the lines from top to bottom of the page. They need to note punctuation and capital letters, and understand that these delineate pauses within the passage. They must learn that titles contain important information (Clay, 1981).

5.2. Phonological Awareness

Phonological awareness is awareness of sounds in words (e.g., rhyme and alliteration). It first occurs at the oral stage, and is an important prerequisite of mastering written language. (Bradley and Bryant, 1983).

5.3. Segmentation Skills

Awareness of rhyme and alliteration in oral language mark the beginning of segmentation skills. The appreciation that words segment into syllables arises from feeling the rhythm and beat of nursery verses. In chanting or singing "Jack and Jill went up the hill" the child becomes conscious of the rhyme "ill" in Jill and hill and then begins to divide words naturally into onset and rime, e.g., p-in, tr-amp, sp-end, etc. (Goswami, 1990).

As a child begins formal reading instruction, he becomes aware of separate letters and that each letter has a sound. Thus his segmentation of words into phonemes is sparked by his beginning to read. Learning to write the letter shape reinforces sound–letter links.

5.4. Blending

Blending is the final skill in basic reading. This is when the child takes the sounds of these letters in order and blends them into a vowel–consonant word (in, at) or a consonant–vowel–consonant (cvc) word (him, log). Once the child can successfully blend separate phonemes into a meaningful word, he has "cracked the code" and established the roots of reading. If there are any gaps in his understanding and skill at this point, they will affect his subsequent acquisition of literacy.

5.5. Terminology

Within the trunk of the tree are other important concepts concerned with the structure of words. The terminology associated with these concepts can be learned gradually and used by most children whose verbal and conceptual ability is average or above. The terms "vowel" and "consonant" can be learned as the child learns the alphabet sequence and the letter names. The term "syllable" can be used in games or oral activities to encourage accurate beating and counting of syllables in words. The concept of a known word with an ending such as *dog(s)* and *jump(ing)* is an additional segmentation skill, and so then the terms "base word" and "suffix" should be learned and used after the other terms are well established. Later the concept and label "prefix" can be taught. If both teacher and student use the correct terminology, then the student is more likely to learn the concepts correctly. Other grammatical terms may be appropriate later: noun, verb, adjective, tense, etc. These terms are needed to augment the work in literacy lessons in school, but the dyslexic child may find the words and concepts hard to remember. It is better to teach the essentials thoroughly, than to try to teach all terminology and create an incomprehensible muddle.

The branches in the figure contain graphemes and word patterns which occur in English, and rules of the language. Literate adults will be able to apply these orthographic regularities in their normal reading and spelling. The special education teacher needs to know them thoroughly so she can recognize, explain and teach them.

5.6. Orthographic Patterns

The branches in the figure represent the orthographic patterns which occur commonly in words. These elements of word structure form the spelling guidelines which apply to English words.

5.6.1. Consonant Blends

Consonant blends are difficult to recognize, segment, and read for most children with reading disabilities. There are many consonant blends in which **r** or **l** occurs after one or two other consonants at the beginning of the syllable: /br/, /gr/, /fr/, /str/, /spr/, /sl/, /bl/, /gl/, /fl/, /spl/. The letter **s** often occurs as the first letter of a blend: /sp/, /sk/, /sw/, /sl/, /spl/, /str/, /spr/, /scr/, /squ/. Three letter blends are particularly difficult for students. Final blends can also cause difficulties, for example, /-nt/, /-nd/, /-lf/, /-lp/, /-lt/, /-mp/, /-ft/, /-ct/, /-sk/, but these are best taught as a rime, with words arranged in rhyming groups: -and, band, sand, stand; -isk, risk, brisk, whisk. Consonant blends are particularly difficult and must be taught carefully and continually.

5.6.2. Vowel–Consonant–e

The vowel–consonant–e pattern occurs with all five vowels as **a–e**, **i–e**, **o–e**, **u–e**, and **e–e**, and is variously referred to as magic **e**, or silent **e**. The **e** itself is not pronounced but has the effect of lengthening the preceding vowel if there is only one consonant in between, for example: cake, hide, rose, tube, centipede. These vowel–consonant–e groups of letters form rimes. Students should become familiar with the words in rhyming groups.

bake	*hide*	*rose*	*cute*	*delete*
make	*side*	*pose*	*mute*	*complete*
lake	*bride*	*nose*	*brute*	*athlete*
flake	*slide*	*chose*	*flute*	*concrete*

Note that the vce pattern includes **e–e** words but these are mainly in longer words.

5.6.3. Endings to One-Syllable Words

The "floss" rule is sometimes used as a convenient shorthand for a group of words of English origin in which the final consonant doubles, as in ff/cuff, ll/kill, ss/cross. This occurs in words of one syllable following a short vowel. The same rule applies to the following letter groups in which an extra unpronounced letter is used: /ck/ (pack, stick), /zz/ (fuzz, jazz), /dge/ (badge, hedge), /tch/ (catch, pitch).

5.6.4. Digraphs

Digraphs are two letters which occur together to represent a single sound. There are consonant digraphs such as sh, ch, th, ph, and vowel digraphs such as ea, oa, ai. Some of these only have one sound when read but others have a choice of sound for reading, for example, *ch* making the sound /ch/ as in cheese or /k/ as in chemist; or ea /ē/ as in dream, /ĕ/ as in head; ou /ow/ as in loud, /o͞o/ as in soup, /ŭ/ as in double. When there is more than one response for reading, then establish the most frequently occurring sound first, before teaching a subsequent sound. So ch should be taught as /ch/ (as in chip, chick, cheese, etc.), which is more common and occurs in English-based words. The sound /k/ occurs in less frequent Greek-based words such as chemist, choral, technology.

5.6.5. Vowels Followed by r

When a single letter **r** follows a vowel, it has an effect on the vowel sound, for example, /ar/ (star), /or/ (storm), /er/ (herb), /ir/ (girl), /ur/ (hurl), /ear/ (pearl). However, this is affected by regional variations. In Scottish, American, and West Country English, the **r** is pronounced. Note that /rr/ doesn't usually alter the vowel sound for example, carrot, lorry, ferret, and hurry, and the vowel merely maintains its short sound.

5.6.6. Soft c and g

Soft **c** and **g** refer to words of French origin. If the letter **c** is followed by **e, i, y**, it is always pronounced as /s/ (city, center, cycle). If the letter **g** is followed by **e, i**, or **y**, it often represents the sound /j/ as in gentle, giant, gyroscope. But in several common words of Anglo-Saxon origin, the **g** is pronounced /g/ as in get, give.

5.6.7. Spelling Choices

Spelling choices have to be made when spelling English words. Knowing the sounds of a word does not necessarily lead to spelling it correctly.

There are about 44 phonemes in standard English. Many of them can be represented in more than one way. For example, the sound /f/ can be spelled f, ff, ph, or gh. Each long vowel sound in particular has several choices for spelling. The teacher should be well acquainted with these from the language program she is using and she should know the circumstances in which each spelling is likely to occur.

5.6.8. Syllable Segmentation

Syllable segmentation is an important skill for tackling words of two syllables or more when reading. It is also useful as a spelling tool and proofreading strategy. Syllable boundaries depend on the position of vowels and consonants in the word. The following patterns are useful to help with spelling and proofreading: vc–cv (kidnap) v–cv (robot) v–v (diet). Once divided in this way the word will yield an open or closed syllable. A closed syllable has a consonant after the vowel making the vowel sound short, for example: ab, seg, stip, lost, shud. An open syllable is left open, having no consonant after the vowel and the vowel sound is, therefore, long (making the sound which is the same as the name of the letter), for example: sta, be, di, glo, stu. When faced with a two-syllable word, the student can divide the word into syllables by noting and marking the position of the vowels and consonants.

vc	cv		v	cv		v	v
cŏn	tăct		sī	lĕnt		fū	ĕl

Another group of syllables occurs at the end of words, and each needs to be treated as a unit. They are termed regular final syllables and consist of -ture, -tion, -sion and the /le/ syllables (ble, gle, tle, etc.). They are divided off from the rest of the word so the preceding syllable can be read separately, for example:

ta-ble	tum-ble	rat-tle
na-ture	den-ture	na-tion
fric-tion	fu-sion	man-sion

5.6.9. Prefixes

A prefix is a morpheme added to the beginning of a word that usually alters the meaning of the word, for example, <u>un</u>kind, <u>in</u>eligible, <u>pre</u>dict. Students need to be able to recognize and segment these elements from the base word or root to aid meaning and spelling.

5.6.10. Suffixes

Another important segmentation skill is the recognition of the suffixes on words. A suffix is a letter or group of letters which change the way the word is used. They are morphemes with a grammatical function.

Students need to spot a suffix on a word as a clue, not only to decoding the word in order to pronounce it, but also as a link into meaning: jump(ing), hand(ed), care(ful), sad(ness). The teachers must know these morphemic elements, prefixes and suffixes, and also the rules which govern them.

These suffix rules are reliable and admit few exceptions. Therefore, they can be taught and learned. There are two kinds of suffixes: consonant suffixes, such as –ly, -less, -ness, which begin with a consonant; and vowel suffixes, which begin with a vowel, such as –ing, -ed, -es. The suffix rules are as follows.

Just Add: Add consonant suffixes, except to words ending in **y**; add vowel suffixes to words ending in a vvc pattern (seem, train), or a vcc pattern (send, cross).

Double: Double the final letter before adding a vowel suffix to a word ending in a vc pattern (hop + ing > hopping; trim + ed > trimmed). This only applies to words of one syllable.

In words of more than one syllable, in which the final syllable ends with a vc pattern, double the last letter, but only if the stress is on the final syllable (oc<u>cur</u> + ed > occurred, but <u>off</u>er + ed > offered). In British English only, the exception is to double that final **l** even if the stress is not on the final syllable (travel > traveller).

Drop: Drop the **e** in a word ending in e (bake, dance) before adding a vowel suffix, (>baking, dancing).

Change: Usually change **y** to **i** before adding any suffix except one that begins with **i** (-ing, -ish).

5.5.11. Root Words

Students should first be aware of the base word where it is easily recognizable in words such as *<u>needed</u>, <u>unkind</u>*. Later, they will be able to tackle the more advanced skill of spotting root words. The term *root words* is used here to refer to recognizable morphemes from other languages, often Latin and Greek, that help us recognize the meaning of the word. For example, *auto* in automatic, automobile, and *graph* in grapheme, graphology, photograph, autograph.

A thorough language program such as Hickey (1992) or the Dyslexia Institute Literacy Programme (DILP) (Walker & Brooks, 1996) will explain these language points fully, and can also suggest how to teach these points in a step-by-step way. If a teacher is thoroughly familiar with this structure she can decide whether a word spelling is irregular or whether it can be generalized to other vocabulary, and is therefore worth learning.

Skilled readers do not need to be taught these language points in such a thorough way. Such spelling rules seem to be absorbed and understood as recognizable patterns by skilled readers and spellers, without conscious effort. However, with the increasing emphasis on structure and grammar in literacy lessons in English schools, the information has greater value for teachers and children alike.

6. STRUCTURED LANGUAGE PROGRAMS

The special education teacher is usually by nature acquisitive and eclectic, ever on the lookout for a good idea to help her students. However, she needs to confine herself to one particular language program around which to structure her teaching. Some programs are based on a set of materials, such as Units of Sound, and this is dealt with in Chapter 7. Other programs provide a structure and methodology which the teacher uses as the basis for an individualized program. A full set of materials is not always provided and the teacher has to select or makes suitable structured materials according to the needs of the student. The latter sort of program will be considered here. Gillingham and Stillman (1956) devised such a program, with Hickey (1977) and the Dyslexia Institute Literacy Programme (1996) being two of its derivatives. They each have a list of letters and letter-groupings which are taught in an orderly sequence to ensure a cumulative mastery of the elements of English word structure.

Single consonants and short vowels are usually taught first, followed by digraphs, regular final syllables, and more esoteric choices. Syllable segmentation, suffixing, and spelling choices are taught throughout the program.

Some basic procedures are usually followed when covering a new teaching point in any of the programs.

- Reading cards
- Cursive handwriting
- Multisensory links
- Spelling cards
- Reading structured words and sentences
- Simultaneous-oral-spelling
- Spelling structured words and sentences

An explanation of each procedure is explained in the following.

6.1. Reading Cards

A reading card is often used to focus the student's attention on the target letter and its associated sound. This card also acts as a memory aid. The student draws a picture containing the target sound and the teacher makes sure that he can segment the phoneme from the word. For the letter **c** he would say carrot /k/. The student needs to be aware of the position of his tongue, teeth, and lips as he makes the sound accurately. In this case the **k** is unvoiced, and if he tries too hard he may make the sound voiced, so producing the sound /g/. The student looks at the letter **c** on the front of the card and says carrot /k/, then turns the card over to check, the picture (Figure 4).

Each letter covered to this point will have its own reading card. These can be practiced at the beginning of the lesson as a fast revision of previous teaching. Once the correct grapheme–phoneme links have been established, they need to be linked to the handwritten form and practiced regularly.

6.2. Cursive Handwriting

Some dyslexic children have poor motor control. It takes them longer than usual to establish a new motor pattern until they can do it automatically. A writer needs to form letters automatically without having to think about it. Therefore, instead of teaching children two forms of writing, print first, and cursive later, it is preferable to teach joined handwriting from the beginning. This is done routinely in France and other European countries. Fully cursive script, on lined paper is easier to learn, because each letter starts, and most finish, on the line, so ligatures between letters are easily made (Figure 5).

6.3. Multisensory Links

The child learns by tracing over the model letter, in this case **c**, and then practices writing the letter on his own, saying the sound of the letter /k/, and its name **c**. Thus, he establishes multisensory linkages at the single letter level (Gillingham and Stillman, 1956; Hickey, 1977).

6.4. Spelling Cards

The more detailed language programs would also make a spelling card so that this response can also be practiced with the reading cards at the beginning of the lesson. To practice the spelling card, the teacher says the sound /k/. The student repeats the sound /k/, names the letter **c**, and writes it in cursive script.

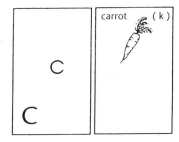

Figure 4. Reading card. (From Walker & Brooks, 1996).

Handwriting

In this style of handwriting, most letters start and finish on the line with an approach stroke and a finishing stroke. This gives a flow to the feel of the patterns in words.

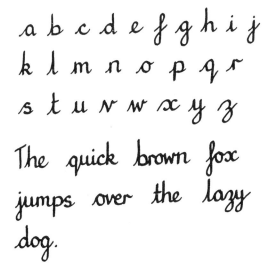

Take care with 'top-joiners'

These alternative forms may be used:

Figure 5. Cursive writing. (From Walker & Brooks, 1996.)

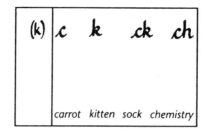

Figure 6. Spelling card for the sound /k/. (From Walker & Brooks, 1996.)

Later as he covers the other spelling choices for the sound /k/ they will be added to the card: k, ck, ch, which also make the sound /k/ in kitten, *trick*, and chemistry (Figure 6).

6.5. Reading Structured Words and Sentences

With the handwriting links established, the child then needs to practice reading words which incorporate the letter **c** and the other letters he has learned. He should be able to easily decode the words and sentences presented to him. Some students may only read cvc words at this teaching point, while others may cope with consonant blends and suffixes. Besides making sure that her student understand the meaning of all of the words, the teacher should check if he can spot any patterns in the presented words, such as rhymes, or words with suffixes. Looking and listening for patterns will be a frequent task in all the literacy activities.

6.6. Simultaneous Oral Spelling

To establish spelling patterns in words, the technique of simultaneous oral spelling (S.O.S.) has been found to be more effective than other methods, such as visual inspection (Thomson, 1991). In the S.O.S method, the teacher or helper says the word, the student repeats it, names the letters, writes the letters in joined writing and then proofreads the letter. The helper says "camp." The student echoes "camp," names the letters **c-a-m-p** and writes "camp." He then looks at the words again and checks it by reading accurately what he has written.

This technique entails several other processes, particularly phoneme segmentation, memory and sequencing, thus making it a valuable multisensory task.

6.7. Writing Words and Sentences

When he has had adequate additional practice in spelling the words (from picture clues, etc) the student should try to write a dictated sentence. This might be dictated by the teacher, but it is better from the student's own voice, recorded on to a Language Master card reader or tape recorder. When he has heard the sentence, the student should repeat it clearly and then say each word as he writes it down. This involves memory, sequencing, and good phonemic segmentation skills. Correct punctuation is an additional chore that the student may need to include in his dictation: "Capital letter. The cat hid in the camp. Period."

These basic techniques ensure systematic and careful teaching of graphemes in a step-by-step way. But rarely are they enough on their own. The special education teacher needs to guide her student through the language program with four points in mind:

1. His general conceptual ability
2. His reading level
3. His spelling level
4. His particular difficulties

In this way she can decide how he should progress through the teaching program, and what extra support he will need for his particular difficulties.

6.8. Differentiating within the Teaching Program

A student who needs a full language program, because he has many gaps in his knowledge of language, should begin at the beginning. This means that the teacher may have students of different reading and spelling ages and of different abilities starting on the program. Although they all may need to cover the same ground, their learning will differ in depth, pace, and complexity.

A struggling student at the basic level may go through the first stages of the structure only learning basic sounds for reading cvc words. He will need to spend time on handwriting, as well as blending and manipulating wooden letters to learn spelling patterns.

A student who has some rudimentary, but inaccurate reading skills will cover the same ground. But the vocabulary he deals with will include consonant blends, simple suffixes, and easily segmented two-syllable words.

A student of average or above average ability, with reading skills at almost functional literacy level, would need in addition, more challenging reading at each level including multisyllabic words and passages of prose to read. He will work on word patterns and word structure, learning syllable-division and suffix rules.

6.9. Reading vs. Spelling

Some students may require a higher level of challenge in the structured reading which they tackle, than in the spelling work. So the reading work may require them to read the more challenging, higher level vocabulary. When writing and spelling, they may be dealing with structured vocabulary and sentences at the simpler level.

A careful list should be kept of the teaching points covered, and notes made on the student's successes and his difficulties.

7. THE LESSON

A lesson with a special education teacher using a cumulative structured multisensory program would ideally take place with a group of one to three students, each on an individualized program, but may be adapted to a wide variety of group situations. The lesson needs rhythm and routine to establish good work habits and practice, but also variety and several changes of activity to ensure maximum attention, concentration, and use of all learning channels. A great amount of input from the teacher is required both to teach the language point and to give close and coherent feedback on the student's performance. However, there need to be times in the lesson when the student must work on his own to establish independence and confidence.

Here is an example of a typical, straightforward lesson to teach the digraph _ee_ for a student whose routines and learning pattern are well established. In a cumulative program, he has learned to read and spell all the letters of the alphabet and use them in cvc words (zip, bag) and also in words with consonant blends (s<u>top</u>, la<u>nd</u>) and simple suffixes (trip<u>s</u>, mend<u>ing</u>). He can read simple sentences and prose using the letters and concepts covered, including high frequency regular words. He can spell individual words and short sentences within the structure he has learned.

A one-hour lesson would aim to contain the following elements:

7.1. Alphabet Work

The student arranges wooden or plastic letter in alphabetical order in a rainbow shape, so he can reach them (Figure 7).

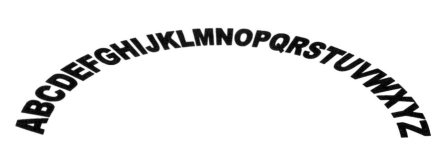

Figure 7. The Alphabet Arc.

Upper or lowercase can be used, although lowercase letters are more difficult for a child to orientate correctly (problems occur with **p**, **b**, **d**, **q** and **n**, **u**, in particular.) The student is asked to spell words covered in the previous lesson (quit, quest) to comment on word structure (quits—has the ending–suffix **s**) and analogous words (best, west, and crest rhyme with quest).

QUIT S   QUEST
B
W
CR

7.2. Memory Routines

1. Practice reading cards containing previously covered letters or letter groups.
2. Practice spelling cards, writing down the spelling of individual letters or letter groups covered previously.

7.3. Review

The student practices spelling words and sentences covered in the last lesson, by writing the word under the picture or by listening to a self-dictation recorded last time.

7.4 Introduction of a New Teaching Point

The student is given a reading card with the targeted grapheme (ee, EE) and a clue word (teeth), and sound /e/. The student practices the card and draws a picture to remind him of it.

7.5 Establish Multisensory Links

The student establishes multisensory links by saying the sound and name as he writes the target grapheme, in cursive script.

7.6 Read Words and Sentences

The student needs to read words and sentences with the target sound using only previously learned graphemes, noting any patterns or word structure.

seen	need
been	feed
queen	seed
	bleed

He rereads the words clearly onto an audio tape for later use.

7.7. Simultaneous Oral Spelling

In simultaneous oral spelling, the teacher says the word. The student repeats it, spells it naming the letters and writes it in his book in joined writing.

7.8. Student Listens to Tape

When the student listens to the tape, which he recorded earlier, he pauses it after each word and writes the words in his book.

7.9. Free Writing

In free writing the student composes his own sentences or prose. He uses one word to write or type a sentence of his own, then repeats this to produce an appropriate number of sentences. Some students can sequence their sentences into a story.

7.10. Game

The lesson is concluded by playing a game. It may be designed to practice reading, spelling of "qu" or "ee" words, or by collecting rhyming words. If there were problems at any stage, then further support work would be given so the student could practice that particular skill (such as noting rhymes, or suffixes, more handwriting practice, or an irregular word).

The pace of the lesson should be brisk while still allowing the student time to process the information and practice the skill. The elements of the lesson should follow a logical sequence of learning, using a bottom up approach at this stage, so that the lessons build the skills carefully and cumulatively. Alphabet work can be done with two or three students in the group (each student building his words at his teaching point). The group can practice the spelling pack and play the game together. See Figure 8 for the timing of a one-hour lesson.

For a younger student who is near the beginning of the program, more time may be spent on alphabet work, on handwriting, and blending sounds into words in reading. For a more competent student, the alphabet work may not always be necessary; he may need more extended reading practice, segmentation of multi-syllable words and free writing, perhaps on a word processor.

8. PROBLEMS AND SOLUTIONS

Teaching dyslexic students is constantly diagnostic and analytical. The learning curve is rarely smooth and the student will present the teacher with many problems which have to be solved. Here are some of the common problems, and some suggested solutions. Firstly, a general approach to all teaching.

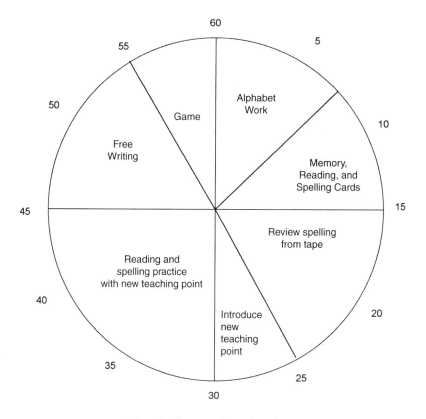

Figure 8. Elements of a one-hour lesson.

8.1. In General

- Move from the concrete to the abstract.
- Demonstrate words with wooden or plastic letters.
- Make it multisensory. Is he saying, looking, listening, and writing *simultaneously*?
- Practice. Give a reminder card for daily practice.

8.2. Student Cannot Perceive Rhymes in Words

- Say or read nursery rhymes or silly poems. Clap or stamp on the rhyming word.
- Sort pictures into rhyming sets (Make sure the sets contrast widely. Have tap, map, cap and dream, cream, steam; but not tap, map, cap with tan, man, pan).

- Sort structured words into rhyming pairs (take care, as above).
- Make words he can read with wooden letters.
- Slide the rime:

HAT

C

S

- Use highlighters to mark the common rimes.
- Make a card "slide" or wheel (Figures 9 and 10).
- Trace the rhyming group in cursive writing while saying the sound of each letter (Figure 11).
- Commercial materials such as Phonological Awareness Training (P.A.T.) (Wilson, 1995) worksheets. The student writes rhyming words from selected onsets and rimes.

8.3. Student Cannot Blend Sounds into Words

- Teacher speaks the word without emphasis; she may say /b/ /a/ /g/ three times. Student tries to identify the word before hearing it the third time.
- Track letters of a word, starting with two letter-word (Figure 12). He says the sounds as he tracks with the pen. What's the word?
- Trace over the letters with a pen or pencil, saying the sounds:

in pin tin

- "Crash" wooden letters together, saying sounds. Include continuant sounds (such as /s/, /m/) to help him at first.

S ← E ← T   SET

- Use the student's own voice. On a good tape recorder, record him saying pure sounds, separately. Use the "pause" button to minimize the gap so the sounds are close together in sequence. Play back to student, several times, so he hears the phonemes, more closely linked, in his own voice.

8.4. Student Cannot Visually Segment Words for Word Attack in Reading

- Highlight structured word lists, noting rime, suffixes.

bag	dogs	helping
sag	tins	mending
rag	rags	bending
drag	pots	
stag		

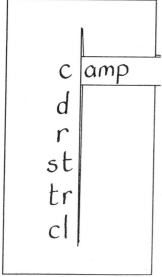

c |amp
d
r
st
tr
cl

Figure 9. A word slide.

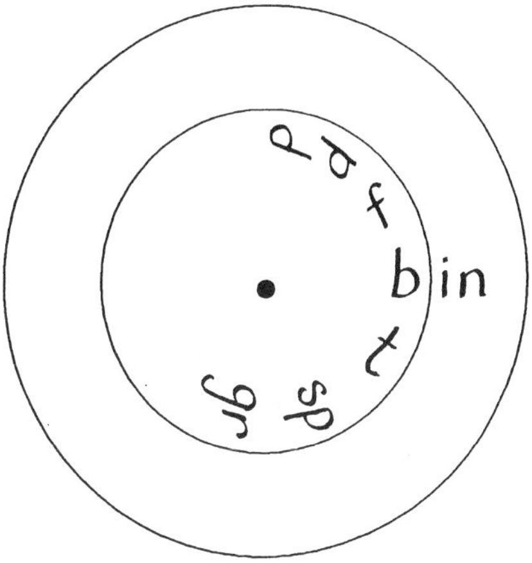

c d f
p b in
gr ds t

Figure 10. A word wheel.

hand
band
stand

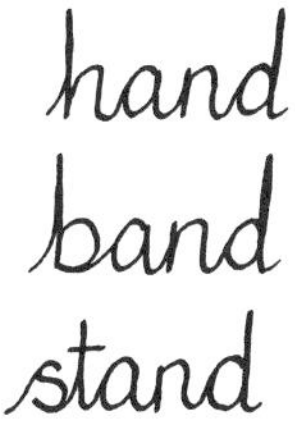

Figure 11. Tracing to hear and see the rhyme.

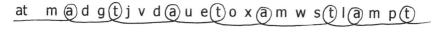

at   m ⓐ d g ⓣ j v d ⓐ u e ⓣ o x ⓐ m w s ⓣ l ⓐ m p ⓣ

Figure 12. Tracking and sounding "at."

- Use wooden letters

SAD LY   PAN S

- Present words hyphenated into syllables, for example, pic-nic.
- Record hyphenated word onto Language Master (Figure 13).
  ban –dit   bandit   help –ing   helping

8.5. Poor Sequencing Skills

- Make tape of alphabet song to take home. Sing or say in rhythm and point to wooden letters in order.
- Put reminder card in reading pack, with the alphabet printed in order.
- Days of the week, months of year: Use rhythm or song. March and chant or clap and chant.
- Put each day of the week and each month on separate card. Student draws significant event (cubs night; swimming day; birthday month; Christmas month). Regularly practices rewriting in order.

8.6. Poor Visual Memory for Words

- Make the words bigger. The student traces words, naming the letters in tray of sand or salt, on chalkboard, or write on paper with a large colored pen.
- Use oral or auditory mnemonics. Record on tape recorder, or on card reader such as a Language Master. "Wed nes day." "Should o–u–l–d oh, you lovely duck."
- Use visual mnemonics (Figure 14).

8.7. Terminology

Learn only one term at a time. Make sure each term is well established before introducing another.

Record and listen to own voice: "con–son–ant."

Games in which the term must be use at every turn. For example, turn over card, name the letter and say if it is a vowel or consonant before moving counter.

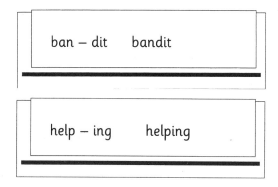

Figure 13. (a and b) Prepared cards for Language Master card reader.

9. CHOOSING OR MAKING MATERIALS FOR DYSLEXIC STUDENTS TO READ

For the dyslexic student, the biggest problem occurs when he needs to read or spell words as part of a sentence or piece of prose. For the teacher who is choosing or designing materials for her students to read, here are some guidelines.

If your student, when reading, is still having trouble with word attack, then be sure to make the sentence easy to understand. The dyslexic student cannot deal with two difficult aspects of reading at once. Therefore if the decoding is hard, the syntax, grammar and sentence length should be simple. The simplest sentence is the Simple, Active, Affirmative, Declarative sentence (SAAD) (Hornsby, 1975), which is usually the easiest to understand and should be used for struggling dyslexic children, e.g., The boy dropped the pen.

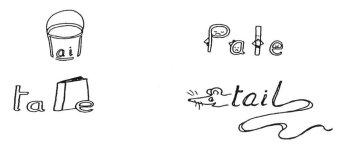

Figure 14. Visual mnemonics.

The other sentence constructions are a little more difficult and are the opposite of each of the SAAD attributes.

1. Simple–Complex.
2. Active–Passive
3. Affirmative–Negative
4. Declarative– Interrogative

The SAAD sentence above could be varied in these ways:

1. On reaching forward, the boy dropped the pen. [Complex]
2. The pen was dropped by the boy. [Passive]
3. The boy did not drop the pen. [Negative]
4. Did the boy drop the pen? [Interrogative]

When the struggling reader puts effort into decoding, he should be rewarded by easy access to meaning. It is not only word length which affects readability: grammar, syntax, and conceptual difficulty have a part to play too. "Tim put his kit in his bag" is easily understood, but "Tim pits his wits at Dan," with words which are similarly easy to decode, is much harder to understand because of poor grammar (one pits one's wits *against*, not *at*, someone or thing), and figurative language. Teachers providing a tightly structured sentences using a limited number of letters should be aware of such major pitfalls.

So the dyslexic student must read for meaning and must feel that the effort is worthwhile. The aim is to have him read material which he needs and wants to know. If it does not cause him to be better informed, to laugh, to cry, be interested, or even amazed, then it is hardly likely to be motivating. It is to demand too much of tightly structured materials that they evoke much emotion in the early stages, but the reader must read meaningful text. He needs to feel that he is progressing. The work must become more demanding and complex, so that he knows he is making progress in basic skills. This improvement will then open the door to more interesting reading.

10. TIMING

We know that dyslexic students appear to have weaknesses in one or more of the sensory modalities through which written language information is processed, and that dyslexic students have trouble with the speed of information processing.

To the observant teacher or helper there is often a feeling of rush, panic or mistiming about the reading performance of the dyslexic student. He may try to read faster than he can process the details of the letters and words in front of him. When faced with the sentence, "The robber tried to hide but the police found him," a dyslexic student may read "The rabbit tripped and hid but the p___ find him."

Clearly, both his orthographic and phonological processing is breaking down. Certainly, the two are not working in synchrony. The student appears to be looking only at some of the letters in the words, and he is saying the words before he has had time to process all the letters. It is noticeable that such students are often not looking directly at the word they are trying to decode. Paula Tallal (1985) alerted us to the slow processing of language impaired children, and showed that, by slowing down the speed of presentation of words, these students were able to access, process, and remember those words.

How often do we hear a teacher saying to a dyslexic student as she listens to him reading, "Slow down, take your time" in an effort to curb the reader's anxiety? The dyslexic reader wants to read as fast as possible. The reason may be:

1.   He wants to read at the speed of a "normal" reader.
2.   He's used to failing and being inaccurate.
3.   He wants the painful task to be over.

The dyslexic learner who is impulsive and distractible, must be made aware that timing in reading is crucial, that he must work out a comfortable speed for accurate decoding. He needs to practice this first of all when reading single words. He should be encouraged to keep his eyes on the word until he has spoken it, and then hold his gaze on it for a little longer, allowing the word's image and sound to be processed together. In this way, he is more likely to retain the word in his memory.

The multimedia version of the Units of Sound program acknowledges the need for this processing time by highlighting each target word for two seconds to hold the reader's attention for long enough for it to be read, repeated, and studied (see Chapter 7).

If the word is long and requires more than one fixation of the eyes, the student should be aware of visually segmenting it according to its syllables or morphological structure: auto|mat|ic, help|ing, in|depend|ent. Previous experience of segmented or hyphenated words and practice in coding the word will be an important precursor to doing this efficiently. Once he has decoded a word, he should then allow his eyes to take in the whole word in one fixation for a split second. In this way he gives himself time to fix the visual representation of the whole word in the lexicon of his visual memory. Similarly, when reading prose, he should practice segmenting sentences into phrases or meaningful word groups as he scans the sentence ahead. He should have practice in doing this, using pencil (Figure 15), to prepare the text for reading aloud, so it will become a familiar activity. He thereby is using meaning and context to segment the prose into semantic units and also into syllables. He should try to match the visual speed at which he can

-ay words with suffixes

Read.
Code any long or tricky words.
Tape and write.

1   She displayed her cards for sale.

2   I am dismayed that all the chocolate has gone.

3   You may find fungus on the trunk of a decaying tree.

4   On Wednesday, planes landed on this runway for the last time.

Figure 15. Worksheet prepared to taping.

perform this process with the speed at which he can accurately decode and understand the words and phrases.

This adjustment of timing seems to improve accuracy and memory for words and takes away the panic, which reading aloud often engenders.

The teacher should of course give her student prose to read that is within his level of mastery and with an accessible syntactic and conceptual structure. She needs to get him to slow down sufficiently to be accurate, even if his reading is very robotic. She must check that he has understood what he read. Then he can reread accurately, adding intonation and phrasing. Then she can praise him for his expression. He finally, perhaps on a later occasion, rereads the passage for fluency, that is, accurately, with expression and at a reasonable speed. Such repetition gives practice but with a different focus each time. We know that the repeated reading of a text improves word recognition, fluency and comprehension for all readers (Adams, 1990). Fawcett and Nicolson (1994) have found that automaticity is harder to achieve for dyslexic students, and so practice and overlearning are very necessary.

11. SPELLING IN PROSE

The most frustrating and often humiliating experience for the dyslexic student is to write prose and deliver it for public scrutiny, whether it is a story at school, a report at work, an essay at university. This is when the dyslexic is at his most vulnerable.

His progress in spelling is likely to be slower than his progress in reading, since the spelling process is more complex and requires greater integration of skills.

When a child is reading from a printed page, at least the symbols are in the correct order. However, when spelling, he starts from a sound (spoken by the writer aloud or silently, or dictated by someone else) and must produce written words. This is a more complex task. He is starting from scratch, with no visual prompts to help him. The writer needs to coordinate more modalities and learning channels and is therefore open to more potential errors. So when composing a sentence, story or essay, the dyslexic learner may only be able to concentrate on two aspects of the task, for example, semantic and phonological processing. This would lead possibly to a meaningful sentence with very phonic spelling. As the dyslexic learner has difficulty in using all the processes in a coordinated way, he needs another layer of checking after writing the work. It is vital that he begins to appreciate the importance of developing drafting and proof reading skills.

12. PROOFREADING

A student's work exemplifies the layers of checking and drafting he must go through.

For his first draft the student wrote:

th monstr rerd with slim drip from boby

He used phonic spelling so that he could get his thoughts on paper before he forgot them. This is when the teacher then needed to encourage him to proofread.

12.1. Sense

First he had to read to make sure that the sentence made sense. He may find that he has missed out words, or got them in the wrong order. At this point the student added "e," "up,"and "its."

the monstr rerd up with slim drip from its boby"

12.2. Punctuation

Then he read for punctuation to make sure that periods at least delineate the end of a sentence where he paused in his reading aloud. He added **T** and a period).

The monstr rerd up with slim drip from its boby.

12.3 Grammar

Next he looked at grammar and syntax, including agreement of nouns and verbs, word endings, particularly suffixes. He adds "ing" to drip.

The monstr rerd up with slim driping from its boby."

12.4. Spelling

Finally, he looked for spelling errors, being aware of his own personal pitfalls. These frequent spelling errors were listed in the back of the student's book as a proofreading procedure. This student had the following list:.

capital letters   *said*
full stops   *before*
suffixing rules   *lick/like*
b/d

Usually if he checked his work for these predictable errors, he could find at least half of his mistakes. He corrected "slime," "body," and "dripping." So he had now written:

The monster rerd up with slime dripping from its body.

The word "rear" was difficult; he got it by analogy to "fear" with the teacher's help. He spotted that the ending was the "ed" suffix.

The monster reared up with slime dripping from its body.

And his parents and teachers wonder why he is so exhausted and frustrated! Clearly, he was in a determined mood that day, but he could not keep up such effort continually. However, because the dyslexic student's work is error-ridden, he needs the knowledge, strategies, and tenacity to go through this sort of procedure, as a proofreading strategy, until some of the procedures become more automatic so that he can apply them at the composing stage.

Of course this whole exercise is very much easier and more rewarding if he can do it on a computer with a spell checking facility, which would alert him to about half of his errors. After the student has done his own proofreading, he needs to have quick feedback from the teachers to reinforce his correct writing and spelling, and correct his mistakes.

Constant but sensitive feedback is needed to help the writer to correct mistakes so that the correct version is seen and written more times than the faulty version.

However, to be nitpicking about a student's mistakes can be soul-destroying for him and may prevent him from composing anything except the shortest sentences and paragraphs, using simple easily spelled vocabulary. So the teacher needs to negotiate with her student whether she will do the following.

1. Correct all mistakes and let him practice a small number which he needs to know.
2. Only correct high-frequency words and given words for that particular topic or subject.
3. Correct only words with the spelling patterns which he has learned and should know, and which will generalize by analogy to other vo-

cabulary. For instance if the teacher corrects "heart" she would be asking him to learn a one-off word as few other words look and sound the same. However to correct "start" if it had been misspelled would be useful; it could be linked to other similar words (part, cart, dart smart), and would be a good reinforcement of the strategy of spelling by analogy.

Proofreading is an important skill and process for the dyslexic student and needs to be appreciated by his teachers as a difficult and time-consuming task. He should make sure that he retains all previous drafts to show to his teachers. It is hoped he can demonstrate to himself that the drafting process has helped improve his proofreading and spelling skills.

13. IS STRUCTURED, CUMULATIVE, MULTISENSORY TEACHING EFFECTIVE?

A random sample was taken of the reading and spelling progress of 184 students taught at the Sheffield Dyslexia Institute between 1979 and 1990 (Rack & Walker, 1994). The students were taught for one or two hours a week for an average of 2.2 years. When they started to receive teaching at the Dyslexia Institute, their improvement ratio from starting school was 0.5—that is, their improvement in reading was only half a year for each year of time in school. After DI teaching the average improvement ratio in reading was 1.3 and in spelling 1. They had, therefore, doubled their rate of progress in spelling and had done even better in reading with an hour or two of special education per week. These results should encourage special education teachers by showing that their skilled teaching is productive.

For the dyslexic student, learning to read and spell is a laborious and demanding task. With a structured cumulative multisensory program and a knowledgeable and sensitive teacher, he can be given learning responses and strategies which will be effective and tangible, and which will give him control over his reading and spelling.

SUMMARY

- The special education teacher is the most important resource for the dyslexic student. She must have a good knowledge of the theory and practice of literacy and dyslexia so that she can help him effectively.
- Instructional methods which work with the majority of students may be insufficient for the dyslexic student.

- The teacher should understand: the normal acquisition of literacy for the skilled reader; the particular difficulties for the dyslexic learner; the principles of multisensory teaching; and the structure of English words.
- The importance of selecting a clear and coherent program was addressed, and the difficulties inherent in choosing or producing suitably structured teaching materials. Some of the common problems of a dyslexic learner were listed, with some practical suggestions for teaching. The difference between reading and spelling was considered, and all these factors are incorporated into a lesson plan.
- The aspect of timing was addressed, as mistiming is a common difficulty in processing for most dyslexics. Teaching should encourage close text and word analysis. This can be achieved by training the student in prereading strategies, and proofreading as a postwriting strategy. Finally, the effectiveness of structured multisensory teaching was considered.

TEACHING RESOURCES

Broomfield, H., & Combley, M. (1997). *Overcoming Dyslexia. A Practical Handbook for the Classroom*. London: Whurr Publishers Ltd.
Combley, M. (ed.). (2000). *The Hickey Multisensory Language Course*, third edition). London: Whurr Publishers Ltd.
Cowling, K., & Cowling, H. (1993). *Toe by Toe*. 8 Green Road, Baildon, West Yorkshire.
Hatcher, P.J. (1994). *Sound Linkage: An Integrated Programme for Overcoming Reading Difficulties*. London: Whurr Publishers Ltd.
Hornsby, B., & Shear F. (1980). *Alpha to Omega*, third edition. Oxford Heinemann Educational.
Klein, C. & Millar, R. (1990). *Unscrambling Spelling*. Hodder and Stoughton.
Lloyd, S. (1992). *Jolly Phonics*. Jolly Learning Ltd, Tailours House, High Road, Chigwell, U.K.
Miles, E. (1992). *The Bangor Dyslexia Teaching System*, second edition.
Stone, C., Franks, E., & Nicholson, M. (1995). *Beat Dyslexia*. LDA, Duke St. Wisbech, Cambs. PE13 2AE.
Walker, J., & Brooks, L. (1996). *Dyslexia Institute Literacy Programme*. Dyslexia Institute, 133 Gresham Road, Staines, TW18 2AJ.
Wendon, Lyn. (1995). *First Steps in Letterland*. Teaching Programme 1. London: Harper Collins.

REFERENCES

Adams, M.J. (1990). *Beginning to Read—Thinking and Learning About Print*. Cambridge, MA: MIT Press.
Borwick, C., & Townend, J. (1993). *Developing Spoken Language Skills*. London: The Dyslexia Institute.
Bradley, L., & Bryant, P.E. (1983). Categorising sounds and learning to read: A causal connection. *Nature, 310*, 419–421.

Bryant, P., & Bradley, L. (1985). *Children's Reading Problems*. Oxford: Basil Blackwell.

Clay, M. (1981). *The Early Detection of Reading Difficulties: A Diagnostic Survey with Recovery Procedures*. Oxford: Heinemann Educational.

Cripps, C. (1988). *A Hand for Spelling*. Wisbech: Learning Development Aids.

Fawcett, A., & Nicolson, R., (1994). *Dyslexia in Children: Multidisciplinary Perspectives*. London: Harvester Wheatsheaf.

Frith, U. (1985). Beneath the surface of developmental dyslexia. In K.E. Patterson, J.C. Marshall, & M. Coltheart (eds.), *Surface Dyslexia*. London: Routledge and Kegan Paul.

Gillingham, A., & Stillman, B.W. (1956, 1969). *Remedial Training for Children with Specific Disability in Reading, Writing and Penmanship*, fifth edition. Cambridge, MA: Educational Publishing Co.

Goswami, U., & Bryant, P. (1990). *Phonological Skills and Learning to Read*. London: Lawrence Erlbaum Associates.

Hickey, K. (1977). *Dyslexia: A Language Training Course for Teachers and Learners*. Private Publication.

Hickey, K. (1992). *Dyslexia: A Language Training Course for Teachers and Learners*. Available from the Dyslexia Institute, Staines.

Hornsby, B., & Shear, F. (1975). *Alpha to Omega*. Oxford: Heinemann Educational.

Orton, J. L. (1967). The Orton–Gillingham approach. In J. Mooney (ed.), *The Disabled Reader*. Baltimore: Johns Hopkins University Press.

Peters, M.L., & Smith, B. (1993). *Spelling in Context: Strategies for Teachers and Learners*. Windsor: NFER Nelson.

Rack, J., & Walker, J. (1994). Does Dyslexia Institute Teaching Work? In *Dyslexia Review, Vol. 6, Number 2, Autumn 1994*. Staines: The Dyslexia Institute.

Seidenberg, M.S., & McClelland, J.L. (1989). A distributed, developmental model of word recognition and naming. *Psychological Review, 96*, 523–568.

Snowling, M.J. (1987). *Dyslexia: A Cognitive Developmental Perspective*. Oxford: Blackwell.

Tallal, P., Stark, R.E., & Mellits, D. (1985). The relationship between auditory temporal analysis and receptive language development: Evidence from studies of developmental language disorder. *Neuropsychologia, 23*, 527–534.

Thomson, M. (1991). The teaching of spelling using techniques of simultaneous oral spelling and visual inspection. In M. Snowling & M. Thomson, *Dyslexia Integrating Theory and Practice*. London: Whurr.

Walker, J., & Brooks, L. (eds.) (1996). *Dyslexia Institute Literacy Programme*. Staines: The Dyslexia Institute.

Wilson, J. (1995). *Phonological Awareness Training*, Parts 1 and 2. Aylesbury: County Psychological Service.

6

Developing Writing Skills

Wendy Goldup

INTRODUCTION

We write so we may communicate. We write so we may convey thoughts, ideas, knowledge, or to enable the reader to reach an understanding of something. The competent writer achieves a state of what Csikszentmihalyi (1975) calls flow:

> You yourself are in an ecstatic state to such a point that you feel as though you almost don't exist. I've experienced this time and again. My hand seems devoid of myself and I have nothing to do with what is happening. I just sit there watching in a state of awe and wonderment. And it just flows out by itself.
>
> Csikszentmihalyi (1975), p.3

Hamilton (1984) describes this state further:

> Watching someone in flow gives the impression that the difficult is easy; peak performance appears natural and ordinary. This impression parallels what is going on within the brain where a similar paradox is repeated: the most challenging tasks are done with a minimum expenditure of mental energy. In flow the brain is in a "cool" state, its arousal and inhibition of neural circuitry attuned to the demand of the moment. When people are engaged in activities that effortlessly capture and hold their attention, their brain "quiets down" in the sense that there is a lessening of cortical arousal.

Contrast this with the struggling dyslexic writer, who is preoccupied with how to hold the pen, where to begin his letters, which direction to push his wrist, whether he should use capital or lower case letters, how to spell the words, where to punctuate. . . . There is little room here for a single idea, let alone any kind of flow.

Wendy Goldup, The Dyslexia Institute, 32 Avebury Avenue, Tonbridge, Kent TN9 1UA, United Kingdom

The dyslexic writer often, though not always, has associated motor difficulties, which hamper his efforts from the very beginning. He might hold his pen too tightly, engraving the paper he is writing on sometimes to the point of tearing it. The huge effort he takes to make marks with a tight, tense hand means that after a line or two his muscles will be completely exhausted. He might need to take a rest after a small amount of writing, or might want to 'down tools' altogether, his fingers, wrist, arm, and shoulder in revolt against such a tiring activity.

Other dyslexic would-be writers might have the opposite problem: very low muscle tone. This means they hardly feel the writing tool in their hand at all. Their grip is loose. Their hand and wrist are floppy. They get no feedback from the paper. They lack control over their hand's movement on the paper.

Whole body exercises which work on loosening, stretching, and general control are helpful in either low muscle tone or associated motor difficulties cases. Gross motor control precedes fine motor control. Thus by starting with whole body exercises before moving on to hand and finger exercises is a sensible approach. Nash-Wortham, & Hunt (1990) and McAllen (1992) propose a range of very helpful activities for the class teacher to use. The advice of an occupational therapist should be sought in extreme cases.

Sidney Chu, an occupational therapist in Walker, et al. (1996), suggested activities to strengthen wrist and hand muscles. These include wringing, squeezing, and crushing either sponges, cloths, or newspaper; or implementing either carpentry skills, such as using a hammer and screwdriver, or cooking skills, such as beating, whisking, kneading, and pressing dough. Fine finger control can be improved by tearing paper, stringing beads, sorting and picking up small objects with tongs or tweezers, cutting with scissors, or sewing.

Chu believes control over the writing implement and medium can be developed with early exercises that focus attention on how to use pencil and paper. He advises using paints, chalks, or bright colored, thick crayons on paper to encourage scribbling, pattern making, and flow while gradually reducing size and range of movements to those closer to those made during writing (prewriting patterns, letter shapes, joined letter shapes).

Posture is important. Children should be regularly reminded they need "six legs down" for good writing: four chair legs plus two human legs, securely planted on the floor. They also need straight backs and shoulders; support for their writing hand just below the wrist, from the table or surface; and support from the other hand to hold the paper still and in place (see Figure 1).

The choice of tool should be the writer's. If we wish him to take control of his writing then he should pick a suitable, acceptable, and comfortable tool. Possibly the tool chosen for improvement of writing skills will not be the same as that used for eventual writing. If the student knows he will use his preferred implement most of the time, he might be less reluctant to do improvement exercises using say, a pencil.

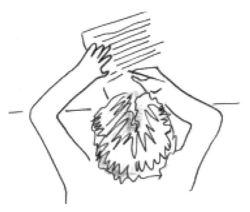

Figure 1. Ready to write.

Pencils are enormously helpful for prewriting and writing exercises because they come in varying shapes, sizes, and degrees of softness. They also give a certain amount of sensory feedback to the writer as they mark paper.

The tense writer would benefit from practicing with a very soft lead pencil. Minimum pressure creates a mark and maximum pressure turns the pencil to dust! He should be encouraged to attempt very soft, flowing shapes regularly for short periods of time, then switch to his chosen implement to practice these shapes.

The student with a slack wrist and poor feedback should try either a pencil grip, three-cornered pencil, or a fountain pen. Either of these will provide better sensory information than say a roller ball which glides effortlessly over the paper. A lead slightly harder than #2 will also help. Again, the student should switch to the pen which he will use for most of his writing and practice his newly acquired skills. This will enable him to maintain consistent improvement.

Writing is a many faceted activity. It can be divided into two main areas: mechanical or secretarial aspect and meaning-based or communication process. It is helpful to deal with these two aspects separately, just as it is helpful to learn and practice the two separately, merging as soon as possible to create a satisfying whole.

1. MECHANICAL ASPECTS

1.1. Handwriting

Handwriting is the making of marks on paper. This definition includes appearance, neatness, spelling, and punctuation, all of which make writing understandable to the reader.

In each of these areas, as with everything else, the dyslexic pupil needs explicit development, that is to say he needs to be taught; he does not pick up skills, rules, and generalizations for himself. In handwriting, the teaching mode should be modeling: The teacher draws the letter shape or word while the student watches then reproduces. This can be done in tutoring, as a small group or whole class activity. It can be a marvelous settling activity when children have just arrived in the morning or returned from recess.

The National Curriculum in England and Wales (DfEE, 1995) states that all children should be taught a range of key skills in handwriting. At Key Stage One (5–7 years), children should be taught how to: hold a pencil correctly; write from left to right; create letters that start and finish correctly; make these letters regular in size, shape, and spacing. In addition, students

> should be taught the conventional way of forming letters, both lower case and capitals. They should build on their knowledge of letter formation to join letters in words. They should develop an awareness of the importance of clear and neat presentation, in order to communicate their meaning effectively.

At Key Stage Two (7–11 years), "pupils should be taught to use neat, legible handwriting."

The National Literacy Strategy in England and Wales (DfEE, 1998) suggests handwriting be taught during the reception year and throughout year one "in a style that makes the letters easy to join later." From year two, term one onwards, pupils should begin using and practicing the four basic joins."

For all children, it is not possible to spend a great deal of time perfecting some kind of printed script, only to change sometime later, perhaps when secondary education looms, to joined handwriting.

For dyslexic children and others who have learning disabilities, any learning should remain valid for the rest of their lives, not just for a year or two. Dyslexia specialists have always begun the remediation process for children who have failed to acquire successful literacy skills by teaching them fully joined cursive handwriting.

Styles of cursive handwriting differ slightly. Some styles lift the pen for certain letters. Other styles join fully from the beginning of a word to the end, as does the version preferred by the Dyslexia Institute (see Figure 2). There are various reasons for teaching handwriting in a fully joined cursive form, rather than individual, separate, printed shapes. They are as follows.

It follows natural movement. Young preschool children love to make marks on paper. They let the crayon or pencil run in free flowing forms. They make

Figure 2. The Dyslexia Institute's style of fully-joined cursive handwriting.

broad sweeps, curvy squiggles and scribbles. They enjoy "taking the pencil for a walk." They do not naturally make abrupt staccato movements. In any kind of teaching it is always better to capitalize on what comes naturally than to go against something which already works well.

Correct letter formation is taught from the start. The correct letter formation is *taught* to the child. He does not have to pick it up for himself. He does not have to abandon a halfway learned print style and learn joined writing at a time when he needs his brain for other things such as ideas, punctuation, grammar, spelling etc.

There is nothing to unlearn later. The child learns from the beginning the letter formation he will use for the rest of his life. The only thing the child has to do after the initial teaching is practice, practice, and perfect.

As the dyslexia specialist teaches, she also makes connections between letter name, sound, shape for reading, and shape for writing. The form of cursive script used by the Dyslexia Institute is designed so that the cursive form is superimposed over the printed form the child reads, for maximum transparency. The child can see the printed form *through* the cursive and realize that this is not a new or separate entity but is linked to his reading and spelling work.

This style aids left to right movement. We read and write English from left to right. The cursive script favored by the Dyslexia Institute begins to the left of the letter and moves to the right in every case, sometimes in an up–down stroke, sometimes up and over, but always left to right (see Figure 3).

There is less load on memory. The children learn two basic rules for mastering the letter shapes initially:

1. Every letter begins on the line.
2. Every letter has a lead in and a lead out stroke.

This prevents students from worrying where to put their pencil on their paper, whether the letter that begins at the top and goes down, or begins in the middle and goes round and so on. This is unnecessary worry, an unnecessary waste of brain space. Every letter begins on the line, be it a real line or an imaginary

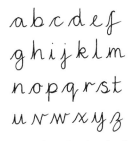

Figure 3. The Dyslexia Institute's style of cursive script.

one—it doesn't seem to bother children, and, as already stated, every letter moves in a left to right direction.

Spacing is helped. Letters don't get crammed together, nor do they roam too far apart. Finger spacing (leaving a space the size of a finger's width), which is often a great distraction to children, is unnecessary. Joins make natural spaces.

Words are seen as separate whole units. Words begin when a pen touches the paper and end when it is lifted. They are separate entities with spaces between. This helps children in the very acquisition of the concept of a word as well as in their writing.

This method helps the child who has persistent reversal problems. The letters **b** and **d** look like mirror images of each other in their printed form. Their cursive formation is different and distinctive, and helps the child to separate them in his mind and writing (see Figure 4).

Other groups of similar letters are also more distinguishable in the cursive form, even though they are still similar in the underlying print. The wise teacher will always teach similar looking and similar sounding letters separately. She will give one form time to settle in and become soundly acquired before introducing the next.

This method increases speed. Fast, fluent writing is essential if a state of flow is ever to be reached. It is rarely possible to print quickly. Also, it is difficult to achieve the 17–23 words per minute required for General Certificate of Secondary Education (GCSE) examination success in print if the pen is lifted at every letter.

This program allows the development of a personal style. This is not a highly stylized form but a naturalistic one, which lends itself to personal interpretation. Once the basic letter shapes are acquired and secure they will take on the personality of their creator. No two people write *exactly* the same.

This takes the focus away from the hand and directs it toward the brain. Fully joined cursive writing, within a structured, cumulative program of literacy acquisition, is a truly multisensory experience. The memory of things heard (sounds), things seen (shapes), and things experienced (the motor movements of the hand) are integrated. They are welded together for security of retention and readiness of retrieval. Fully joined cursive writing makes full use of the kinesthetic memory, the strongest modality for learning.

Once the agonizing over where to start the letter, which direction to move in, and which letter comes next is over, the writer is then free to get on with the business of communication. Practicing cursive letter shapes to automaticity has been found by one researcher in the United States to "free up mental resources for other activities. (Leutwyler, 1998)

Figure 4. Distinctive cursive formation helps separate letters that are easily confused.

Monday
Learn a basic cursive stroke.

Learn these letters.

l t i n m h k

Tuesday
Learn these letters.

b p r u y j

Wednesday
Learn a second basic cursive stroke.

Learn these letters.

c a g q o s d f

Thursday
Learn these odd letters.

e v w x z

Friday
Start to join!

main rain again Spain

Next Monday
I always write in fully joined cursive script now!

Figure 5. Switching to cursive script.

It improves spelling! The dyslexia specialist has long been convinced that sound writing skills are crucial foundations for later learning, that welded words last better in the memory than those made of separate entities which can so easily drift apart or change places.

Any teacher, who has a mixed ability class, can enable all her students to share in this good fortune by implementing fully joined cursive writing alongside a spelling program which builds cumulatively in word families. In both the National Curriculum and Literacy Strategy, spelling work on common letter patterns and in word families is recommended.

Students or whole classes, who learned printed letters and need to switch to joined up for writing, can do so swiftly and easily. The teacher can group the letter shapes into those which begin with the same entry stroke. She can teach a batch a day and provide lots of opportunities for reinforcement and practice. One week is enough to do the initial teaching. The students then know that from then on, they are to write only in cursive. They then have the rest of their school careers to practice and perfect (see Figure 5).

Teachers, particularly those who teach young children, often say, "but what about reading? Children read print. Won't they become confused?" When students are taught the sound–symbol relationship between the printed form of a letter and the sound it represents in reading, then they are just one small step away from learning how the cursive form superimposes over the print for writing (see Figure 6).

The teacher should demonstrate this, so the students can see for themselves that the original, printed form remains and can still be seen through the cursive shape. It is not necessary to show this every time, just the first few times while the student is learning the basic letter shapes.

Recent initiatives in education might lead us to think that joined writing is a new or radical move. Paillasson told us over 200 years ago that:

> The links in handwriting should not be neglected; they are to this art as the soul is to the body. Without these links there would be no movement, no fire, none of the vitality that lends quality to handwriting. (Paillasson 1763, in Jean, 1992)

British school children were taught joined handwriting until 1922 when school inspectors issued a pamphlet on print script. This script style was believed to be easier for young children to learn than the various copperplate-type scripts in use at that time. School children in many continental countries are taught joined handwriting from school entry today.

1.2. Punctuation

Punctuation marks are tiny. They represent abstract concepts. They often elude the dyslexic pupil altogether, both in his reading and his writing. The teacher needs to think about how to make these marks real, and how to make them bigger and more noticeable for a period of time until the student understands.

A good way for teachers to begin to make punctuation meaningful is to attempt to read a piece of prose without emphasis or allowing for punctuation. Do *not* use a piece of prose produced by the student but use an artificially manufactured piece. This is quite easy to do on a word processor, or by photocopying text, eradicating punctuation marks, and re-photocopying.

Students can have great fun trying to read this piece. They can do this one to one, in a small group, or in a larger group or class, clustered round a big book during the literacy hour. They can listen to their teacher try to read it without breathing. They must then decide where the reader can take a breath and mark this place with the felt tip pen. They should do this several times until they reach the end of

Figure 6. Cursive script superimposes over print script for writing; the print can be seen through the cursive writing.

the piece. That might be enough for one day. The group might also decide to continue thinking about restarting reading after a breath and marking this place with a capital letter.

Subsequently the individual or group might read through the piece—now more easily—and cluster separate ideas together. They might cut the piece where one idea ends and another begins, and mount these on another sheet of paper, leaving a space between ideas. Thus they begin to develop a feel for paragraphs. Subdividing the piece further with enlarged, colored commas will draw attention to smaller breathing spaces. Punctuation needs to be meaningful and highly visible for learning and reinforcement. It can resume its normal size once the pupil has acquired the necessary skill.

Appreciation of the need for punctuation in this way has to be tackled and understood for speaking and reading if the pupil is to have a chance of using it correctly in his writing. Quotation marks can be taught on a listening and speaking level by using a "talking hat." This is a top hat or something similar that has large quotation marks drawn on (see Figure 7). The teacher orchestrates a little game where she says, "Today John says . . ." and drops the hat on to John's head as he answers. She lifts it when he stops and moves on to another child, perhaps altering the vocabulary to, "And Sheila replies . . ." and so on. The game uses different speech labels (exclaimed, shouted, whispered, etc.) each time it is played.

At some stage it will be necessary to move this work into the written form. After playing the game with the talking hat, the teacher then writes what the children said on the board:

John says, "I am playing for the school football team tonight."

The group can then be asked what they notice, i.e., that when John was speaking he was wearing the talking hat with special marks on it, and what he said was written in between the same special marks.

Activities like those described above can be adapted and extended in many different ways. Arbitrary symbols not only come to life, but they have meaning

Figure 7. The "talking" hat.

and purpose. Students will need this kind of understanding if they are to learn how to use punctuation successfully.

Even with good understanding and plenty of practice, the student might still require a memory aid. The student might make a bookmark and put the main punctuation marks and their purpose on it. He might laminate this and keep it on the desk when he is writing and editing, as a concrete reminder of former learning.

2. WRITING TO COMMUNICATE

When the dyslexic pupil is given a writing task: *Write a story entitled . . . Find out about . . . Do a project on . . .* one of two things can happen. At worst, a couple of pieces of paper, crumpled, crossed out or erased, is produced or even "lost." Priscilla Vail (1997) describes this as "litter." It is entirely unsatisfactory and irritating for the expectant teacher, but is many times more so for the would-be writer.

Or the opposite may occur: Lots of writing may be produced. Chunks may be copied from a textbook, a friend, Encarta, etc., which the teacher is unable to follow and the pupil is unable to read back. This, too, is an unsatisfying experience for all parties but it is an empty and humiliating experience for the writer.

The huge task of producing a perfectly written story or piece of prose is too large to be tackled all at once. The struggler needs a system of diminishing support, which allows him to learn the process or processes involved. He then begins to take control of them.

2.1. Story or Creative Writing

The idea of a story is not immediately obvious to the dyslexic pupil who may not have read many stories for himself. His struggle to read stories often involves 99 percent effort on the decoding side. This leaves him with little brain space to round up and make sense of the meaning or even notice the structure the story followed. Even if he has been read to a great deal, he may not have grasped many of the rules of written language for himself. Those rules will need to be taught.

The Dyslexia Institute Story Hump serves this purpose. It portrays the stages that build into a rounded story. At the earliest level a six-stage hump is drawn, and each stage is talked about with the child (see Figure 8). Work at the speaking, listening, and reading levels sets the scene for later composition and writing.

The child might make his own story hump, or a set of story cards, and follow a story with his finger as his teacher or helper reads it to him (see Figure 9).

By taking a piece of plain paper, folding into six parts and numbering each in the same way as the story hump, the child can create his own satisfying story. Perhaps he can begin with just a picture drawn in each space then build gradually to

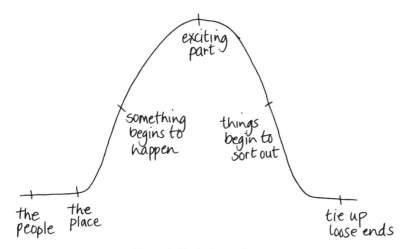

Figure 8. The basic story hump.

a picture and single word, from there to a picture and a phrase, then a picture and a sentence, and finally to a couple of sentences.

In the very early stages the teacher or support assistant might actually transcribe the child's words. She can invite the child to read back his story at the end, gradually encouraging him to perhaps write in the final box himself, then the last two boxes and so on until he is confident enough to do the whole thing by himself.

Once the student is competent at this level, he can then move on to a supported story writing sheet where date, title, etc., might be provided. The student chooses some essential vocabulary and uses the boxes that mirror the story hump to create his story (see Figure 10).

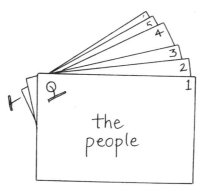

Figure 9. Story cards.

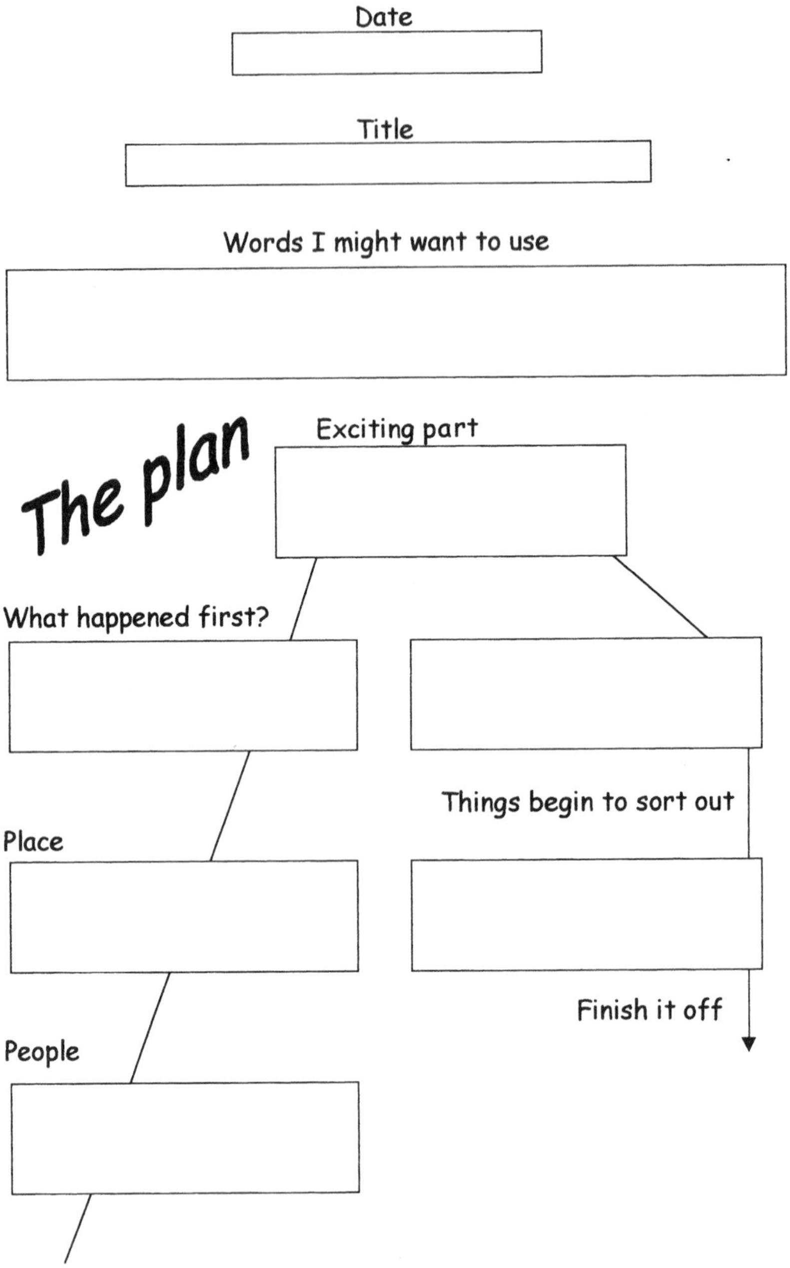

Date

Title

Words I might want to use

The plan

Exciting part

What happened first?

Things begin to sort out

Place

People

Finish it off

Figure 10. Framework for supported story writing.

Again, the possibilities for support are endless. The teacher might supply some of the writing, gradually giving over more and more responsibility to the student until he is confident enough to do it by himself. In the classroom setting, this work might be supported by a paraprofessional.

It is important to note, however, this sheet is not intended to be a worksheet that is filled in and forgotten. It should be an aid to the creative writing process. Once the sheet is filled with ideas, those ideas should be written up as a rounded, linear piece of prose. The sheet should be used for organizing the ideas for that final piece of writing.

As the student feels confident and competent, he should be encouraged to move around the hump in varied directions; perhaps he can use the "exciting part" as a starting point, then touching back to explain the characters once his story is underway. There are many possibilities.

Eventually the student will do the whole thing for himself. He can seek spelling of key vocabulary from his teacher, her assistant, or a dictionary. He can decide the direction for his story. He can plot his main ideas on the sheet, and he can use the sheet to support his writing. The student's growing confidence will dictate the degree and timing of support—from full to diminishing to none. Eventually, the story's shape and stages will be built into the student's mind. He will then have no further need of the sheet.

2.2. Advanced Creative Writing

The ideas described in the previous section can be adapted for a student at any level. The GCSE student for example, might be encouraged to design a creative piece around the headings:

Exposition

Complication

Crisis

Climax

Resolution

Denouement

Further complexity could be added if "false crisis" and "false resolution" were built in. The student who did story hump-type work in his early years will be more amenable to this way of structuring ideas than the student who begins this a few months before essay exams.

Writing is a richly rewarding experience; creating a rounded and satisfying piece of prose which a reader can understand, appreciate, and comment on is its own reward. Artificial reward *and* sanction systems rarely have a lasting effect because it is rarely making an effort that is the problem, but more often knowing what kind of effort, and in which direction, that undermines the struggling writer's efforts: for example, Where am I going wrong? What do I need to do to put it right?

The process of writing begins with an idea. Students who verbally work through their ideas are likely to be more successful when they put those ideas into the written form.

Czerniewska (1992) quotes Bloomfield (1935) to illustrate the primacy of speech as a precursor to writing:

> Writing is not language, but merely a way of recording language by means of visible marks.

Czerniewska herself states that "writing practices are intertwined with talk and reading."

The National Curriculum (DfEE, 1995) outlines Speaking and Listening, Reading and Writing as separate programs of study. At the same time they acknowledge that "Pupils' abilities should be developed within an integrated programme of speaking and listening, reading and writing."

Students who find it difficult to express themselves in writing need to talk first. They need to explore their ideas in a range of ways: discussion, debate, art, dance, drama, etc. Students who find they cannot "get started" should get help from someone else who will start for them. This person can provide an opening paragraph or sentence to help the student get over his particular block. Any student who finds the task just too huge will be helped by the scaffolds described previously, and also by the slimming down of the task.

Recreating history is often a satisfying experience. Students can follow early human's attempts to communicate. They can learn how to make pictograms, short messages on clay or wax tablets, recorded events on "scrolls," or short stories in seventeenth century type booklets. Manguel (1997) and Jackson (1981) are useful sources of information for this type of work.

Today, short e-mail messages might ease the reluctant writer gently into the writing process. This can be done by building up slowly through small cards containing a simple message, or writing postcards recounting events, or considering short books written for a younger reader, perhaps with illustrations and so on.

When doing longer pieces of writing, students can use the analogy of building a wall starting with a single brick (a word), then a row of bricks cemented together (a sentence), then row upon row producing a wall (a paragraph).

Aitchison (1994) quotes Chand (date unknown) with saying:

> Words are like glamorous bricks that constitute the fabric of any language.

2.3. Writing for Different Purposes

Writing for different purposes takes various forms. This will be obvious to the successful student writer; he will internalize it with experience. The dyslexic or struggling writer will not necessarily do this and will need explicit development of each of the forms, or genres.

Text level work within the National Literacy Strategy begins at Key Stage One (age 5–7 years) with simple captions or labels, extended captions, simple questions, lists. It goes on to simple recounts, sequential instructions, note-taking, reporting, and simple story writing.

At Key Stage Two (7–11 years) there is further development in the form of instructions, messages, letters, summaries of text and reports. Students move on to connected, persuasive, and recounted prose, explanatory texts, commentary, argument, biographical writing, and journalistic reporting as well as poetry and extended story writing.

The dyslexic writer will be helped enormously if he has a clear idea of his purpose for writing. He needs to know the intended audience and the type of writing required. Each form, or genre, will need to be carefully explored and explained.

Many ideas for helping the dyslexic or struggling writer to generate and write factual information in a range of genres are contained in the work of David Wray and Maureen Lewis on the Exeter Extending Literacy Project (EXEL) at the University of Exeter and their publications (1997,1998).

Above all, the dyslexic writer will need to know that writing is about communicating thoughts and ideas, rather than covering paper or pleasing the teacher. This is helpful for all writers and *essential* for the dyslexic would-be writer.

2.4. Note-Taking

Note-taking is an activity that can be fraught with dilemma. It is hard to decide what to write down and where. This can result in time lost actually writing down. The first crucial part of the talk gets lost and nothing else makes much sense afterwards. The skills involved in note-taking are:

1. Understanding the language
2. Selecting what is important
3. Organizing the information gained
4. Reorganizing that information and presenting it in a different way

None of these are easy. None come naturally to the dyslexic student. He will have to begin by finding a note-taking style that suits his own personal style. Linear notes may not work for him. Alternative layouts such as diagrammatic notes or a mind map might work better. He will need explicit teaching and help to find his best strategy. (See Chapter 8.)

He will also need explicit work on deciding between relevant and irrelevant aspects. He will need lots of unpressured practice at making these decisions from reduced pieces of prose, newspaper or magazine articles, or very short talks. This will teach him the skills he will later need to employ at speed.

The student might organize and reorganize his ideas, after note-taking, by employing the support of a set of headings which will direct his thinking:

Main point > Supporting points > Summary

This, or a similar framework, might be useful.

Of course the onus for successful note-taking rests not with the student, but with the teacher who conveys the information. She might use a set of headings or questions as guidelines for her talk. This may help achieve maximum understanding and competence from her students.

These might be:

- What is the main message of this lesson?
- Can I state that clearly and unambiguously at the outset and perhaps several times during my talk?
- What are the key points I want my students to understand, to listen out for, to note?
- Can I make these points at the outset, during the talk, and again at the end of the talk?
- Can I issue the main message and key points as a handout for the students to follow, or write them on the board at the outset either as linear notes or as a flow chart?
- Are there any unusual names, place names, etc., that will be unfamiliar, and can I add these to the handout or write them on the board?
- Are there any other words that I would hate to see misspelled, and if so, shall I provide them?

Special education teachers supporting a dyslexic pupil in curricular subjects might talk to subject teachers about the importance of this kind of presentation for all their students, and the absolute need of it for the dyslexic and struggling student. If this is not possible, the special education teacher can still help by advising her student that each piece of work has a main point and supporting points. She should give him lots of practice at listening for and noting them. This will have to begin at a low level and build as the student becomes confident and competent.

2.5. Marshaling Ideas

Students who struggle with writing might have ideas that are so many, so varied, so wonderful, yet too many and too random ever to nail down into some kind of presentation form. Other students may not be able to think of a single idea because their vision is clouded by the awfulness of what to do with them, namely to write them down! In either case what hits the paper is unlikely to be satisfying to writer, or subsequently, reader.

The dyslexic student, struggling to produce ideas or to bring his ideas under control, needs some kind of concrete support within which to organize. The use of headings or labels will help enormously. Many special education teachers use "magnets" as a means of eliciting their student's thoughts and ideas, and then organizing them.

Magnet headings for the young or inexperienced student begin with the five senses:

- Sight
- Hearing
- Touch
- Smell
- Taste

A concrete object can be explored under these headings. An orange, apple, cabbage or similar is a useful stimulus—whole or cut in two—for the student to talk about under those sensory headings. He considers how it looks, smells, feels, and so on. The student transfers this information to a diagram and then has the basis of a short piece of factual writing (see Figure 11).

Again, this is not the end of the writing activity, but the beginning. The student should be encouraged to write up his ideas as a short piece of prose, either straight away or at a later time. His ideas will be there on the planning sheet for him to return to.

The student who has had previous experience with the five senses magnets can move on to a more advanced set of "thinking" headings. The teacher can take any subject and encourage her students to brainstorm using these headings as a guideline.

- Art
- Geography
- History
- Economics
- Psychology
- Religion

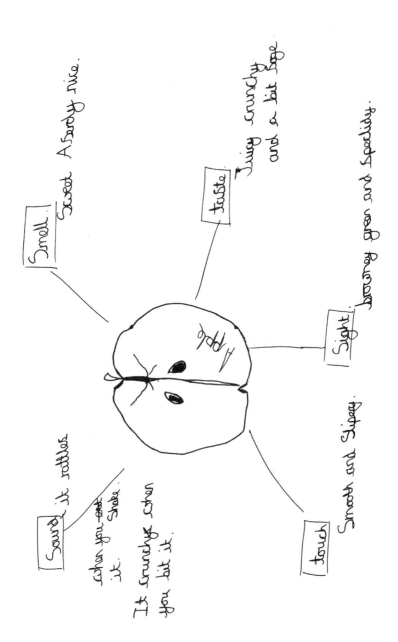

Figure 11. Magnets to *draw* thoughts from the brain.

Suppose a new superstore has just opened on the outskirts of town. By using the thinking headings, the teacher can generate these, and more, questions:

Art:
Who designed and built it?
What colors predominate?
What shape and style of architecture is it?
Is it pleasing to look at? Does it fit in with its surroundings?

Geography:
Where was it built and why?
Who can get to it easily, and how would they travel?
Is its position advantageous to other traders in the town?
Can items sold in the store be traced to their country of origin and journey to England?

History:
What was on the site before?
How has land use changed?
What is the story behind the store's originator?

Economics:
How do prices compare to other superstores, smaller stores, village stores?

Psychology:
How does this store persuade shoppers to part with their money?
Where are slow-moving products placed, and why?
What sensory mechanisms are used to persuade shoppers that bananas are ripe, or bread is baked in-store?

Religion:
What has been the impact of Sunday opening?

The students can brainstorm aloud first with the teacher writing their ideas on the board. She can do this in a linear form or as radiating spokes with both the central image and store name in the center and headings at the end of each arm for her to group students' comments around. This enables her to go back to a subject heading if a student thinks up something new. Ideas which needed stimuli or were out of control are now marshaled and organized and ready to be written. Early mind-mapping skills have begun. For further ideas see Chapter 8.

2.6. Checking Strategies

Work can be checked or edited in one of two ways. Some students prefer to get their thoughts and ideas on to paper without thinking about spelling, grammar, punctuation, etc., and then return to their finished piece and check each aspect separately using a "MAPS check" (to follow). Other students find this impossible and need to edit their work as they go along.

Regardless of how the student chooses to check and edit his work, he must know vital components, such as the use of capital letters, verb agreements, spelling and punctuation. These need to have been thoroughly taught, practiced, and used, and he needs access to any possible memory aids. It is impossible to know whether any work is correct without having had explicit teaching and learning of each of the concepts involved.

Direct instruction is necessary to help the dyslexic student to check his work. There are those students who prefer to get their thoughts on paper and then check afterwards. Figure 12 has useful suggestions for them.

For other students, this way of working will be uncomfortable. They prefer to undergo the same process, but only as they go along. In this case they should have a concrete reminder of areas that need to be checked, perhaps in the form of a small version of a MAPS check, such as a bookmark with a note of the main areas:

> **M**eaning
> **A**greement
> **P**unctuation
> **S**pelling

This can be as minimal or as detailed as the student needs. If it is beside him as he writes, he can glance at it per paragraph or per line to help him to collect his thoughts.

3. WRITING WITH INFORMATION COMMUNICATION TECHNOLOGY (I.C.T.)

In this technological age many reluctant writers have been "won over" to writing by the use of personal computers, laptops, etc.

The same two aspects of the skill need consideration as with manual writing: the mechanical aspect and writing to express thoughts and ideas.

Students need accurate, fast, and fluent word processing skills if they are to be successful in this medium. These skills take a long time to build, requiring much repetition and practice to gain competence. Some students who have poor fine motor skills or illegible handwriting have been switched to a computer as a "cure all." Switching to a word processor, alone, will not help.

Priscilla Vail, speaking at the Fourth International Conference of the British Dyslexia Association in York, U.K., in April 1997, said that many American schoolchildren arrive at eighth grade with three semideveloped systems: print, cursive, and keyboard. This is also often true of the British secondary

A Strategy for Success in Written Work

First, the most important thing about any piece of written work is that it reflects the wonderful *you*ness of you. It is a translation in writing of the thoughts in your head, a *downloading* of your brain on to paper! Don't ever forget that this is the reason for writing.

Next, you need to ensure your audience can get your message by making it readable, and that means making it as clear, sensible and well presented as possible, with spelling as near as you can get to the way that everyone else spells. So, to maximize your chances of success, get into the habit of following this simple strategy for success:
1. Get what you want to say on to paper and don't think about anything else. Let the ideas flow.
2. Take a break.
3. Return to your manuscript with a different colored pen, make yourself comfortable, and check your work FOUR TIMES.
4. Each time you check, look for something different. We call this the maps check. The **MAPS** check looks at:

> *Meaning
>> Have I said said what I meant to say?
>> Have I left anything out?
>> Have I repeated myself?
>> Have I kept the same tense all the way through?
>
> *Agreement
>> Do the verbs match the subject?
>
> *Punctuation
>> Do I need CAPITAL LETTERS?
>> Do I need to punctuate?
>>> . , ? ! " " '
>
> *Spelling
>> Which words do I always get wrong?
>> Are there any words that I am uncertain of?
>> If so, how shall I tackle them?

IDEAS
Underline any I am not sure of.
Ask a friend, teacher, parent.
Look up one or two in dictionary or on a spellchecker.
Have my spelling book handy—these are the words I have learned.
Approach my teacher beforehand and ask for a list of the main spellings, including names, places, technical terms, etc. (Julius Caesar/Egypt/distillation).
Also ask my teacher—Are there any words which, when spelled wrong, drive you bananas, and if so, would you please write them down for me now?
Look for things such as silent e (lak<u>e</u>, tim<u>e</u>, tub<u>e</u>), or double letters (ru<u>nn</u>ing, tri<u>pp</u>ed).

Finally. . . . Rewrite your work to look its best. It may not be absolutely perfect, but it will definitely be close.

Figure 12. The MAPS Check: A strategy for success in written work.

school entrant whose print was barely acquired before he switched to joined-up writing; too little practice meant that this remained illegible for him and his teachers, so he is given a keyboard but not given the accompanying training which is necessary for his success. Thus the student enters an important phase in his education *without a single, reliable recording system.*

Thoroughly and carefully taught word processing skills must accompany the provision of any technological aid. There are many published packages that can help with organizing and communicating ideas. Microsoft Creative Writer is one example which has motivational ideas and frameworks for the young student. Redrafting facilities, spelling and grammar checks on personal computers and laptops take much of the sting out of perfecting a piece of writing for public consumption. These serve to motivate and encourage. Handwriting practice needs to continue alongside computer skills practice because a back-up system will be needed whenever technology fails, batteries run down and hard drives do crash.

4. LEARNING TO WRITE: WRITING TO LEARN

Our students are apprentice writers who need to be taught writing skills. They need good models, step by step instruction at every stage and in every aspect of the skill. They need a diminishing system of support from people and from resources. They need to practice individual aspects of writing separately and eventually bring these together into a satisfying whole.

They need to write because as they learn to write, they write to learn. In the National Writing Project of 1989, Margaret Wallen said:

> There is no doubt that learning occurs during the writing process as writers organize and recreate knowledge on the page. (Czerniewska 1992)

They need to write well for to help them achieve a good self-image and high self-esteem. They need to write to take part in, and influence, their own culture. Manguel (1996) says

> The child learning to read is admitted into the communal memory by way of books, and thereby becomes acquainted with a common past which he or she renews, to a greater or lesser degree, in every reading.

The child who learns to write gains the opportunity to shape the future—his own, and that of the society in which he lives.

REFERENCES

Aitchison, J. (1994). *Words in the Mind.* Oxford UK. Blackwell.
Bloomfield L (1935) *Language* London: George, Allen and Unwin.

Cripps, C., & Cox, R. (1990). Cambridge. *Joining the ABC.* LDA.

Csikszentmihalyi, M. (1990). *Flow: The Psychology of Optimal Experience.* London. Harper and Row.

Csikszentmihalyi M (1975) "Play and Intrinsic Rewards" *Journal of Humanistic Psychology 15*, 3.

Czerniewska, P. (1992). *Learning about Writing,* Oxford UK. Blackwell.

Department for Education (1995). *The National Curriculum.* London. HMSO.

Department for Education & Employment (1998). *The National Literacy Strategy* London. DfEE.

Goleman, D. (1996). *Emotional Intelligence.* London. Bloomsbury.

Hamilton J, Haier R & Buchsbaumm (1984) "Intrinsic Enjoyment and Boredom Coping Sales: Validation With Personality. Evoked Potential and Attention Measures" Personality and Individual Differences 5(2):183–93.

Jackson, D. (1981). *The Story of Writing.* London. Barrie & Jenkins Ltd.

Jean, G. (1992). *Writing: The Story of Alphabets and Scripts.* Thames & Hudson. London.

Leutwyler, K. (1998). Reading, Typing and 'Rithmetic, *Scientific American.* Volume 278 Number 4 page 17 April 98.

Manguel, A. (1997). *A History of Reading.* Flamingo. HarperCollins. London.

McAllen, A.E. (1992). *The Extra Lesson.* The Robinswood Press. Stourbridge.

Nash-Wortham, M., & Hunt, J. (1990). *Take Time.* The Robinswood Press. Stourbridge.

Paillasson (1763) in Jean, G. (1992)

Sawyer, C.E., Gray F. and Champness, M. (1996). Measuring Speed of Handwriting for GCSE Candidates, *Educational Psychology in Practice,* 12(1) p. 19–23.

Vail, P.L. (1981). *Clear and Lively Writing.* Walker & Company. New York.

Vail, P.L. (1997). Theory's fine, but what do I do on Monday? Speech given at Fourth International Conference of the British Dyslexia Assocation, York, April 1997.

Walker, J., & Brooks, L. (1996). *Dyslexia Institute Literacy Programme.* The Dyslexia Institute. Staines.

Wray, D., & Lewis, M. (1997). *Extending Literacy.* Routledge. London.

7

Using Literacy Development Programs

Helen Moss

1. INTRODUCTION

The aim of every teacher must surely be to equip students adequately so that they not only have a mature and fully balanced approach to life and the world but also sufficient tools to use in a literate society. Many children absorb these skills with little apparent effort by following their school's reading program and making progress. It is only when this development does not take place that the concerned teacher should question how the child is learning and what methods and programs of remediation could be used. What course would be suitable for the student depends not only on the needs of the child but also on school resources—both financial and human.

Therefore a literacy program should contain the necessary equipment for a teacher and a student to work and develop the student's ability to cope with all reading and writing requirements in a living and working environment. Such a program should be structured and cumulative in order that the student can make progress. It should be presented so that the teacher knows how to use it without going to great lengths to understand and interpret it. It should require as little teacher preparation as possible. It should also be structured in such a way that it builds on the student's current achievements, has the capacity to fill gaps in the student's current knowledge, and that it works in a cumulative way, thus develop-

Helen Moss, The Dyslexia Institute, The Huntingdon Centre, The Vineyards, The Paragon, Bath, BA1 5NA, United Kingdom

ing language use (written, read, and aural). Most children would benefit from a multisensory approach to learning but for dyslexic students, this approach is crucial. Information processing problems and the consequences that arise when retrieval of information is slow necessitates the need for strong literacy skills. They should be as automatic as possible thus freeing the student to work with the task at hand. For example, in essay writing a student should not have to be concentrating on sentence structure and spelling. He should read for comprehension rather than word attack analysis.

Peter Hatcher (Dyslexia Institute, 1993b) made the following recommendations for a successful reading program:

1. Reading and spelling must be integrated.
2. Text should be read at an instructional level with 93 to 94 percent accuracy.
3. Students must have help with sounds.
4. Letter names and sounds must be taught.
5. Direct relationship–link between letter sounds in words.
6. Ability to cross-check these strategies.

This chapter examines three case studies using literacy programs developed by Walter Bramley. Each case study is preceded by a description of the relevant program. In all three cases there is an overlap of one program with another as each student has either needed to have gaps in his learning filled or has moved on to the next stage.

2. DEVELOPING BASIC LITERACY SKILLS—ACTIVE LITERACY KIT

This program was designed initially for students aged 11 or younger, who are resisting remedial measures implemented by class teachers. Often, because of their awareness of failure and, emotional factors which developed, these children lack confidence and have a low self-esteem. At times they may even be unwilling to attempt anything with which they are unfamiliar, especially if they think they might fail the task. Students suitable for using this program have low reading and spelling levels (6½ years and lower), poor phonological awareness, insufficient alphabet knowledge and an inability to decode or encode consonant–vowel–consonant (cvc) words. If any reading happens, it is labored and halting with much content-based guesswork. At this extreme level, the student is spelling phonetically and his spelling can outshine his reading ability. Spelling processing speed is considerably slower than that for reading. Motor skills are required for writing words, and this being a slower process gives the student greater time to think about the sounds he is using. In addition, reading at this level is more difficult because sound processing of cvc words needs to be automatic, and this response has not yet established itself. Many children at this level have become totally stuck and seem unable to make further progress.

2.1. Assessment

The program includes a diagnostic *interview record sheet.* The teacher uses this to pinpoint specific areas of disability and implement exercises and timed targets which enable the student to reach an automatic level of response.

The interview record is easy to work with. It contains suggested dialogue to use when conducting the interview and has a sheet for recording the findings. There are 16 short tests. At the end of each test there is a bracket containing numbers indicating which exercises need to be worked if the student has not managed the task adequately. There is also a teaching guide onto which the teacher can score the results of the tests so at the end of the interview a summary of the work needing to be covered is already in place. This would form the basis for future lessons. In this way, the student works only on these areas of weakness as the lessons progress.

The tests include:

1. Alphabet work, i.e. oral sequencing: naming and sounding in random order, writing the alphabet, laying out the alphabet sequence with lower case letters, naming and sounding vowels and the use of letter "y" as a vowel
2. Sequencing days of the week; months of the year; counting to 20 by twos, and writing 1–26
3. Reading 20 cvc words and 20 long and short vowel words—both are timed exercises
4. Eleven sentences, all at a 5 years 9 months to 6 years reading level
5. Spelling 15 words at a basic spelling level; all the alphabet letters are included
6. Short rhyming tasks

The manual advises how to interpret and understand the nature of the problems. also, in dialogue form, it explains how to approach specific exercises.

2.2. The Program

The introductory exercises include basic alphabet work and sequencing exercises. These are timed targets where necessary. The main group of exercises develops the early alphabet skills and reinforces the association between the names and the sounds of letters.

There is a battery of exercises which contain groups of 25 cvc words of increasing difficulty. They begin with rhyming words with one vowel per page moving on to keeping the same vowel on each page but gradually changing the final consonant and onset letter. The pages slowly increase in complexity until the cvc words are in random order with mixed short vowels. The same groups of words are then used in a multisensory way for spelling

The next group of exercises contains a list of 20 pairs of words, some of which rhyme. The student is asked to listen and decide which pairs rhyme and which do not. There is also a record sheet for the student to record his results and perform a self-check. The group that follows works on alliteration using the same style of exercises.

By this stage the student should be working with a literacy program, such as Units of Sound (described later in this chapter), and should have an automatic response when reading cvc words. The exercises at this level strengthen the student's ability to hear the different short vowels. They can be worked with the teacher reading the words while the student gives the vowel sound, or they can be read by the student, who extracts the vowel sound as he reads: "mat"—/<a>/, "bed"/<e>/, etc.

After this, the student moves on to similar exercises which focus on long and short vowel sounds.

All the reading exercises are timed so the student can see how his own performance is increasing. The target for each exercise is 30 seconds.

The final group of exercises concentrates on spelling, and the structure for this is based on the progression of the sounds within the Units of Sound Program Stage One. The first five exercises practice the use of cvc words, encouraging the student to listen for either the beginning or the end sound of a word.

The whole program centers around the importance of alphabetic skills in reading and spelling, and on developing an automatic response to early reading skills. The demands needed in phonological awareness are well covered thus responding to current thinking about early literacy requirements.

3. CASE STUDY 1: LUCY

3.1. Background

Lucy was 7½ years old when she was assessed at the Dyslexia Institute. At this time her parents were concerned about her progress in reading, writing, and maths (arithmetic) at her local primary school. She appeared to lack in confidence because she preferred to keep quiet and say nothing rather than risk saying something which might be incorrect. Lucy tended to fidget, and she had trouble concentrating for any length of time. She was also reported as having particular difficulty in sounding out words.

Her school thought she was of below average ability and this ability varied from day to day. Lucy cooperated well. She was friendly and responsive but sought approval and was easily distracted.

The educational psychologist used the British Ability Scales Second Edition to assess Lucy. This showed Lucy had an above average general conceptual ability of 112, at percentile 79. Her greatest strengths were in terms of her reasoning skills, both verbal and nonverbal. She experienced a significant degree of difficulty with regard to phonological processing skills: Although she could hear and repeat polysyllabic nonwords, she found it very difficult to manipulate the sounds within words. The formal assessment showed:

		(Approximate Expectation)
BAS11	Word reading age: 5 years, 7 months	(7 years, 6 months)
WORD	Reading comprehension: 6 years	(8 years)
BAS11	Spelling age: 6 years, 1 month	(7 years, 6 months)

Lucy showed a significant degree of under achievement in her reading and spelling compared to what was expected for her overall level of cognitive ability.

When reading, Lucy relied heavily on auditory strategies. She tried to decode letter by letter, often giving the correct sound, but she was unable to encode to make a full word.

When spelling Lucy relied heavily on phonic strategies. As she wrote she said the sounds aloud. Unfortunately although what she sounded and wrote were the same they did not correspond with what was actually within the word. In both reading and spelling she made no recourse to her memory storage for words. Lucy held her pencil in a poor way in her right hand. Many of her letters were incorrectly formed. She had developed circuitous tactics: writing capital **B** to avoid lower case **b/d** confusion.

3.3. Intervention

The Placement Test from the Active Literacy Kit (ALK) was administered to Lucy. It was used to identify specific areas of weakness that needed to be addressed.

Lucy did not know there were 26 letters in the alphabet. She was only able to sequence part of this. **A–k** was accurate. She then continued **l o, m o, p q r s t**, proclaimed "I am getting muddled," and she stopped. When writing the sequence she produced a mixture of uppercased and lowercased letters that were incorrectly sequenced after the letter **k** (see Figure 1). When using the lowercase wooden letters in sequence she followed a different order (see Figure 2). The letter **l** was not included.

She knew the names of the alphabet letters in random order but gave reverse names for **b** and **d**, gave the sound /ū/ for /ŭ/ and called **q p**. In sounding out the letters in random order she again reversed **b** and **d**, **k** was /kī/, **y** was /ŭ/ and she was unable to attempt **x**. She did not know how vowels were used.

She thought there were ten days in the week. She gave Tuesday, Friday, Saturday, and then she stopped.

Lucy had no ideas about either the names of the months or their sequential order. Although she was able to count to 20, she was unable to count in twos up to 20. When writing 1–26 she reversed 3 and 9 but after writing "1P, 20," went on to 22, 30, 40 (the 4 was reversed).

When reading five blocks of four cvc words with a target time of 30 seconds, Lucy took almost five minutes. The italicized words are her erroneous attempts. **R** indicates a refusal; * indicates a correct response:

Sob	*don*	dog	*	hot	*	hen	*han*	pal	*pot*
Cat	*	set	*sore*	tax	*down*	hum	*hot*	big	*
Cut	*cup*	rat	*ran*	sum	R	not	*on*	yet	*
Mum	*men*	pen	*pushed*	win	*	pin	*pan*	beg	R

In the light of these results she was not given the Foundation Reading test.

When her spelling test was begun, her writing was slow. She managed the first line accurately but wrote SISX for six.

As Lucy's basic literacy skills were so insecure it was decided to begin her lessons using ALK (Active Literacy Kit) and work through relevant exercises as indicated from the initial assessment and recorded on the test record sheet. Her lessons also included supporting material from Sounds Abound, SRA (Science Research Associates, a branch of McGraw-Hill) School House and Stile (initially Early Phonics program). Once these skills were established Lucy would then be at a point where she could begin the Units of Sound program.

Lucy came for tutoring twice a week for one hour each session. She was always motivated to work. She presented as a lively, bubbly, chatty little girl who had an enormous sense of humor and a great capacity for saying what work she liked and what she did not like. Her self-confidence completely astounded and silenced (for a while!) a nine-year-old boy in the class. After three lessons the boy

a b c d e F 9 h i J K n L m o q p r s t y v w x z

Figure 1. Lucy's attempt at writing the alphabet.

v added

abcdəf ℮hⁱⱼk n m qprstu ∧ wxℓ≤

Figure 2. A record of Lucy's placement of lowercase letters in alphabetical sequence.

had the courage to join in the conversation and a healthy repartee developed between the two. For several months she had assistance from "Seal" or "Bunbun" or "Dogdog," soft toys who accompanied her to her lessons.

The lessons began with her using the *no name picture cards*, a set of 26 cards illustrating each letter of the alphabet, from ALK. These were placed in an arc on the table. Lucy said what each picture was and gave its initial sound, apple /ā/, boat /b/, cat /c/, etc., six /ks/ being the exception.

She was asked to put each lowercase letter under its respective picture card and say the sequence, touching each letter as she named it. This activity was followed by joining together both aural exercises so Lucy touched the picture, said apple, gave its initial sound /ă/ and then its name /ā/ boat /b/ **b**, cat /k/ **c** etc. All exercises were timed and their results recorded.

Various games and memory exercises were developed using the no name cards and lower case alphabet while these were out on the table. Lucy was also asked to say how many letters were in the alphabet, how many vowels, to select those from the arc, put those out in front of her naming as she went and then to add the extra vowel, **y**.

Letter **a** was then kept out and other consonants added at the end: a + t, **a** + **g**, **a** + **b**, **a** + **d**, **a** + **p**, etc. All the time Lucy was saying the sounds and reading "at," "ag," "ab," etc. These vc patterns were then written onto small cards 2 cm × 5 cm and Lucy began to say "at," "ag," "ab," "ad," and "ap," etc. An individual kit was made for Lucy similar to that in ALK. The alphabet card from the ALK was also used to build cvc words aurally. It was initiated with vowel **a** and used rhyming exercises from the program: bat, cat, fat, hat, etc.

Over the weeks, as these skills became more automatic, Lucy began to read rhyming cvc patterned words from the ALK. The timed exercise was always recorded, Lucy being in charge of the stopwatch. These words were also written into her notebook and the method of spelling followed the Repeat, Spell, Write, Check (RSWC) spelling routine. A soft pencil grip (known as "my squidgy") had to be used and even so Lucy had to be reminded regularly to hold her pencil correctly. After five months Lucy was able to write cvc words without any problem naming the letters as she wrote with a reasonably well formed fully cursive handwriting script.

As vowel **a** became secure the other vowels were introduced sequentially, in a similar manner, into the reading. All the vc patterns were added to the small reading pack. Lucy was eventually able to read this pack of cards within one minute which meant that the response had become an automatic one. The reading exercises were worked through systematically. Lucy had particular problems with changing from rhyming patterns to nonrhyming ones. She was gradually able to cope with the additional expertise needed, and she managed the timed element involved (30 seconds). It took 12 months to get this far.

While all this was in progress, work continued with rhyming exercises, number tracing, and sequencing the days of the week—later months of the year. The rhyming exercises from Sounds Abound were used as well as SRA School House Violet Band in conjunction with the long and short vowel exercises from ALK.

Cards were made for the days of the week. Lucy was encouraged to put these out in number sequence and name them. Discussion and questions followed to strengthen her knowledge of before and after, e.g., "What day do you have PE at school?", "What day was it yesterday?", "What day do we begin school at the beginning of the week?", "What comes after Saturday?" Lucy had a standardized sheet, covered with tracing paper, which had numbers 1–26 on it. She was asked to trace over the numbers, saying each number as she went. She was reminded to begin writing each number at the top.

3.4. The Lesson

A typical one hour lesson at this early stage was composed of:

1. Put out the no name cards, add lowercase letters and give picture sound and name response—all timed
2. Reading pack (vc) timed
3. Build cvc words using alphabet cards
4. Work with SRA violet card
5. A reading exercise from the ALK Program
6. Write cvc words as appropriate
7. Phonological awareness game, syllable counting game, Stile exercise

Once the picture–sound name routine was established, Lucy laid out the lower case letters without picture assistance and timed the exercise (aiming for one minute). She then moved on to an exercise called "Find the Letter" (ALK). She was required to say the alphabet sequence as she followed the line of alphabet letters putting in the letters which were missing. This developed into the tracking exercise sheets from *Letter Tracking Book* (Ann Arbor).

Eventually she began to use the Units of Sound Program, which she had initially started to reinforce her current learning and build up her confidence with using a tape recorder. The aural–oral response of the tape machine helped Lucy to focus. There is a long way to go with her yet. After one year of tutoring at the Institute she is holding her own well at school and is more confident in the classroom.

4. UNITS OF SOUND: AUDIOVISUAL PROGRAM

4.1. Introduction

Although this program was created 25 years ago, its multisensory approach, structure, and cumulative format are so well thought out that it continues to have a noticeable impact on a student's literacy development. The whole program holds up well against current research into teaching dyslexic students; it is a program that fulfills students' current needs.

4.1.1. Headphones

The use of headphones—both with a tape recorder and when using the CD ROM—is supported by current research on the sound processing delays dyslexic people experience when listening to incoming information and processing it for oral response (Shaywitz, 1996).

4.1.2. Phonological Awareness

Phonological awareness is developed throughout the program especially at the beginning when cvc words are used. One page may have blocks of words that contain the same vowel letter where the rime remains constant but the onset letter changes. The next page will have the same vowel letter but the blocks of words will have differing rimes while the onset letter in each block remains the same.

4.1.3. Overlearning

It is known that dyslexic students need continual overlearning in their lessons and the program supports this by, for example, introducing sound checks at regular intervals. These help to revise the more difficult sounds the student encountered earlier in the program. Any sounds the student is uncertain of are made into reading pack cards similar to those used in other literacy programs.

Probably the most important aspect for the busy teacher is that no preparation is necessary once he or she knows how to use the program. The books, tapes or CD ROM are all ready for use. The program is designed to develop a student's independent learning. Each new page is worked alone by the student before it is worked with the teacher.

Units of Sound is intended to be used to teach basic reading and spelling skills. It can be used with a "9-year-old student whose reading development is inhibited and it can be used in its upper stages with teenage examination students as well as with adults wishing to improve or extend their reading or spelling abilities." (Bramley, 1995).

The program has three stages. Each stage has a 48-page book which has been recorded either in tape form (one tape for each four pages) or on to CD.

4.2. Testing

Each stage has its own screening test:

- First stage screening test—for reading age approximately 6–8 years
- Second stage screening test—for reading age approximately 8–10 years
- Third stage screening test—for reading age approximately 10 years plus

The student can home in on the program at the point he has reached in his own literacy development and does not need to start at the beginning of the program. However, once a starting point has been found and fixed, the pages must be followed in sequence to build in a cumulative way for the student. If the student's reading ability is at the junction of two stages, i.e., 8 years or 10 years then the screening test for the lower age group can confirm if there are any gaps in the student's earlier learning skills.

The screening tests can be used for both reading and spelling.

When using the test face to face with the student, the teacher needs to record carefully on the teacher's record form all the hesitations, inaccuracies, and refusals made. Once the test has been stopped the teacher can immediately circle the errors on the sheet. These numbers relate to the numbers at the bottom of the page which again need to be circled if appropriate. There may be one or two isolated pages which need to be addressed by a face to face check read with the student but once a cluster of difficulties arises then that will be the starting point for working. With Stage Three, where no numbers are printed at the bottom of the screening test, the starting point is the page where the earliest error shows. It is advisable to be slightly cautious in placement as it is always easier to move a student forward in the program than back.

4.3. The Program

Stage One is essentially built on words of one syllable with only a small percentage having two and two words having three syllables. Words include all the basic consonant sounds, short vowels, long vowels with silent **e**, words with final vowel **y**, elementary consonant blends placed initially and finally, and first level diphthongs or vowel digraphs.

Stage Two uses many words of one syllable. It requires higher level decoding skills than Stage 1 and has more difficult combinations such as "ei," "ie," and "gh" words.

Stage Three shows the influence of Latin–French origins. It also has some words of Greek foundation and almost none of Anglo-Saxon origin.

Each page of the book except for Stage One (pages 46–48) and Stage 3 (47, 48) contain the new units for the page. Under these are blocks of words containing the unit of sound.

Some pages have a series of sentences, sometimes linked together by a theme, that are built to be read at the specific level of the page. Some pages have checks of the units of sound previously met with and often those which present more difficulty. Other pages contain groups of words with no pattern which are intended to reinforce words and sounds met earlier in the program.

4.4. The Procedure

Standard procedure is for the student to listen to the tape and read the words in the book as directed. Most pages also finish with comprehension questions so that the student is brought back to the word blocks after completing the whole page. Each page takes approximately seven minutes to work through.

In the next lesson, which can be up to a week later, the teacher and student sit at right angles to each other while the student reads the page to the teacher. The teacher records any problems and works on them immediately. This check read page is crucial because it signals to the teacher how the student is reading and whether he is reading adequately at that specific level. The teacher must ask the student questions on the blocks of words he is reading to develop his comprehension and extend his vocabulary. It is with the teacher's imagination and involvement at this point that the program comes to life. More advanced students can be introduced to syllable counting and etymology.

After every four pages in each book, there is a yellow page with **a** in the right-hand corner. Underneath this is a number referring to a reading age. Each page contains a passage of strictly controlled vocabulary to that particular reading level based on the Fry Readability Graph. These pages are not on the tape but are an essential part of the program. If the student has reached a yellow page in the program he should be able to read it aloud to the teacher with few, if any, errors. This signals to the teacher if the student has reached a satisfactory level and can continue to the next page. At the end of each stage the teacher administers the screening test for the stage just completed. This will identify any remaining problems and these can then be worked on.

Students reading in Stage One are unlikely to be sufficiently motivated to pick up a book at home and attempt to read it. This usually happens when they approach the halfway mark in Stage Two. At this point the student's reading ability is usually more competent and fluent. He is developing decoding skills and has a greater vocabulary to use.

Although primarily a reading program, Units of Sound is successfully used for spelling and writing activities. It is possible to use the tape for spelling following a screening test similar to the reading one.

1. The student prepares the page by writing the numbers of the blocks of words relation to the appropriate page he is working with (Teachers' Manual 6.5)
2. The student turns on the tape, listens to the word, and writes it in the appropriate block.
3. The student checks his own work once the blocks of words have been completed.

The normal procedure though, is to use the Repeat, Spell, Write, Check routine and for the student and teacher to work together. Spelling rules can be taught if appropriate and as necessary. It is important not to overload the student. A spelling pack can be built for a student having trouble with spelling choices.

Because spelling comes from sound it is important to establish the pattern of the sound the student will be using. For most students, the appropriate way would be for the teacher to read several of the words from a designated page (not in order) and ask the student to identify the common sound and name the letter(s) giving that sound. Afterwards, the page can be worked. Sometimes it is necessary to introduce finger spelling (Teachers' Manual 5.8.2).

The spelling completion exercises (ALK) is another spelling activity based on this program. Each exercise consists of five or six lines of words with five or six words in each line taken from a specific page in Stage One. The student's copy has a number of dashes relating to the number of letters in the word with one letter given as a clue. The teacher's copy contains the correct order of the words. The student is asked to find the place along the line where the given word will fit and then write the word, naming the letters when writing. Clues involve initial and final consonants and recognition of vowels. This is an enjoyable activity which develops listening skills and phonological awareness.

Once a student has progressed in his spelling beyond page 28 of Stage One (and usually his reading level will be in Stage Two at this point) he can begin sentence writing. The student should be one page ahead of his spelling at this point; so if he is spelling on page 40, he will be writing from page 41. He will choose one word from each of the blocks and put each one into a sentence. Thus from US 1 page 41 he will be writing five sentences. In this way he looks at and uses the words before the next lesson when he will be spelling them.

The groups of check words at the bottom of the pages can be used for paragraph writing. Once a student is spelling in Stage Three he can begin this process. The student is asked to write the first ten check words in his book. He then is asked to put each of these ten words into different sentences but the theme of the writing must be linked, so he writes a passage which does not need a beginning or an ending. This is the first development from sentence writing into essay writing.

The yellow pages can be used for dictation once the student is spelling well into Stage Two. When this activity is introduced the spelling page should be at least half a book ahead of the dictation. The student is asked to read this passage slowly onto the tape and include punctuation and paragraph changes. In the next lesson, he uses the tape for his dictation and after writing out the passage he checks with the original in the book.

The visual memory training cards exercise is another way to extend and reinforce problematic patterns of spelling (ref. Teachers' Manual 6.12). This has proved invaluable to many students because it develops their visual short-term memory capacity, extends their ability to develop and organize work, as well as encourages self-checking and correcting.

The program manual gives a sample two hour study session for a student based entirely on the Units of Sound program. The value in developing independent learning activities is that these free the teacher to work with other students at the same time.

The Word Bank is a valuable resource activity which is bought independently of the program but works in conjunction with it. Stage One has been operational for many years but Word Bank 2 covering Stages Two and Three is shortly to be published. Word Bank 1 has a variety of comprehension exercises, cloze procedure, mixed sentences for the student to rearrange, spelling activities, crosswords, and other exercises which are planned for each page of Stage One. These act as useful overlearning activities reinforcing what has been learned already. They are also designed to encourage students to approach and look at words in a way they may not have done before.

5. UNITS OF SOUND: MULTIMEDIA VERSION 2

5.1. Introduction

With the increasing use of computers and computer programs in education the development of Units of Sound for use with multimedia has presented a new facet to the program. It was essential to maintain the strong emphasis on the aural–oral work within the program. The addition of an active visual impact, which the student feels in complete control of, has opened up new possibilities to many. It has extended the multisensory approach. The program's simplicity benefits dyslexics because, unlike other programs on the market, it is not crowded out with busily moving figures, shapes, and colors. Thus the easily distracted dyslexic student can concentrate better.

There is insufficient research into the progress of students using the CD-ROM compared to those using the audiovisual program. For students who respond well to a visual stimulus, the use of the screen and its novelty in a reading program is a strong motivater.

Some students do not benefit from the stronger visual impact. These students often need to develop listening skills and the visual impact of the screen distracts them. For a student such as Philip (See case study, Section 6), however, the CD-ROM was particularly helpful. Initially, he was using his finger to cover parts of words when he was reading. The highlighting on the screen encouraged his tracking and visual recognition of sound patterns.

There are three CDs, one for each stage. Each one has a screening program for each stage, student management file, teacher's tutorial, teacher's manual, along with the relevant program for that stage.

5.2. Teacher's Tutorial

The teacher's tutorial explains the screening test. It tells how to work in the student management file, how to set up a student on the program, how to use the pages and what to expect, how to conduct a check read and what to look for. The teacher's manual, which can be printed out from the CD, gives a good start to using the program if the teacher has no prior training.

5.3. Student Management

Student management is the means by which the teacher keeps an electronic record of her students and their progress. It enables the student to find his place on the CD very easily.

5.4. Screening

The screening test is on the CD, but many teachers may prefer to test the student directly. This is because the student can track ahead and anticipate if he has the whole sheet in front of him. In some cases the student may even go back to a word and correct it. A teacher can monitor this process.

For some students the mere fact that the teacher is writing indicates a misread word and can be very off putting if this is not performed discreetly. So the use of the screen can be an added bonus. Here the teacher only has to move the mouse minimally to record an incorrect word. Also the student has a two second time span in which to read each word; it disappears from the screen after that. There is the opportunity to recall it if necessary.

The computer will print out test results and will also transfer these results onto the student's management file and set up the starting point. This is helpful to the busy teacher.

However the teacher can also set up a new student onto the file if necessary or change the number of the page manually. The program was designed to be easy to use for the teacher with minimal computing knowledge.

5.5. Stages One, Two, and Three

The sound track has remained almost untouched in the CD-ROM production. The pacing between words in the blocks and in the text has not been altered from the audio program. Thus the student still retains the space in which to make a vocal response and can correct if he read the word incorrectly.

When a student is using a page from Units of Sound the CD-ROM cannot show the complete page and often there will be five or six screens making up the whole which will require scrolling. The student must wear headphones to maintain a strong sound input whenever working on a page.

When the student clicks onto a page, the teacher's hat icon changes color automatically and the vocal input for the introduction to the page begins. When the hat icon reverts to black the student must click either onto the unit of sound or onto the icon for sound. Clicking onto the unit of sound will highlight the units in all the blocks of words on the screen. This gives the student the ability to overview if he or she wants to and hear the sound again.

Once the sound icon is clicked, the recorded voice reads the words in the usual way. Each word is highlighted just before the word is read. The student is encouraged to read the word as it changes to blue and before the voice reads it. After the word has been read by the voice, if the student reads incorrectly he still has the opportunity to self correct.

One of the benefits of this program is that the student can repeat each block of words as often as required if the practice is needed. So it becomes proactive.

The student controls scrolling from screen to screen by clicking onto the right-hand blue arrow. The left-hand arrow goes back to the previous screen, and the middle arrow returns to the student index. The units of sound checks are worked in the same way: by clicking on the sound icon and working along the line as the unit changes to blue.

The procedure is the same for the check word groups at the bottom of the page, but the passages for reading are differently organized. When these passages or sentences come onto the screen a group of green arrows appears at the bottom. A click onto the right-hand single arrow lights up the whole first sentence. The student can either read this to himself or look at it before clicking onto the middle double arrow which releases the text for that sentence. Thus each sentence is looked at and read individually. The left-hand arrow enables the student to go back over the passage as many times as necessary.

On the comprehension questions pages there are blocks of words which have one or more question marks at the left-hand side of the block. The student clicks a question mark to release the sound. The student answers questions by clicking what he or she believes is the correct word. A red check shows up if this is right. If incorrect a horn sounds. The student is given three chances and on the fourth the correct answer is shown.

The increased interaction by the student using the screen helps to maintain concentration. A page can be worked more than once before the teacher goes over it with the student. For example, on the first lesson the page could be prepared by using the screen and the CD-ROM. On the second lesson the same page could be repeated using the tape recorder and book with the audio program.

6. CASE STUDY 2: PHILIP

6.1. Background

At ten years old, Philip was having considerable problems with his literacy skills. When Philip was almost eight, an educational psychologist assessed him and found him to be of average intelligence with a weakness in his auditory short-term memory. He had a lower score on the WISC III for his performance (non-verbal) abilities than his verbal abilities, despite his being above average in visual organization and visual material retention.

At this stage his score on WORD was 6 years, 6 months, and his spelling age was 6 years, 9 months. His small private school offered help, which continued for the next two years. This help was expected to be adequate.

Philip was described by the psychologist as having good oral ability and good verbal reasoning skills. He enjoyed drawing and art work. He was a sociable boy, having many outside interests, and was well coordinated and good at sport. He was full of life and had a good sense of humor. He was described as having a moderate degree of dyslexic difficulty.

6.2. Intervention

Almost three years later Philip was brought to a specialist center for assessment and teaching because his mother was still concerned about his reading and spelling. Tests showed he was significantly underachieving in his reading. The gap between he and his peers had widened considerably. During his two years and six months remediation at school, his reading in context had only progressed by five months and his single word reading by a year.

The teacher who worked with him noticed that when he read, he covered up the letters of each word with his finger and gradually moved his finger along the word revealing one letter at a time. He had problems reading lists of words at speed and made many inaccurate guesses and assumptions. When reading single words from left to right across the page he managed familiar one or two syllable words but had no decoding strategies for unfamiliar ones ("junus" for journey, "cardy" for carry and "turul" for terror). When reading in context he was unable to use the clues to decipher the more difficult vocabulary. This was surprising because his comprehension and vocabulary on the WISC III were above average.

His spelling ability was unusually well ahead of his reading—it had increased by two years during the two years and six months since the psychological testing. He could spell simple, phonetically regular words but struggled with vowel digraphs: "somer" for sooner, "joun" for join. He showed a lack of common spelling rules and showed some weakness in auditory discrimination.

The special education teacher recommended Philip be taken to an optometrist for a thorough examination. He had already visited two. The first one prescribed tinted lenses (described by one of his friends as "cool") but these did little to alleviate the problem in reading. The second optometrist gave him a series of eye exercises to try for six months, and these helped considerably. This work has been supported in his lessons with tracking exercises.

Philip attended twice a week for one-hour lessons. Although he is generally well motivated there are times when it takes tactical skills to encourage him. Philip was given the screening tests for Stage One of Units of Sound in both reading and spelling. He managed the whole of the test for reading but had errors scattered throughout the whole test. There were numerous self corrections and hesitations. It became obvious that his knowledge of long vowels was nonexistent, e.g., note being read as "not," bake as "back," dune as "done," etc. He had problems with various consonant blends and the use of y as a vowel.

Because his problems were scattered, he was placed just over a third of the way through Stage One and given the CD ROM program. It was hoped the highlighted words on the screen would help his focusing and prevent his finger from covering over the word when he read.

A reading pack was built which initially included the long and short vowel sounds and the letter y both as a consonant and a vowel. The use of y as a vowel was explained, and a chart was built at the beginning of his book to help him to understand this. It was referred to over a period of lessons to make sure he knew this thoroughly and could explain it himself.

He was screened for spelling using the same sheet as for reading. Spelling errors were fewer than reading ones—particular mistakes coming with settle, silk, and even. Because of this the spelling completion exercises from ALK were used, beginning at a fairly early stage. This was chosen for two reasons: (1) Philip was still experiencing phonological awareness difficulties and the clues in the exercises would encourage him to listen, look, and think; and (2) his handwriting tended to bunch together; such an exercise would encourage an easier flow. The exercise was worked with the multisensory RSWC spelling routine.

The use of SRA School House cards beginning with orange band were a helpful tool in working with long and short vowel sounds. This work also continued with long and short vowel sheets from ALK, which were used with both modes, i.e., oral–aural with the teacher and Philip together, and mode two with

Philip reading the word and giving the vowel sound. These were always timed exercises (30 seconds).

Alphabet tracking exercises were given at every lesson. Philip was encouraged to keep his pen on the line all the time he was working—not just to identify the letter of the alphabet. Selected exercises from Sounds Abound using final consonants were practiced. Philip rapidly became more secure with the ability to hear end sounds.

At every lesson, one page of Units of Sound would be worked on the CD ROM, and the page prepared with the computer at the previous lesson would be gone over with the teacher. Any problems were worked on. The units of sound that were problematic became a part of his reading pack.

One exercise from the spelling completion exercises was completed every lesson. Word Bank cards were introduced because these focused on comprehension, looking and analyzing, developing thinking skills, and organization.

Although his spelling was not the weakest point in his learning, additional written work was needed to develop sentence writing skills and to rehearse spelling patterns. Philip used sentences for dictation to develop this skill. These sentences had been prepared from the pages in Units of Sound and concentrated on the vocabulary up to the specific page required. Philip was asked to read the sentences on to the tape at one lesson. At the next lesson he used this tape-recording for dictation. Afterwards he would use the original and check it against his own work.

As the program of work continued, Rate Builders from SRA were introduced. Philip would again self check the answers. The 2a level was used because of his reading age and chronological age.

When Philip began reading in Stage Two and once he finished the spelling completion exercises in Stage One, he began spelling in Stage Two.

During one session, Philip would use a page from Units of Sound for sentence writing. This required him to choose one word from each of the blocks and write a sentence with the chosen word in it. If there were seven blocks of words on that page, he wrote seven sentences.

At the following session he wrote six sentences from the next page, reinforcing previous work. For example, if he wrote six sentences from page 4, with the /ai/ sound in them, he would also be spelling the "br" and "str" words worked from page 3 at the previous lesson. The spelling completion exercises for Stage Two reinforced this knowledge.

Philip still does not enjoy the process of reading and balks at a page of print. Considerable progress has been made. In just under a year, his context reading ability has improved by two years. His confidence in his own ability has changed beyond recognition. Most important of all, Philip is happy with what he is doing and achieving. His percentile score in reading has moved from the 2nd to the 13th percentile.

6.3. A Typical Lesson

A typical lesson would include:

1. Rate builder (SRA Schoolhouse), 2c, Aqua 5
2. CD-ROM Units of Sound (UoS) Stage 2, page 21
3. Check read UoS Stage Two, pages 20 and 20a, and reading pack
4. Spell UoS Stage 1, page 47
5. Sentence writing UoS Stage 1, page 48
6. Tracking exercise
7. Dictation exercise
8. Stile exercise or game

7. DEVELOPING LITERACY FOR STUDY AND WORK: A PROGRAM FOR TEENAGERS AND ADULTS

7.1. Testing

Before planning any special education program it is necessary to establish not only the student's starting point but also his level of difficulty and if there are gaps in his knowledge. Developing Literacy for Study and Work (DLSW) has five tests which can be easily administered and interpreted by the teacher. There are three reading tests, one spelling test, and one writing test. These are not normed tests. All these are explained in Section 2 of the manual, and the actual tests are found in the appendices. The test solutions and the analysis and interpretation of the student's work are found in Section 3.

7.1.1. Sentence Reading Test

The sentence reading test is a context reading test to be read aloud. It measures approximate reading levels ranging from a base level of seven years to a top level of 19 years.

7.1.2. Silent Reading Comprehension Test

The silent reading comprehension test is an individual test of silent reading–comprehension. It is timed. Its range is from a base level of six years to a top level of 20 years.

7.1.3. Isolated Word Reading Test

The isolated word reading test has no context. The student's ability to sightread, and synthesize and analyze syllabic constructions is identified as he reads the words aloud. The test's range is from a base level of seven years to a top level of 20 years.

7.1.4. Spelling Test

The spelling test is a list of words where no context is used except if there might be a misunderstanding due to homophones e.g., reign, rain, rein. The range is from a base of seven years to a top level of 18 years.

7.1.5. Timed Writing Composition

The timed writing composition is designed to help the teacher understand how the student composes sentences and whether he is able to write to the same level that he speaks and correctly spells the words used. The manual has a full explanation of how to use this test.

7.2. The Program

Often the student has a great disparity between reading sentences or paragraphs, reading single words, and reading silently for comprehension. Section 4 of the manual is devoted to developing the techniques to improve reading accuracy. Within this section is a reference to the use of Units of Sound. It tells how to extend a student's word ability. Section 5 considers the improvement of silent reading with comprehension and refers to the use of SRA material. Section 5.9 explains the use of the valuable Listening Skills Material. Probably the most valuable aspects of the manual are the complete programs within it:

1. The Spelling Program and Dictations (Sections 8 and 10)
2. The Verb Exercises (Section 7)

These are all ready for use and there are instructions for their application.

As spelling is one area that causes problems not only to dyslexic students, but to many other people as well, it is invaluable to find a complete program covering the spelling rules. This program does more than that. It is backed up with the etymological background to the development of the rules. For example, Section 10.3 covers the -y ending rules and the connection of letter **y** with **g**, **i** with **j**, **i** with **y** and **j** with **y**. Students may find the history of words interesting. This often helps them to relate one word with another and so understand their spelling.

The historical explanation is always followed by a section beginning "We teach that. . . ." This needs to be read through with the student until the teacher is certain the student fully understands it. There is a rule explanation followed by an oral exercise in which the student responds to the teacher's questions e.g., "What is a suffix?" and then "What is a consonant suffix?" etc. After this series of questions is an exercise that applies the rule just addressed. This is approached with the RSWC routine.

At the end of the manual is a photocopyable spelling program/dictations guide (SPDG) and a record sheet which should be used in conjunction with the spelling program. If this is carefully followed according to the instructions, then overlearning takes place. The program thus becomes cumulative as well as being multisensory and structured. The record sheet also reminds the teacher when the student should prepare and use a dictation exercise. This way, the teacher monitors whether the student is able to use the spelling rule he has just learned as the dictation contains words just covered by the rule. The student prepares his own tape recording one lesson and uses it the next and self-checks and corrects as necessary. There are 40 dictation passages of increasing complexity.

The spelling rules begin with the basic vowel–consonant -**e** base words plus consonant and vowel suffix, e.g. lately, through to the difficult doubling rule for multisyllable words.

Section 7 has a useful exercise called Exercises with Verbs. These cover non-regular verbs, past to present and present to past tense, identifying verb bases from derived words, mixed regular and irregular verb bases to past tense and work with synonyms and antonyms. Some of these stretch not only the student! Some examples will show the high level at which the student is now working:

- Write down the verb base for the past tense verb "let"
- Identify the verb base of "compulsion," "revolution"
- Write down an antonym for the past tense word of "assumption"

There is a record sheet which helps the student to identify how to follow from one exercise to another in numerical order because the different groups of exercises are not intended to be worked in sequence, e.g., Group A has Exercise 1, Group B has Exercise 2, and Group C has Exercises 3 and 4. In this way there is continuing usage of present and past tense and base word derivation. There is also a small section covering paragraph and essay writing and a list of topics on which to write.

8. CASE STUDY 3: GEORGE

8.1. Background

George is 35 years old and in school for building surveying. He quit school when he was 16 and began working in the construction industry. For more than 12 years he worked either as a bricklayer or as a mason. He then decided to pursue a degree and got a B.Tec National Diploma in construction at his local technical college. Following this success, George took a one year Access Course and then entered the university.

George came for an assessment after his first year at the university, when a tutor felt his exam answers indicated he might have dyslexia.

The assessment showed George to be within the low average range of ability. His strengths lay in his aptitude to recall information, his use of vocabulary, his social awareness and general comprehension. He was of average ability in reasoning and temporal sequencing and in analyzing the components of a design.

His specific weaknesses lay with his auditory short-term memory, identifying relevant from irrelevant information when presented visually and spatial organization. His reading level was the 14th percentile and his spelling at the 10th percentile. George's literacy weaknesses lay in his reading capacity and comprehension, spelling, writing, and organization of thoughts and ideas. His reading speed was well below that necessary for a university graduate. His writing speed (including thinking time) was at 11 words per minute, half of what it should be for ease in note taking at lectures. George is unassuming. He has great tenacity, motivation, and determination, and it is largely this which has brought him through to the level he is at today.

8.2. Intervention

When he first came for tutoring (one two-hour session per week) he was asking for help with his essays. However, it became obvious that George lacked the necessary tools for essay writing. He was committed to regular tutoring for the next two years so it was possible to work to fill in the gaps in his literacy weaknesses before moving on to the more difficult areas of essay writing and exam answers. In order for an essay to be written the correct tools need to be readily accessible, so it was absolutely necessary to build firm foundations prior to this.

George's lessons were planned based on the information from the educational psychologist's report and from the five tests which were administered from the appendix at the end of DLSW. These latter tests are invaluable for targeting teaching to the needs of students 14 years and older. They showed George was still having difficulty in reading for accuracy. Sometimes he would make contextual guesses, hesitate or reread words and sometimes miss out syllables. Occasionally he would read a word which looked similar to another one, detective/defective, despot/deposit, for example.

George showed specific problems with spelling. He relied heavily on the sounds within words and often followed a strong phonetic approach. He showed incorrect letter placement in words; syllable difficulties; lack of knowledge of spelling rules; and limited understanding of the uses of prefixes and suffixes.

Initially his sentence construction was basic. They showed grammatical and spelling inaccuracies and style immaturity.

1. The man had createted a masterpiece of a house in the woods.
2. There are many people who live together, but have seperate lives when they are apart.
3. The man's head had been chopped off by the train but was rushed to the emergency department of the hospital.
4. The surface of the moon has many lumps and bumps on it, due to the lack of atmospher_ around it.

When lessons began it became obvious that George's information processing abilities were very slow and that he would not be able to achieve as many activities during his two-hour lesson as originally thought.

At every session, George read either one or two Rate Builders from SRA Level 4a. This is the most advanced level and is suitable for students in high school and college. This exercise originally took George up to 25 minutes to complete. Over a period of 18 months, he has cut this time in half. He used to take work home, usually Reading for Understanding Level 3—published by SRA and designed to develop the reading comprehension skills of the older student. Sometimes he would take dictation passages home to write out.

He also read a page from Units of Sound Stage Three with his teacher at every session. This was to develop his fluency and confidence as well as extend his use of vocabulary, help him make connections etymologically, and develop his syllable count. For example:

From Units of Sound Stage Three, page 5
    Independence—Find base word, prefix, suffix
    Show how words like pendant, pendulum, perpendicular, suspension,
        suspender etc. connect through Latin *pend* or *pens*.
From Units of Sound Stage Three, page 6, block 10
    Destruction—base word, structure
    Change prefix—instruct, restructure, construct
From Units of Sound Stage Three, page 20, block 4
    Words can be used in different forms of speech
    Delegate, intimate, and advocate

In this way his reading development was covered, i.e., comprehension, fluency, word analysis, syllable understanding, and a growing awareness of etymology.

George's spelling ability was addressed through the Units of Sound and DLSW. Although his spelling age was shown as 10 years, 9 months, it was clear George needed help at a much lower spelling level. Following a screening test for spelling in Units of Sound Stages One and Two, George started working at the beginning of Stage Two.

One page, sometimes two pages, of word blocks were worked with at every session. George used the RSWC routine. Initially this was a painful exercise for him and he was very slow but gradually he increased his pace, and his confidence grew. He had little understanding of the terminology of vowels, consonants, prefixes, or suffixes. While he was working on one page for spelling he would use the following page for sentence writing. In this way George used words within his spelling ability, constructing sentences by using vocabulary of his level and at the same time familiarizing himself with the vocabulary on that page which would be used in the following lesson for spelling. As this exercise in writing became more familiar George became confident. His use and development of language grew. He had several ingrained grammatical errors which needed addressing, e.g., confusing "as" and "has" Has he was walking down the road. . . , mixing singular and plural within a sentence, and mixing the verbs. Other common errors such as "there" and "their" were also evident. He had trouble with syllables in words: "integral" became "interigal."

George needed to learn spelling rules. These were taught through the use of DLSW Section 10. The logical, multisensory way in which these rules are taught enables a student to become familiar with them through oral responses with the teacher and regular practice. George had initial difficulty in identifying long and short vowel sounds within words (exercises from ALK were used) and understanding the difference between consonant suffixes and vowel suffixes. Through learning and applying the rules, he now makes fewer errors, works out polysyllabic words for himself and frequently gets them right. His own confidence in word analysis has grown. He even spotted a spelling error in his lecturer's notes.

The spelling program includes a series of dictations which are introduced at regular intervals to help the teacher understand whether the student needs to have the spelling rules reinforced. George would read slowly onto a tape the required passage reading on the punctuation, such as "period," "comma," "exclamation mark," "new paragraph." Thus the exercise not only reinforced spelling but also developed punctuation and text layout.

George was writing sentences but also becoming familiar with writing longer passages, because having recorded one lesson, the next lesson the passage was used for dictation. After completing the assignment in his notebook, George checked the original with his own work in order to identify any mistakes. This dictation exercise was also used in conjunction with Units of Sound.

Sometimes a yellow page from Units of Sound would be used for dictation. George always kept about half a book behind his spelling page and occasionally used sentences for dictation which his teacher had constructed with words from that particular page and from further back in the program. In this way reinforcement took place and any problem spelling patterns were worked on again.

With George's growing confidence it became possible to introduce paragraph writing—the next stage up from sentence writing. He was asked to select 10 of the check words from the bottom of Units of Sound Stage Two, page 4 and write them into his exercise book. George was to put each of these ten words into individual sentences but he was told they should all fit together with a common theme thus creating a paragraph. The words could be used in random order. Surprisingly, this was an exercise George enjoyed, and he has written quite fluently. Initially his speed of writing, including thinking time, was very slow at seven words a minute. After 14 months of this exercise, he was working at a speed of 13 words a minute. While this is not a comfortable speed for examination purposes, it is considerably quicker than when he first began.

Another helpful exercise, but one George found difficult, was the verb exercises from DLSW Section 10. George found changing verbs from past to present and vice versa and identifying base words a very demanding exercise. For example, he gave "compulse" as the base word for "compulsion" and "permit" for the present tense of "allowed."

As George's reading, spelling, and writing skills developed his confidence grew, and it became possible to address the needs of essay writing. Many lessons were spent working with mind maps and essay planning. George insisted he understood what it was all about yet he found trouble selecting key words and phrases, homing in on specifics, and adding detail to the mind map.

Initially he was given general topics to work on that required no specialized knowledge. Then he was asked to write opening paragraphs on selected topics. Finally, he was asked to attempt the whole essay. George's thought organization will always benefit from further development but he has learned the basic skills needed for essay writing. During his tutoring session, he managed to pass the next stage of his examinations—not a high mark, but a pass. This was the first time during the whole of his university career that he had passed without having to retake the exam.

8.3. A Typical Lesson

A typical two hour lesson would be

1. Rate Builder Level 4a, Tan 5 and 6
2. DLSW Spelling (four exercises)
3. DLSW 2, verb exercises
4. Sentences Units of Sound Stage 3, page 19
5. Spell UoS Stage 3, page 18
6. Paragraph writing UoS Stage 2, page 48 (ten check words)
7. Word Bank 2 (Units of Sound unpublished support material) No. 95
8. Dictation DLSW
9. Reading for Understanding Level 3, no.3

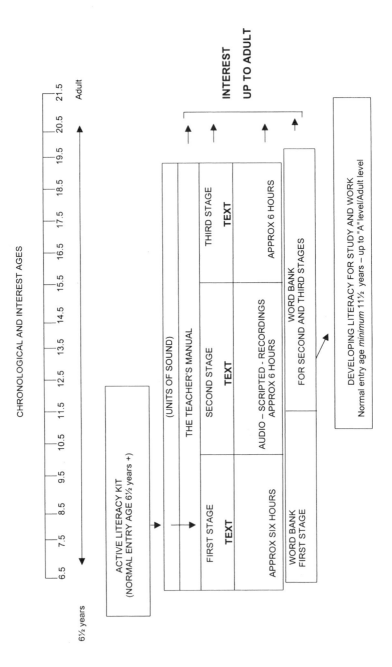

Figure 3. Materials for the development of literacy (The Dyslexia Institute/Walter Bramley)

9. CONCLUSION

In all three case studies, it was critical to identify the student's needs prior to starting any remedial help. The problems then needed to be prioritized in relation to the literacy difficulties and logical progress.

With Philip, it was essential that the Units of Sound program be followed sequentially, without interruption, to improve reading and spelling ability. For George, both spelling programs and verb exercises, as well as the SRA material, needed to be sequential to achieve a cumulative effect.

Lucy's program focused on the difficulties she was experiencing. It was not necessary to implement the whole program. However, she worked each different exercise thoroughly from beginning to end and her work was carefully monitored and timed.

All programs, however good, are beneficial only if they are correctly used. It is the teacher's skills that brings these programs to life.

RESOURCE MATERIALS

Units of Sound—tapes, books and multimedia for Stages 1, 2 & 3 and teachers' manual by Walter Bramley. 1st published 1972. published through Dyslexia Institute 1995
Developing Literacy for Study and Work by Walter Bramley. published 1993
Active Literacy Kit by Walter Bramley published 1998.
Stile Exercises—Early Phonics Programme pub 1995 Lowercase wooden letters.
Available from—Learning Development Aids (LDA) Duke Street, Wisbech, Cambs PE132AE U.K.
24⁰⁰, Turner Avenue N.W. Grand Rapids MI 49544 U.S.
School House Word Attack Skills pub. 1973
Reading for Understanding Levels 1, 2 & 3. pub. 1990.
Reading Laboratories 2c, 1978 3b—1988 & 4a (if still printed) pub. 1959.
Available from Scientific Research Associates (SRA)
McGraw-Hill Book Company Europe, Shoppenhangers Rd, Maidenhead, Berks. U.K.
Letter Tracking by Ann Arbor pub. 1975
Available from Ann Arbor Publishers. Learning Programs Engineered to Behavioral Specifications
Lakeland Press Inc. Dexter Michigan. ISBN (1) 89039-153-x
Solving Language Difficulties by Amey Sture, Caroline Z. Peck, Linda Kahn rev. Ed. 1984.
Available from Better Books, 3, Puganel Drive, Dudley DY1 4AZ U.K.
Educators Publishing Service Inc. Cambridge, Mass. 02138 U.S.
Sounds Abound by Hugh Catts and Tina Vartianinen
ISBN 1-55999-394-4. pub. 1993
Available from Better Books (see above)
Lingui Systems Inc. 3100 4th Avenue, East Moline IL 61244 U.S.

REFERENCES

Bramley, W. (1972 and 1995). *Units of Sound*, LDA, Grand Rapids, Michigan.
Bramley, W. (1993). *Developing Literacy for Study and Work*, LDA, Grand Rapids, Michigan.

Bramley, W. (1998). *Active Literacy Kit*, LDA, Grand Rapids, Michigan.

Dyslexia Institute (1993a). *Developing Literacy for Study and Work, Vol. 2: Overlearning*, Dyslexia Institute, Staines, United Kingdom, p. 159.

Dyslexia Institute (1993b). *Peter Hatcher Lecture on Reading*, Easter Conference at Royal Holloway College, Dyslexia Institute, Staines, United Kingdom.

Shaywitz, S. L. (1996). In: *Scientific American*, November, 1996.

8

Higher Level Literacy Skills

Clare Elwell and Janet Townend

1. INTRODUCTION

Some children acquire early literacy skills without apparent difficulty, but exhibit problems later, maybe during middle school or late high school. Others, having struggled in the early stages, learn to decode and become functionally literate, but have trouble with more complex literacy tasks. Both groups need continuing support so their literacy skills will develop to a level that enables them to meet the demands of school, work, or college. The principles of teaching at this level are broadly similar to those that are pertinent at an earlier stage (see Chapters 1, 4, and 5).

2. WHAT ARE THE HIGHER LEVEL LITERACY SKILLS?

The term, higher level literacy skills, suggests that these skills are hierarchical and their attainment occurs in a linear, sequential manner. However, the process of becoming literate is not equivalent to being taught to read or write in a step by step process (Webster, Beveridge, & Reed, 1996). We use this term to include those skills that need to be developed beyond decoding skills and early encoding, encompassing the production of reading and writing beyond the sound, word, and sentence level.

Clare Elwell, Virginia Lodge, Blacknest Road, Virginia Water, Surrey GU25 4NU, United Kingdom   Janet Townend, The Dyslexia Institute, 133 Gresham Road, Staines, Middlesex, TW18 2AJ, United Kingdom.

Higher level literacy involves the integration of a number of different skills as well as an ability to adjust processing strategies during reading and writing. The individual has to learn to think about what he or she is doing during reading and writing activities, and at secondary school level, where different writing tasks make different demands, then they also have to learn how to determine how to approach the various literacy tasks they are faced with (Beveridge, 1989).

The teaching of higher level literacy skills is a complex process. It must take into account those experiences the individual had outside the classroom in addition to what happens in the learning process. The student's social and cultural experiences, as well as his previous subject or domain knowledge, influence his development of reading and writing skills.

Within the school environment the development of these skills will be affected by any discussions that may occur before reading or writing, as well as whether the student has any knowledge of strategies used during the process. Other factors to consider include physical processes, such as eye movements, or if an individual has poor motor coordination skills; the individual's cognitive processes, including comprehension, reading speed, fluency, accuracy, and strategies the reader uses to deal with errors or noncomprehension, or how to overcome spelling problems or a limited vocabulary.

The acquisition of higher level literacy skills requires that students be taught the process of review or reflection when they complete either a reading or writing activity. They must ask: What did I learn during the process? Do I need to take or make notes to ensure I understand and retain the requisite knowledge? Do I need to reread the text to evaluate its information or to proofread for written errors? Teaching higher level literacy skills involves teaching pupils these strategies and how to use them, introducing students to ways that help them retain information and to methods that enable them to communicate information to others, such as by writing.

The teaching of higher level literacy skills therefore involves not only teaching students to decode print, but also allowing them to develop the ability to access text in a fluent manner so that they understand what is written, gain knowledge, and enjoy this process. It involves teaching students to plan their written work and to think about what they wish to communicate before they start to write. Students need to be taught how to access and use those tools that will increase their written vocabulary, to understand the need for drafting, proofreading, and editing and to allow sufficient time in which to complete a piece of work. The teaching of higher level literacy skills also involves the teaching of spelling, not in a rote fashion, but from a structural perspective by studying word origins and relationships and by using strategies to check spellings without relying on a dictionary. Beyond this level of instruction, it is also necessary to teach metacognitive strategies to ensure that both thinking about their learning while it is happening and reflecting on the process afterwards are included as an integral part of becoming fully literate.

The development of higher level literacy skills is a process that takes place across the whole curriculum, not just in English lessons or the Special Education department. An inability to read competently, and therefore to comprehend, is a block to the student's learning throughout the school. Poor reading causes poor performance not just in English, history, religious knowledge, geography, and so on, but also in mathematics, chemistry, physics, and biology.

Webster, Beveridge, and Reed (1996) consider it important to address the development of literacy skills in a systematic and regular manner within the recurrent teaching contexts of the mainstream curriculum. They do not suggest that teachers be merely involved in taking on more responsibility for raising the standards of spelling, handwriting, reading, or writing, but argue that the consideration of literacy as an intrinsic part of every subject helps understand more about effective teaching and learning. Literacy skills should not be considered an activity separate from the work students do across the curriculum. Their development should be an integral part of the learning experiences students have. This approach to literacy enables students to take increasing control over the texts they use or construct; the importance of using different kinds of texts in different subject domains can be stressed, beginning with the student's own awareness and experience; and it enables the student's learning experience to be modified from that of receiving information to learn to a more constructive learning process in which the student gains understanding, and becomes an independent learner.

3. LITERATURE REVIEW

Prior to the development of formal schooling as a method of education, an apprenticeship was probably the common way knowledge was passed from one generation to the next (Collins, Seely Brown, & Newman, 1989). Language acquisition is just one learning activity that takes place in the home or other similar social environments. Much of this occurs by apprenticeship, where the more capable members help and guide the child's performance, but not necessarily by direct instruction (Tharp and Gallimore, 1991).

In the secondary school, much learning is based on direct instruction methods where students, 11 and older, are expected to learn and remember facts and concepts without their understanding what is being taught or why. Not much time is devoted to teaching strategies that facilitate greater retention of subject specific facts or help with the transfer of useful strategies from one domain to another. Many dyslexic pupils have trouble applying what they learn to new or unique situations; research has investigated how those students who do achieve good understanding of what they are taught transfer and apply their skills in different domains (Collins, Seely Brown, and Newman, 1989). This work was done to develop strategies that could be taught to other individuals who did not have such skills.

Collins, Seely Brown, and Newman (1989) looked at applying the observation, scaffolding or fading, and practice aspects of apprenticeship to reading, writing and mathematics in the formal school setting. They proposed their model of *cognitive apprenticeship*. This concept encompasses two main issues: teaching students the processes used by experts when dealing with complex tasks; and learning through guided experiences, with emphasis toward cognitive and metacognitive processes. With regard to the latter point, the authors believe it is necessary to identify and define those cognitive and metacognitive processes that occur in a learning situation so they can easily be applied to other domains of learning.

Cognitive apprenticeship, as described by these authors, is an important method for teaching younger students how to read, write, and do arithmetic. These subjects underpin all other school learning. With regard to higher level literacy skills, teaching students to think about their learning, the active participation of the student in the learning process and the transfer of skills across the curriculum are essential.

Palinscar and Brown (1984, 1989) developed a set of strategies based on the principles of cognitive apprenticeship to achieve improved reading comprehension. Their teaching method, known as reciprocal teaching, is a method of cooperative learning that introduces group discussion techniques to aid and improve understanding and retention of text content.

Reciprocal teaching involves the teacher helping a group of students learn to use four skills or strategies: formulation of questions based on the text; summary of text; prediction; clarification. The teacher and students read a given text together and then spend time discussing the contents of the text, practicing the four strategies while they do. Initially the teacher takes the lead: formulating the questions, preparing a summary, clarifying areas of difficulty, and making predictions as appropriate. The teacher then coaches the students on how to take on and develop these strategies themselves. In subsequent sessions the students themselves take on the role of group leader, with the teacher only providing guidance and feedback as necessary.

The practice of reciprocal teaching encompasses the concept of *scaffolding* as suggested by Wood, Bruner, and Ross in 1976. Scaffolding is a metaphor to describe the kind of support the teacher gives during the education process: the teacher's support is flexible and tailored to the actual needs of the student, and capable of being withdrawn as appropriate and in tune with the student's increasing expertise. It explains how a task can be reduced to a number of manageable smaller tasks and support can range from actual formulation of questions through to the provision of hints for guidance. It can further fade until the student masters the necessary skills and uses them independently. This adjustable and temporary support during which transfer of responsibility occurs from teacher to student is an interactive form of instruction.

Each strategy is geared toward promoting comprehension and comprehension monitoring. Prediction requires the students to formulate an hypothesis about what will take place next in the text, which means they must activate any relevant background knowledge they already have, and then link this with new knowledge encountered in the text.

In question generation, the reader identifies the salient information in the text and formulates questions; the reader must be an active participant in the reading process and not just a passive recipient of teacher-generated questions.

Clarification directs the students' attention to what they may find difficult to comprehend in the text and why. Teaching students about clarification helps them to realize the purpose of reading extends beyond the ability to decode with accuracy. Clarification helps them recognize the problems that arise with text, including, for example, meeting unfamiliar vocabulary or unclear reference words or having to deal with new and complicated concepts. Discussing the text for clarification requires that students go beyond recognizing what causes lack of comprehension and also demonstrates the importance of taking the necessary measures to overcome the difficulties they meet.

Palinscar and Brown claim to have successfully used this method of teaching with individual students and in small groups. Their students showed improved recall of information and better transfer of the skills of summarizing, question generation, and error detection to other areas of their curriculum. Palinscar and Brown believe their method helps students appreciate reading as a complex activity beyond the practical aspects of scanning, pronunciation, and word recognition. In addition, they consider the four strategies to be metacognitive activities in which the learner is involved in thinking about what is being learned from text, alongside the development of self-monitoring skills.

Bereiter and Scardamalia also applied the practice of cognitive apprenticeship to the teaching of writing in 1985. They designed an approach wherein the expert practices involved in writing strategies were modeled by the teachers, who also gave the students as much support as they needed and withdrew the help as the students' expertise increased. In addition, the students had to evaluate and reflect upon their work, as well as that of other students in the group.

Bereiter and Scardamalia (1987) define novice writers as those who simply write down ideas when given a topic to write about. Their written work is simply a sequential record of their thoughts, which ends when they cannot generate any more new ideas. Expert writers are considered to be those who plan, organize their ideas, review, and revise what they write in addition to producing written work. After studying such expert writers, Bereiter and Scardamalia produced a set of prompts called "Procedural Facilitations," available for use by the student during the writing process. These prompts were meant to provide the student with specific help, similar to the help given by the teacher in the reciprocal teaching method.

As with reciprocal teaching, the teacher initially demonstrates how to use the prompts, and then the students learn to use them without the teacher's support. Students are expected to question, criticize, and evaluate what is happening during the writing process. They examine their own work as well as that of other students. As they become more experienced, they rely less and less on using the written prompts.

Bereiter and Scardamalia also developed a technique called coinvestigation, where the students are expected to think out loud, and discuss their use of existing strategies and the new ones they are acquiring. These methods, which have also included revision of the written work, are reported to have produced significant changes in the nature and quality of student writing. The coinvestigation techniques help solidify processes that occur during the writing process. The students are not expected to learn from the modeling alone. It is the making explicit of the processes that is considered to be a crucial factor in the success experienced using this method for producing written text by students. In addition, by constantly revising and assessing his work, the student participates in a self-regulatory process.

The teaching programs outlined report improvement in the areas being studied and also address the need to teach cognitive strategies in both domain specific and general areas of the curriculum. Later research by Rosenshine and Meister in 1996 showed that the improvements recorded in the studies they reviewed were less significant if standardized tests were used as measurement tools. Still, it is the practical significance of this work that is important. The development of the cognitive apprenticeship model, and teaching programs based on it, is a move away from considering education to be the building of a base of factual knowledge and a move toward education being the acquisition of knowledge, plus understanding, plus the ability to use that knowledge appropriately. This is particularly appropriate when considering the needs of those who manifest literacy problems beyond the primary school or when considering those who have struggled with the acquisition of literacy skills throughout their school career and continue to do so.

The dyslexia literature sheds some light on the spelling and writing difficulties of the older or more able dyslexic student. In *Phonological Skills and Learning to Read* (page 61) Goswami and Bryant write:

> The contrast between the work on children's reading and on their spelling strikes us as being quite remarkable. It was difficult for us to find any direct and convincing evidence that children use phonological awareness in order to read…but we find abundant evidence that children depend on a phonological code when they are working out how to spell words.
>
> (Goswami and Bryant, 1990)

In view of this "abundant evidence," it is unsurprising that even able students with phonological difficulties should have a problem with spelling.

Frith (1980) looked at the problems of good readers who are poor spellers; this is relevant to some of the people in the group we are considering in this chapter, particularly as she defines good readers as those who have no difficulty in single-word decoding. Frith discovered the errors made by the good readers who were poor spellers were similar to those made by the good readers and spellers, but there were more of them. Their errors were "phonetic," that is, the symbol selected preserved the sound of the word, but was often the wrong symbol. On repeat testing, their errors showed a high degree of consistency. Arguing that this difficulty may be due to an inability to remember what words look like, she then presented a reading task including many misspelled words. The poor spellers who were good readers had more trouble with words which sounded right (nite) than those which looked right (night). She concluded that although this group of subjects used visual strategies for reading, they spelled by phonological strategies, a practice dropped by good spellers by the age of eight years.

Perrin (1983) carried out an important and rather unusual study of 14- and 15-year-olds. She divided her subjects into three groups: good readers and spellers; good readers, poor spellers; poor readers and spellers. She gave two phonological processing tasks and found that the groups containing poor spellers did less well than the good spellers group. The good reading skill of the "discrepant" group was no advantage in this task. The conclusion, though the cause and effect relationship is not clear, is that phonological processing skill continues to be an important factor in spelling mastery.

A rare study of morphological awareness in dyslexic teenagers (Elbro, 1989) concludes that, while these students are "morphologically aware" in many situations, they often failed to use their morphological knowledge to assist them in literacy-related tasks. Elbro points out that effective teaching may need to begin by showing the student what he or she already knows. Morphology is word-structure; a morpheme may be defined as a unit of meaning, which may or may not be a whole word. For example, the word "careless" consists of two morphemes, "care" and "less," both of which are words, but in the word "careful" the second morpheme, "ful," cannot stand alone as a word. The practical implications of this for teaching spelling are discussed later in this chapter, and in Chapters 4 and 12.

A number of studies examined the characteristics of poor written work; when the work of those with low academic ability and the socially or culturally deprived are removed from consideration, the remaining group may be labeled "the poor organizers." Many dyslexic students fall into this group. These pupils characteristically fail to acquire spontaneously a knowledge of text structure and are thus unable to use it in writing (Martlew, 1983); the organization of written work could be dramatically improved by training such students in awareness of text structure. (Fitzgerald and Teasley, 1983) (Taylor and Beach, 1984).

A writing task consists of three stages: planning, translating, and reviewing (Hayes and Flower, 1980). Martlew found poor writers spent less time in planning, failing to collect and organize their information. In the third (review) stage, they fail to perceive deficiencies in their work. Furthermore, they lack the necessary strategies for making corrections. Bruce et al. (1977) describe the phenomenon of "downsliding," which is a gradual deterioration of written work during the translation stage, because of spelling, grammar, and handwriting problems. This will be a familiar pattern to anyone who has graded the written work of dyslexic students.

The literature contains innumerable studies which demonstrate the effectiveness of remedial instruction. The common thread through these instructional procedures is task analysis, organization, and a structured approach to the teaching and learning situation. The importance of metacognition is emphasised. This approach has much in common with the teaching of other skills to dyslexic students.

4. THE LATE MANIFESTATION OF LITERACY DIFFICULTIES

One feature of secondary school education is the increasing emphasis on the learning of complex ideas through reading and writing. Students who have no previous history of literacy difficulties may well have skills that are insufficiently developed to deal with the increasing demands made on their literacy during their secondary education. Reading and writing are multitask activities requiring the integration of a number of skills concurrently, with variable processing strategies. The student must be willing and able to reflect on the reading and writing processes—this does not come naturally to the dyslexic pupil.

Higher level literacy skills have been defined as those skills that need to be developed after a student has grasped the alphabetical principles and has learned the relevant strategies for decoding and, to some extent, encoding written language. Beyond this development, individuals read and comprehend for themselves, in addition to producing their own text. It is the teacher's role to scaffold a student's learning, directing the process along the paths that mediate learning. The process must be supported in a structured manner.

The teaching of higher level literacy skills requires that we, the teachers, approach the difficulties experienced by the dyslexic individual from a dynamic and flexible perspective. To help someone become literate means we have to teach them to acquire more than just the ability to read books. They need to learn that the possession of literacy skills provides the true means of accessing knowledge. Teaching principles need to be adapted according to the needs of those we teach. For example, when faced with text that needs to be studied for examination purposes, the student rather than trying to adapt the content, should alter the manner of accessing the content. We also need to understand the different requirements that various texts make.

At the secondary level, students are faced with dealing with a variety of styles and genres. It is assumed that the literacy skills acquired in primary school will be sufficient to deal with this range of differing styles of reading and writing. For the dyslexic student, this creates even greater problems than it does for those students who do not have literacy difficulties. Dyslexic students need explicit teaching of how to recognize and deal with the differing demands made on them. We need to be aware of these differences ourselves and be always ready to try new routes to deal with the problems the individual has, whether teaching in a one-to-one, small group situation, or in a classroom environment. It is important to develop reflective teaching styles and assess what we do on a practical basis in a dynamic fashion rather than teach in a rigidly structured manner. It is pointless to follow a slavish program if the student is not being helped to learn.

5. READING

5.1 What are the Higher Order Reading Skills?

Once a student has mastered accurate decoding skills and is able to read at the word and sentence level with some degree of accuracy and fluency, then we must teach higher order literacy skills. Higher order reading skills include comprehension skills—skills that help readers become active participants in the reading process; and skills that develop efficient reading.

There are three major kinds of comprehension: literal, inferential, and judgmental. These have been summarized as follows.

Table 1.   Kinds of Comprehension

Comprehension Skills	Activity Involved
Literal	Select significant detail
	Identify main ideas
	Read for specific information
	Understand text organization
	Describe, explain, compare, and summarize
Inferential	Prediction
	Understanding what is not in the text
	Vocabulary
	Reasoning
	Detecting relevance
Judgmental	Appreciating style
	Detecting bias
	Authenticity
	Adequacy
	Appropriateness
	Voice: ambiguity, metaphor, and audience

Comprehension is an interactive, constructive process that involves the skills of synthesis and inference. Skilled readers construct meaning from text as they read, testing their partially constructed understandings against their expectations and existing knowledge. This is an ongoing activity during the reading process and is influenced by many factors: vocabulary knowledge; inferencing ability; knowledge of text structure; personal motivation and what is seen as the perceived purpose for reading; metacognitive strategies; and time spent reading and rereading when understanding requires it. It is important that students interact with the text continuously during the reading process. We can teach readers to do this by (1) demonstrating and having them practice skimming and scanning techniques; (2) encouraging question generation prior to and during the reading process; and (3) by teaching students to reflect on information gained from their reading. This reflection is a metacognitive activity and encourages students to think about what they have gained; for example, have they acquired new knowledge, or have they gained an improved understanding of a difficult concept?

The teaching of these strategies needs to be balanced. The skills instruction must be accompanied by engaging the student in the reading process.

5.2 Teaching Higher Order Reading Skills

To improve the quality and quantity of an individual's reading, we need to find practical ways to help them access text by exposing them to different media. There needs to be a variety of texts for students to read so that in addition to their subject-related text, they read text that interests them.

By establishing areas of personal interest to the student, the teacher can arrange for both the student and teacher to collect relevant material for use at a later, pre-arranged meeting. Involving the student in providing text informally introduces the concept of active participation and allows the student to be instrumental in his or her own learning. The texts collected by teacher and student can be compared and can be used for teaching comprehension skills. Research has shown that direct instruction in vocabulary is most effective when words are clearly defined then used (Oakhill and Garnham, 1988). Direct instruction to help vocabulary development and teaching students how to interact with text will be better assimilated when using texts that interest students.

In the same way as fluent readers enjoy reading material that is amusing or cleverly written, students who struggle with text must also be helped to enjoy humorous writing. In the quest to increase reading output, both humor and enjoyment are important factors to consider, whether they are found through reading short stories or articles, magazines, or computer-generated prose. The text should be at a level the pupil can cope with, but at the same time is not patronizing. Increased reading output, and its commensurate exposure to increased written vocabulary, ensures improvement in both written and spoken vocabulary for the individual.

5.2.1. Main Idea Identification

We can teach main idea identification in texts of different structures and thereby help overcome difficulties that dyslexic students may have in this area (Carriedo and Alonso-Tapia, 1996). The main idea can take several forms, be it single words, titles, topic sentences, or summaries. Comprehension failure may be manifest at any or all of these levels. It is critical to identify exactly what needs to be taught and not to expose students to the unnecessary teaching of concepts they already understand and utilize. As with all teaching of higher level literacy skills, the previous knowledge that a student brings needs to be recognized and used when dealing with text at any level. This may require the development of strategies to activate such previous knowledge, both in the classroom and the individual tutoring environment. Understanding the most important text information can be improved by working on the following:

1. Expanding students' knowledge of the different types of text structures by providing examples and encouraging discussion about the similarities and differences between them.
2. Teaching the students clues that will help identify where, when, and why different text structures are used, for example identifying the differences between analytical and historical prose.
3. Teaching students to categorize characteristics of a text by the events that take place in the text or by the facts included in the text will help them learn to identify main ideas.
4. Identification of the topic or main sentence in a paragraph can be improved by providing practice in writing support sentences for existing topic sentences.
5. Students need practice in the skills of summarizing to help them identify main ideas. This can be achieved by introducing the use of conceptual maps or "spider plans."
6. It is important that adequate opportunities are provided for practice and return further practice occurs regularly.
7. Main idea identification must be taught in a way that enables interactive discussion between teacher and student to take place prior to and during the learning experience. The teacher can model the skills and encourage students to identify and reflect upon the cognitive strategies they are learning and employing.

5.2.2. Identification of Flag Words

Students can be taught to identify *flag words*—words that are clues to important details in the text and express enumerations, superlatives, or transitions in the text. There are four common types of these words.

Enumerative flags. Enumerative flags are those that indicate lists, quantities and sequential placement, for example "first," "in addition," "several," "many," "few," "last," "finally." If a paragraph or sentence begins with the word "first," the student can be shown that there will be at least one or more related concept or commodity to follow, and this must be found and identified. Additional concepts or commodities may themselves be prefaced by enumerative markers. On a practical basis, the student must be taught to annotate these markers in the margin or write them in a list and not trust themselves to remember later.

Superlative flags. Superlative flags show the quality, as expressed by the adjective, is possessed to the greatest or least degree, for example "most," "least," "best," "worst," "highest," "lowest," "largest." When students identify these flags, they must then find the concept or commodity that the comparison relates to.

Transitional flags. Transitional flags mean there is an important link between the concepts preceding and following the flag, for example "however," "therefore," "thus," "additionally," "consequently." Once the flag has been identified, then the related concepts must be found and identified and their relationship understood.

Other flags. Other flags can also point to a special or significant concept or piece of information, for example "unique," "supreme," "universal," "alone," "singly," "everlasting," "only," "other."

In addition to teaching students to identify the flag words, we must go farther and help them engage in analytical thinking about the text in to enhance information retention in their long-term memory.

On a practical basis, this skill can be taught by providing the student with text that can be marked using highlighters. It works well as a class or group activity, with a plenary session at the end of the exercise to compare outcomes. In view of the dyslexic student's difficulty when faced with multiple tasks, it would be more beneficial to tackle each category of flag words on separate occasions before asking them to deal with all the categories together within a piece of text.

5.2.3. Cloze and Comprehension

The cloze technique was developed by Taylor in 1953 to help teach inferential skills (Ashby-Davies, 1985). A text, usually 250 words long, is changed by omitting words at regular intervals throughout it. For example 5th, 8th, or 10th word omissions are common. The first and last sentences of the passage are left intact. Omissions are signaled by lines of equal length. The student provides the missing words without having any hints to the correct answers. The original purpose of cloze was to assess the readability of a passage, so technically only exact answers were considered as correct. However, when the activity is used to improve comprehension and develop inferential skills, then modifications can be made to adjust the exercise suitability according to the needs of the students. Clues to the missing words can be provided. Words may be omitted, but not at regular intervals, but for alternative reasons, for example to support a recently learned rule (such as identifying adverbs). Synonyms could be allowed. Alternatively, correct answers can be chosen from a list of words provided. In these instances it is more correct that we call these "cloze-type exercises."

With strict cloze, the reader is unable to decode meaning at normal reading speed—the process is usually much slower. It also prevents the development of longer eye spans in the way normal reading activities do. Additionally, strict cloze also causes more backward eye movements. On a positive basis, however, those readers who are familiar with cloze are encouraged to read the first and last sentences of the text to help them determine the main gist of the text. Such experience also teaches them the benefit of reading the complete passage when attempting to determine the omissions. They learn how context clues can be helpful to them. They also learn to read the passage more than once, filling in words and guessing at others, and to check or complete their answers. These are beneficial techniques the dyslexic student can use in all reading activities.

Under normal circumstances, there are no omissions present in a piece of prose or text and so the reader can guess for meaning using the word or its phonic pronunciation. Whereas, in cloze, meaning is used to determine the word. This is more akin to encoding than decoding, so a cloze exercise is more than comprehension; it is both reading and writing activity. During the reading process, once a meaning has been attributed to a word, the reader moves forward to continue to process text, which may well consolidate the new meaning. With strict cloze, once the guess has been made, the reader has no way of checking whether the word inserted is that of the author or an acceptable synonym. This aspect of cloze must be brought to the reader's attention prior to, during or after the exercise. Although it is a shortfall, it does afford further opportunity for the student to develop metacognitive and reflective activities.

Cloze also helps readers discover they have more than one meaningful synonym in their long-term memory. Such a realization provides an opportunity for encouraging vocabulary development: The words must be matched taking into account the overall meaning of the passage, inter- and intrasentence meanings, style of writing employed in the passage, and language used by the author. These are all skills not often used in the ordinary reading process.

Cloze strategies not only require students to learn to draw inferences, but also engage them in other thinking tasks. They provide a variety of opportunities to develop those skills that are important in the acquisition of higher-level literacy skills. Inferential skills and a more interactive style of learning can be achieved by engaging in discussion, expecting students to make predictions, encouraging self-monitoring and reflection, asking the students inferential questions, and by employing a flexible teaching style that allows knowledge to be transferred from one learning environment to another. Cloze procedure has the inestimable advantage of being relatively easy to prepare.

5.2.4 Metacognitive Strategies

Research work by Paris and Meyers has shown that poor readers, when reading aloud, do not engage in as much accurate monitoring as do good readers, nor do they evaluate anomalous material as incomprehensible to the same degree as do good readers (Paris and Myers II, 1981). Further, poor readers have less accurate comprehension and recall of stories. Most teachers who have taught poor readers can verify this is so. The study also showed that poor readers engaged in fewer spontaneous study behaviors: They did not ask questions, take notes, or use a dictionary as often as the good readers did. They also did not notice and resolve the comprehension failures of unknown words.

The dyslexic student needs to be taught the range of strategies that good readers use when reading. Such students need guided practice in the use of these study aids and they need to experience their benefits in order for them to become part of their learning.

The active monitoring of comprehension while reading is an important skill and the level of understanding achieved while reading can be evaluated by asking questions such as: Does this make sense? Do I understand this word? Do these ideas fit in with previous information? Initially, the teacher can generate questions, but, at the same time, encourage students to think of their own questions. As the process becomes easier and their self-confidence grows, students take on more responsibility.

Prior knowledge and experience affects learning, but to increase comprehension, and therefore learning, such knowledge must be activated. Asking questions is a means of activating this knowledge, but we must take care to ensure that this does more than promote text recall. Promoting the use of "why" questions enables students to use their prior knowledge and experience to make the relationships between facts more understandable and more memorable.

Because poor readers tend to spend more time concentrating on decoding individual words, they attend less to constructing the meaning of sentences. They must be shown the positive benefits of constructive strategies, such as consulting a dictionary, while reading. Prior to reading text, unusual or new vocabulary included in the text can be presented or highlighted by the teacher, the structure, spelling, and contextual use of the words discussed, and the definitions of this vocabulary confirmed. This sequence of activities introduces concrete associations for the vocabulary and use of the dictionary serves to consolidate the new knowledge. At the same time this provides an opportunity for students to concentrate on the content of the text prior to reading.

Rereading text is another strategy that improves comprehension and information retention. Main idea identification has already been mentioned, but other strategies that build upon this work include deletion of trivial information, making summaries and transforming linear prose into nonlinear form (such as flow charts or spider plans). These skills entail deeper processing on the part of the student for them to achieve the reorganization of the material in these forms, all of which foster better comprehension and recall.

The construction of spider plans or maps is an organizing activity that can be done as a class or in an individual or small group tutoring environment. In this technique, the main idea is written in the center of the page. Lines radiate out from this main idea, connecting to what are determined to be the supporting points or relevant ideas. The advantage to this is the sequence of thought is not interrupted by having to put the information down on paper in a linear fashion. Discussion between teacher and student to determine which facts are salient and worth recording is built on the student's understanding of what has been read. Increased comprehension arises from the student's listening to others' suggestions and from the interactions between teacher and students and between the students themselves.

Graphic organizers are another means of organizing information in a concise fashion. These can be prepared by the teacher prior to reading a text to serve as an overview for the teacher. They can also be referred to when reading, or they can be revisited later as necessary.

Reflective thinking is an important component of reading that is often overlooked. Thinking about our learning is the aim of teaching metacognitive strategies. Much of what we read is often forgotten, thus learning to reflect after reading is a means of helping retain the information presented in a text. Again, this is an activity that requires modeling and guided practice by the teacher if the dyslexic student is to benefit from the process.

By posing relevant questions the student can be guided to reflect upon what has been read. This helps improve comprehension and recall by directing the student towards the author's main points. Questions that require the student to determine what information the headings convey help identify the main ideas and provide the basis for writing summaries. As with the process of question generation to activate knowledge prior to reading, when engaging in reflective thinking, students must learn to formulate their own questions about the information in the text, or any difficulties they have had with the text. It is at this reflective stage that the students are encouraged to relate what they have read to what they already know and to consider how relevant this information is to them and what they are learning.

6.   HIGHER LEVEL SPELLING SKILLS

In light of the research findings, previously mentioned in this chapter, that reveal persisting phonological processing difficulties, it is not surprising older dyslexic students continuously struggle with spelling, even if they have overcome other difficulties. Such students have responded well to a teaching approach which links explicit teaching of spelling rules and strategies to the development of high-level phonological awareness (Townend, 1995).

Older students learn about written language as long as it is interesting and moves away from previous approaches to learning to spell, such as rote learning for spelling tests, or copying errors numerous times. Root words, word origins, clear teaching of complex phoneme–grapheme correspondences, word families, affixes, and individual memory techniques for spelling awkward words help older dyslexic students. These students are often aware their spoken vocabulary is far more sophisticated than their written vocabulary. Early on in their school careers they begin to choose to use simple words rather than risk making further spelling errors. Teaching specific strategies for them to adapt and practice in their use can help them confidently increase the size of their written vocabularies.

6.1. Dictionaries

Metacognitive strategies include using a dictionary, spell checker, thesaurus, and referring to the text for correct spellings. Problems arise, however, when students are not able to use these tools during examinations. Moreover, a dictionary will be of no use to any dyslexic student with a sophisticated oral vocabulary if he makes spelling errors with the first three to five letters of a word. In such circumstances the student's usual response is "it's not in this dictionary." For such students it may as well not be; choosing a simpler word, they avoid yet another failure. Some dyslexic students are greatly helped by the use of an ACE dictionary (Moseley, 1998, 2nd ed.) which does not require good spelling to access a word. Still, dictionary skills need to be taught, using a regular dictionary; this requires work beyond the use of quartiles and guide words. All students can gain much more insight into language if they learn how to decipher those codes found beside the words in the dictionary: how stress in a word is depicted, where syllables break, where information regarding word origin can be found, etc. By observing their teacher frequently consult the dictionary, students can overcome their reluctance to use it. This act goes beyond explicit teacher modeling, to serve as an ordinary event in the course of producing written work.

With regard to higher level literacy skills, producing written work requires more than just writing neatly and attempting to use the punctuation introduced in the previous lesson. Drafting and redrafting need to be taught and modeled by the teacher, then refined, practiced, and used by the student. Using the dictionary for choice of vocabulary and as a means to improve written vocabulary is but the first step in this process. A well produced and accessible thesaurus is an even more effective tool for vocabulary selection; we like the ones which use two colors. Several publishers offer a selection; choose the one that best suits the level at which your student is working. Much practice is necessary before dyslexic students are confident enough to use these tools in their own studies.

6.2. Simultaneous Oral Spelling

The Simultaneous Oral Spelling (SOS) method for spelling errors or awkward words encompasses the principles of multisensory teaching. It is a method that is easily deployed in a one-to-one, small group, or classroom environment. If it is introduced as a method for committing words to memory, it can then be used as the example for expanding the concept of multimodal study skills for revision. As is the case for learning spelling corrections or vocabulary, SOS can be used across the curriculum. Hard-to-grasp words used in chemistry or physics are just as effectively learned using this method as are those used in a piece of creative writing for an English lesson.

Because it is not always practical to speak aloud, dyslexic students should learn to *subvocalize*, or mouth the words. This is infinitely more effective than just *thinking* the word.

6.3. Spelling Strategies

Books, magazines, newspapers, subject texts—even the student's own work—may be used as resources for work on spelling extension. There is a wide range of published material available, some of which is listed at the end of this chapter.

The following is a list of some of the strategies for spelling that we, and our pupils, have found useful for different words at different times. It is by no means an exhaustive list, and we (the two of us and our students) believe that the best spelling strategy is probably the one you thought up yourself. Visual thinkers will like the pictorial strategies, while auditory–verbal thinkers will prefer the ones that rely on sound.

Table 2

Simultaneous Oral Spelling (SOS)
Student looks at word and says it aloud.
Student names letters in word.
Student covers word.
Student writes word *while naming letters as they are written*.
Student checks spelling against original.

6.3.1. Syllables

This is probably the most useful thing to learn about spelling; it builds up confidence and increases the chances of being correct. It is, of course, totally dependent on being prepared to say the word aloud in the usual way, then again, one syllable at a time. Many of the words that are tricky to spell are short; long words are often regular, and the problem is one of memory and confidence. A syllable is easy to spell if the student understands the concept of long and short vowels, and open and closed syllables. A long word may be viewed as a series of such syllables. For example, information is in—for—ma—tion (two easy words, open syllable "ma" and regular final syllable "tion"). (For more detail about syllables, see Chapter 11.)

6.3.2. Little Words in Big Words

A word such as "secretary" gives away little in the pronunciation of the vowels (try saying it now), but if secretary is linked to the word "secret," the spelling becomes obvious. We remember the sentence: "His secretary knows all his secrets."

6.3.3. Affixes

This includes prefixes and suffixes. Having established that confidence is an important element in mastering spelling, we can develop this by introducing our students to the "learn one, spell lots" approach. Affixes are probably the best example of this. Take a simple word such as "help":

Add a suffix—ful—helpful
Add a prefix—un—unhelpful
Add another suffix—ly—unhelpfully
Go back to "help" and try other suffixes: helpless, helping, helped, helps.

By applying these affixes, according to a set of simple and fairly consistent rules (see Chapters 4, 10), to a wide range of known root words, students increase their vocabulary, without putting an extra load on the memory.

6.3.4. Word Families

This is another "learn one, spell lots" technique. It uses association and analogy to access less familiar words. For example, if you learn the useful chunk a–n–a–l–y by saying it aloud often enough, you can easily complete a family of often misspelled words: analysis; analyse; analyst. Similarly, the ending –ine, pronounced "een," helps with the spelling of several elements in chemistry: chlorine, bromine, fluorine, for example.

Another way to use related words is to use the pronunciation of one word to inform the spelling of another. For example, the second vowel in "politics" is unstressed (this unstressed vowel is called a schwa—see Chapter 1). It is impossible to tell from the pronunciation which vowel it should be. However, in the derived adjective, "political," because the second vowel is now stressed, it is possible to hear the (ĭ) sound, and because root words do not change, it is safe to assume the same letter in the noun.

6.3.5. Silly Sentences

This is a variation on the above. Link a group of words with the same spelling pattern into a sentence, for example:

The vicar found a burglar in his cellar stealing vinegar.

The many possibilities are limited only by the imagination of the student and the bounds of decency!

6.3.6. Mnemonics

Tip: Do not expect your student to spell it! This is a sentence in which each word begins with a letter of the word to be spelled. It can be a useful device if the student can remember the sentence, and particularly so for tricky words which are not too long. The best sentences are those that the student makes up, but encourage sentences which are easy to understand and remember.

For example: Yachts Always Come Home Together (yacht)
                  Big Elephants Can't Always Use Small Entrances (because)
                  Rhythm Has Your Two Hips Moving (rhythm)

and our favorite, made up by 13-year-old Guy:
                  Never Eat Cod, Eat Smoked Salmon And Remain Young.

6.3.7. Auditory Clues

Auditory clues may be used when one part of the word is causing problems. In a word such as "necessary," the main confusion is the c and the ss, so "one collar and two socks" or "one captain and two soldiers" can be an effective memory trigger. Guy's mnemonic came into being when the group protested that the vowels in "necessary" were tricky, too!

Another auditory clue is "spelling pronunciation," which is a personal and private way of saying a word to remind oneself of the spelling. (Although I am not dyslexic, I can remember doing this and finding it useful as a very small child). Typical examples would be "Wed–nes–day," "shep–herd," "com–mit–tee," "Feb–ru–ary," "mort–gage" (second syllable rhymes with cage).

6.3.8. Visual Clues

Some students find these helpful, though because they need to be kept on paper they are less portable and more easy to lose than memory aids carried in the head. Figure 1 shows some examples.

6.4. Teaching Spelling

As with all teaching, particularly with dyslexic students, the imparting of information and skills must be clear and thorough, repeated and revised as often as necessary. Just because you have taught it, you cannot assume your student has learned it. The principles of teaching have been clearly laid out in previous chapters, and they apply equally to the older and to the very able student, for whom the kind of work previously described will be appropriate. Effective teaching is multisensory, cumulative, thorough, and interactive. It is particularly important that this group is actively involved in their learning, and that they are in partnership with the teacher in finding—and using—effective solutions to their difficulties.

Of course, there is still the problem of transfer and application of new learning which the dyslexic student faces; the only answer to this is to make the application explicit, preferably by encouraging the student to work it out for himself and then practicing this knowledge. The teacher's skill and ingenuity will need to be applied to maintaining motivation during this practicing time because repetition can be tedious. Amusing or interesting dictation passages are more motivating than boring ones. The interests of the student must be considered.

Group work can be motivating and fun provided that each participant has something to contribute and there is not an individual who is worse or better than the rest of the group. Groups need to be organized to include: revision of recent work; an opportunity for students to share spelling triumphs and disasters since

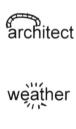

weather

Figure 1. Visual clues to spelling.

the last session, so everyone can contribute ideas for sorting it out; new work taught to the group; and individual work on paper, so the teacher can give one-to-one help where it is needed. Not everyone will work at the same speed, so it is advisable to include some optional extension work, such as paragraph writing or vocabulary exercises for those who have finished. We link the extension work to the same spelling topic for additional reinforcement.

7. HIGHER LEVEL WRITING SKILLS

The literature survey described near the beginning of this chapter outlines the main characteristics of poor writing, which can be summed up as a difficulty in the organization of information—and this is basically a summary definition of dyslexia! It has been our experience in teaching dyslexic teenagers that all their difficulties seem to come together to thwart their attempts to put their knowledge and their ideas down on paper.

The principles of teaching still apply: multisensory, structured, cumulative, thorough, and above all, interactive. We suggest that the key to improved written output is task analysis. This process will not come naturally. Breaking down the writing task needs to be demonstrated and practiced by teacher and student together. This may be done effectively in a small group, or in a classroom. Dyslexic students are not the only ones who would benefit from such an approach.

7.1. Task Analysis

Consider how many different tasks there are in the writing of one essay:

- Understanding the title
- Remembering the title while writing (to keep writing relevant to title)
- Selecting the information
- Arranging it in order
- Remembering which points you have covered already (to avoid repetition)
- Organizing into paragraphs
- Selecting the words that best express what you want to say
- Grammatically correct sentences
- Spelling
- Punctuation
- Handwriting

This list contains 11 items, most of which the writer is trying to do at the same time. In an examination, there is the additional burden of trying to remember the

The topic was placed in the middle. Starting at *, and moving clock-wise, ideas were written as they emerged, but it is possible to start any-where and move in any direction, or even dart around.

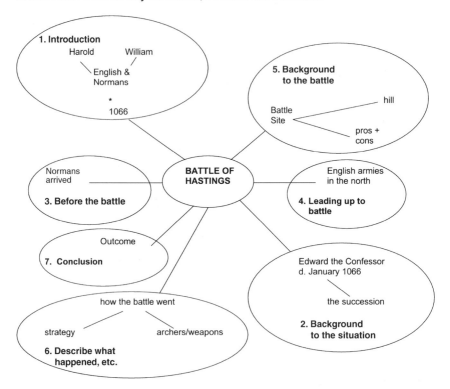

Points must then be numbered in the order they will be placed in the essay.

The end result is an instant essay plan—remembering and sequencing have been done before the student starts to write. This method can be adapted to fit the age and abil-ity of the writer and the complexity of the topic. It works best if the student uses a big sheet of paper. For a superfi-cial treatment, have the student write from the plan. For more detailed work, have the student either develop the legs out from each point or write a linear plan, adding de-tails uunder each point.

Figure 2. Essay planning: Task analysis leads to improved writing.

stuff. No wonder it is difficult! Figure 2 showed a tried and tested way of analyzing the task. It broke up the first six and got them out of the way before the actual writing began, leaving only the five technical elements to be handled during writing.

Task analysis includes breaking down an essay title or examination question into content words (what is the subject matter: photosynthesis, a character in a novel, the causes of the Great War, for example) and process words (what do I do with the subject matter: define, discuss, compare, and so on). This can lead into essay planning—and it is sensible to present a wide variety of methods for this, because different students need to find the ones that best suit their learning style, and to learn to select a method that is appropriate to the work in hand.

Purposes in writing are a useful area to tackle. Many dyslexic students are not widely read, or they have failed to pick up stylistic differences in their reading. They are therefore unaware of the range of styles they can employ for different writing tasks. A popular exercise is to study the prose style of several newspapers and then to take a news item or a familiar story and write the story in two or three different styles to suit those newspapers. This could be extended into writing scripts for news broadcasts of different lengths and radio stations. You will need to have some examples prerecorded.

Chapters 6 and 9 contain much that is relevant to the group of students we are considering in this chapter. You will find many practical ideas there, and in the study skills books which are now widely available.

8. SUMMARY

We have identified the characteristic difficulties in literacy experienced by many dyslexic pupils of secondary school age (11–18 years), once they have mastered the basic skills. Some of the most effective teaching methods, as demonstrated in the research literature, are described. We have attempted to explain some of the ways in which we have used them with our students. It is particularly important to remember, when working with this age group, that there is never only one right answer. The special education teacher must be prepared to work in partnership with his or her students, and to be willing to listen to and learn from them. We have both found this to be a rich source of professional development.

RESOURCES

English to GCSE Revision Guide, Geoff Barton (1999), Oxford: Oxford University Press. ISBN 0-19-831289-X

Grammar to 14 Skills and Practice, Don Shiach (1998), Oxford: Oxford University Press. ISBN 0-19-831442-6

Comprehension to GCSE Focus on Non-fiction, Geoff Barton (1998), Oxford: Oxford University Press. ISBN 0-19-831447-7

Writing Skills for the Adolescent, Diana Hanbury King (1985), Cambridge, Massachusetts: Educator's Publishing Services, Inc. ISBN 0-8388-2054-9

Writing with a Point, Jeanne B. Stephens and Ann Harper, Cambridge, Massachusetts: Educator's Publishing Service, Inc. ISBN 0-8388-2054-9

Developing Literacy for Study and Work, Walter Bramley, Staines, Middlesex: The Dyslexia Institute. ISBN 0-9503-9155-7

Write in Style: A Guide to Good English, Richard Palmer, London: E & FN Spon. ISBN 0-419-14640-7

Study Skills: A Pupil's Survival Guide, Christine Ostler, Godalming: Ammonite Books. ISBN 1-869866-10-X

Learning Skills:

How To Write Essays. Cambridge: Collins Educational. ISBN 0-00-322349-3

How to Manage Your Study Time. Cambridge: Collins Educational. ISBN 0-00-322364-7

How to Improve Your Memory, Robert Leach, Cambridge: Collins Educational. ISBN 0-00-322365-5

How to Succees in Exams and Assessments, Penny Henderson, Cambridge: Collins Educational. ISBN 0-00-322346-9

How to Study Effectively, Richard Freeman and John Meed, Cambridge: Collins Educational. ISBN 0-00-322345-0

Clear Thinking, John Inglis and Roger Lewis. Cambridge: Collins Educational. ISBN 0-00-322347-7

SRA Reading Laboratory 4a, Don H. Parker, Chicago, Illinois: Science Research Associates, Inc.

REFERENCES

Ashby-Davies, C. (1985). Cloze and comprehension: A qualitative analysis and critique. *Journal of Reading, 28(7)*, 585–589.

Bereiter, C., and Scardamalia, M. (1989). Intentional learning as a goal of instruction. In L. Resnick (ed.), *Knowing, Learning and Instruction*. London: Lawrence Erlbaum Associates.

Beveridge, M. (1989). Literacy in primary and secondary schools: The educational context. In K. Mogford & J. Sadler (eds.), *Child Language Disability: Implications in an Educational Setting*. Clevedon: Multilingual Matters.

Brown, A.L., & Palinscar, A.S. (1989). Guided, co-operative learning and individual knowledge acquisition. In L.B. Resnick (ed.), *Knowing, Learning and Instruction*. London, Lawrence Erlbaum Associates.

Bruce, B., Collins, A., Rubin, A., & Gentner, D. (1977). A cognitive-science approach to writing. (Technical report no. 89) Champaign, Illinois: university of Illinois Center for the Study of Reading.

Carriedo, N., & Alonso-Tapia, J. (1996). Main idea comprehension: Training teachers and effects on students. *Journal of Research in Reading, 19(2)*, 128–153.

Collins, A., Seely Brown, J., & Newman, S.E. (1989). *Cognitive Apprenticeship: Teaching the Crafts of Reading, Writing and Mathematics*. London: Lawrence Erlbaum Associates.

Elbro, C. (1989). Morphological awareness in dyslexia. In C. Von Euler (ed.) *Brain and Reading*. London: Macmillan.

Fitzgerald, J., & Teasley, A. (1983). Effects of instruction in narrative structure on children's writing. Paper presented at the National Reading Conference, Austin, Texas, November 1993.

Frith, U. (1980). Unexpected spelling problems. In U. Frith (ed.), *Cognitive Processes in Spelling*. London: Academic Press.

Goswami, U., & Bryant, P. (1990). *Phonological Skills and Learning to Read.* Hove, Sussex: Lawerence Erlbaum Associates.

Hayes, J., & Flower, L. (1980). Writing as problem solving. *Visible Language, 14*, 388–399.

Martlew, M. (1993). Problems and difficulties: Cognitive and communicative aspects of writing. In M. Martlew (ed.), *The Psychology of Written Language.* New York: John Wiley & Sons.

Moseley, D. (1998). *ACE Dictionary, 2nd edition.* Wisbech, Cambridgeshire: Learning Development Aids.

Oakhill, J., & Garnham, A. (1988). *Becoming a Skilled Reader.* Oxford: Blackwell.

Palinscar, A., & Brown, A. (1984). Reciprocal teaching of comprehension-fostering and comprehension -monitoring activities. *Cognition and Instruction, 1*, 117–175.

Paris, S.G., & Myers II, M. (1981). Comprehension monitoring, memory, and study strategies of good and poor readers. *Journal of Reading Behaviour, 8(1)*, 5–22.

Perrin, D. (1983). Phonemic segmentation and spelling. *British Journal of Psychology, 74*, 129–144.

Rosenshine, B., Meister, C., & Chapman, S. (1996). Teaching students to generate questions: Intervention studies. *Review of Educational Research, 66(2)*, 181–221.

Taylor, B., & Beach, R. (1984). The effects of text structure instruction on middle grade student's comprehension and production of expository text. *Reading Research Quarterly, 19*, 134–146.

Tharp, P., & Gallimore, R. (1991). A theory of teaching as assisted performance. In P. Light, S. Sheldon, and M. Woodhead (eds.), *Learning to Think: A Reader*, London: Open University.

Townend, J. (1995). Towards a whole-school approach to dyslexia. (Master's thesis,) *Kingston University.*

Webster, A., Beveridge, M., & Reed, M. (1996). *Managing the Literacy Curriculum.* London: Routledge.

Wood, D.J., Bruner, J.S., & Ross, G. (1976). The role of tutoring in problem solving. *Journal of Child Psychology and Psychiatry, 17(2)*, 89–100.

9

The Learning Skills

Mary Flecker and Jennifer Cogan

This chapter looks at the skills which underpin learning and facilitate the integration of new learning into all aspects of study. The skills are explored under two main headings: organization and memory.

1. AN INTRODUCTION TO ORGANIZATION

1.1. Automaticity

Most of the big skills in learning—reading, taking notes, writing, understanding, remembering—depend upon the simultaneous operation of a cluster of underlying processing skills. Satisfactory note taking, for instance, relies on the student's ability to digest his teacher's current point, while remembering and handwriting a note about his last one. Amazingly, most of us can do this (see Figure 1).

However, if these skills do not function together automatically, they induce an overload in the student. By making a conscious effort in several directions at once, he loses control over one or more of his weaker skills. This situation is demonstrated in Figure 2, which shows the handwriting of a 17-year-old, who is taking dictation.

1.2. Research

Researchers, notably Albert Galaburda (Galaburda, 1991) and Paula Tallal (Tallal 1991), indicate that the visual and auditory processing systems in the brains of dyslexic people are frequently as much as 27 percent smaller than in so-called

Mary Flecker, 34 Burnaby Street, London, SW10 OPL, United Kingdom   Jennifer Cogan, Westminster School, 17 Dean's Yard, Westminster, London, SW1P 3PF, United Kingdom

"normal" brains. Correspondingly, they work more slowly and less efficiently, although the dyslexic person's understanding may be as acute as anyone else's (Tallal, 1997).

1.3. In the Classroom

The dyslexic student compensates for this lack of automaticity by consciously listening and looking, while his peers do so subconsciously and with greater speed and much less stress. No wonder he is tired out at the end of a school day.

His problems may finally be compounded by the fact that neither his teachers and peers nor he himself understand why he struggles when others in the class manage with such ease. Often no one knows that it is not his capacity as a scientist or historian but the lack of automatic function in his underlying processing skills which is frustrating his impulse to learn.

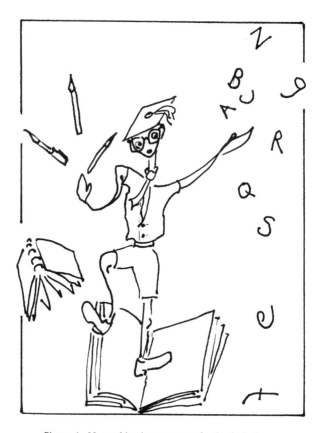

Figure 1. Note-taking is not so easy for the dyslexic.

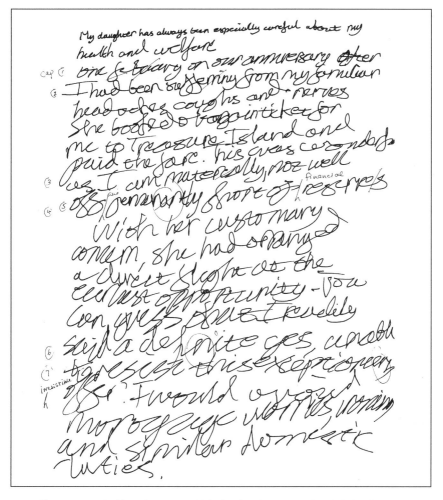

Figure 2. Handwriting of a 17-year-old during dictation. The weaker skills break down.

2. THE ORGANIZATION OF READING

2.1. Problems

Reading is one of the major learning strategies used by schools as part of teaching all but the youngest age. The decoding of words is only one of several essential components of reading. This list shows a breakdown of the subskills typically involved in a school curriculum task:

- Decoding words—fast
- Knowing alternative word meanings
- Holding decoded words in short term memory
- Building meaning in text
- Checking meaning against own experience
- Keeping sequence straight
- Detecting inferences
- Detecting bias

The dyslexic reader who cannot automatically integrate these skills may find that one or other of them breaks down; perhaps he is so busy and so slow at decoding individual words that he cannot take in their aggregate meaning. He may decode inaccurately, reading "per" for "pre," omitting "not," adding "ed" and so distort or even reverse the meaning of the passage. So much processing effort may go into puzzling out individual words that the reader may not be able to respond to meaning implicit in the syntax or in little linking words which so often carry signals about

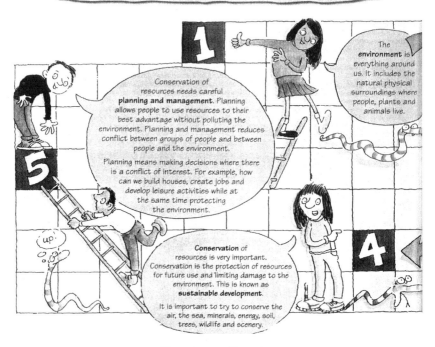

Figure 3. A reading task.

emphasis or direction, such as "however," "finally," "meanwhile," "surely" (usually implying the opposite). The overload on his reading skills may be such that he cannot stand back and consider the writer's style or purpose and when he comes to do that later, his weak short term memory has already forgotten which was the significant phrase and where it was on the page. In rescanning the text, he may forget what he is looking for and become seduced by another aspect of the reading task.

This problem of overload, arising from inefficient subskills, dogs the dyslexic student in every reading task. His classmates, by contrast, appear to read without effort, retaining detail and significance as they speed along. It is discouraging, if not embittering, for a reader to be denied several times a day the power and pleasure which others so obviously enjoy.

2.2. Organizing a Solution

If the dyslexic student cannot trust his brain to manage its own reading subskills automatically, he should consciously take over the responsibility for that organization.

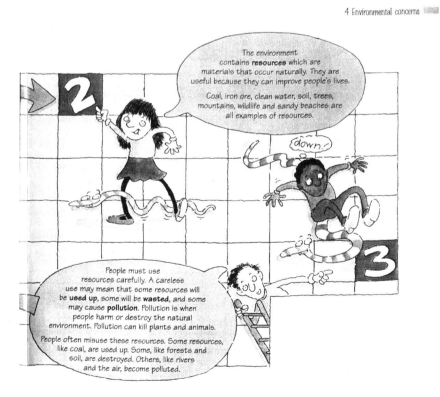

He can interact with his text, question and visualize the ideas, analyze and practice the language. The method chosen for this is determined by his understanding of the way his brain works best.

Problems

In addition to the dyslexic's customary difficulty with reading, this apparently student-friendly presentation of information, though stimulating for many students, might be distracting and confusing for the dyslexic reader:

- It is laid out on a familiar game board, but it isn't a game.
- Are the ladders and snakes significant or not?
- The orientation of numbers, figures, speech bubbles may confuse.
- The physical sequence confuses the semantic sequence.
- The bubbles are densely packed with abstract information.
- Although the figure is meant to have a visual impact, there are no supporting illustrations to the texts.

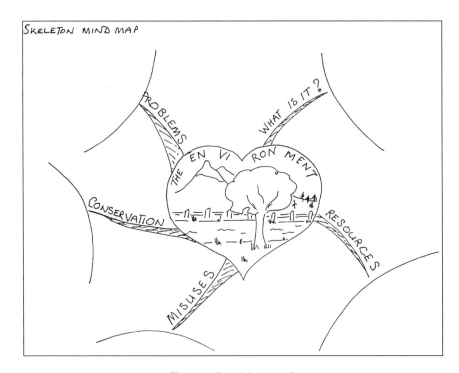

Figure 4. Organizing to read.

The solution is multisensory and step by step

With the help of his geography teacher, a poor reader whose strengths are visual (or even a whole class), might tackle the reading task like this:

- Student reads the text—decoding.
- Teacher provides skeleton mind map which invites categorization (see Figure 4).
- Class discusses each branch.
- Student reads again, sorting out information for each branch.
- Student draws symbols for selected information in the spaces.
- Student talks a fellow student through his mind map, using appropriate vocabulary.

This may look time-consuming, but dyslexics who lean on their visual strength learn to draw quickly. In the end, the inadequate reader should be able to digest the material and be able to talk or write about it, using suitable technical language.

2.3. Teaching Ideas for the Classroom

2.3.1. Organizing for Reading

1. Know the dyslexic student in your classroom:
   - Know his level of reading ability.
   - Find out his difficulties in reading for your subject.
   - Make sure you and he know his best approach to reading.
2. Anticipate the difficulties:
   - Preview the class' knowledge of a new topic on the board before expecting the dyslexic to read.
   - Teach names in a set book: recognizing, saying, and writing.
   - Use only the best quality photocopied reading material.
3. Provide a focus for independent reading:
   - Provide a skeleton mind map with the key ideas drawn in.
   - Offer a question to relate the text to while reading.
4. Look for multisensory reading strategies:
   - Teach visualizing.
   - Give access to complete texts on tape.
5. Foster any individual approach to reading which looks constructive:
   - Have crucial sections of a textbook on tapes to take home.
   - Investigate computer material which is text out loud.
   - Provide alternative textbooks to the one used in class.

3. THE ORGANIZATION OF WORDS

3.1. The Problem

Current research suggests that "the most general information processing deficit in developmental dyslexia lies in phonological processing." Poor phonological processing constantly undermines a dyslexic's control over words. Unusual, often slow, processing, combined with unreliable perception and hesitant grapheme to phoneme correspondence, hampers the dyslexic student's ability to hear, say, read, spell, or handwrite words. He may also have problems with knowing alternative word meanings, understanding inferences, or recalling words accurately to order; naming is a particularly familiar problem. "That thing you go out of; it begins with **e**," is typical of what a dyslexic person might say when searching his memory for the word "exit."

3.2. In the Classroom

A problem with managing everyday words is not insurmountable. People with dyslexia become adept at finding alternatives, though they may be inhibited from naming a book title or telling a joke. Mastering subject-specific vocabulary in school is a different matter altogether. Dominic says he cannot remember the Old Testament stories recounted to his class because he "cannot get hold of the names." Liam, despite an obstinate interest in his science class, cannot recall the word "evaporation" to represent the process he perfectly understands. Alice, so frightened by the look of the word "prescriptivism" in her English textbook, was convinced it stood for a really abstruse idea. Once she could say it, she could see it meant pedantic formal English, as in "up with which I will not put."

These classroom examples illustrate how a specific problem with processing words can block a dyslexic student's mastery of his subject, however interested in it he may be. Words in the classroom, which to the ordinary student are a channel for understanding and communication, are, for the student with dyslexia, a barrier to both.

3.3. Organizing Solutions

One way to tackle the dyslexic student's difficulty with words is to translate them into the individual's stronger modality. This means changing writing into speech, description into diagram, notes into mind maps, facts into symbols, and handwriting into word processing.

A second way is to develop a whole school policy in which the members of each department *deliberately* teach their own subject-specific vocabulary. Teachers instinctively do this. How would they not? But wherever lack of automaticity in low level skills causes dyslexic pupils to underachieve, a possible amelioration may lie in the word "deliberately." If teacher and student deliberate over the difficulty, they may organize multisensory strategies to combat it.

An understanding of Dominic's weak auditory perception and memory prompted his teacher to rehearse Old Testament names with the whole class, before using them in the stories. He then left a list of them on the board where they served as pegs to hang his stories on. The next day, Dominic could say and write the names. He could also recount the stories. Liam tackled his "naming" difficulty by visualizing and saying "vapor" to prompt the term "evaporation." Alice knew it would help to practice segmenting and synthesizing the syllables of tricky words aloud: (pre–scrip–tiv–ism, prescriptivism) before she attempted to understand them.

3.4. A Multisensory Approach

Each subject causes the dyslexic student to deal with a different facet of language difficulty. The words may be technical (circuit, hypotenuse, medieval). They may be used figuratively ("love-devouring Death," "the sauce to meat is ceremony"). They may be archaic or in dialect, homophones (key, quay), tongue twisters (quantitative), foreign, or just too long. Furthermore, the problem of mastering single words takes no account of the higher skills involved in literacy. Mastery of single words is, however, so much a *sine qua non* for an adequate use of those higher skills that it is worth all teachers taking a deliberate and multisensory attitude to teaching the language relevant to their subject.

3.4.1. Word Patterns

Inadequate phonological processing will cause dyslexic students to see a word as a string of letters (frequently too long for his working memory to hold) without segments, shape, or relation to other words. Figure 5 shows how words with "sign" as their root can be recognized in the form of a pattern where affixes build visual and semantic chunks onto the root. Dyslexic students who learn the habit of looking for and recognizing word patterns reduce the problems of complexity and incoherence they have with language.

3.4.2. Playing with Words

The words listed here all appear on one page of a science examination paper for 13-year-olds:

ammeter	beaker	irregularly
heart	thermometer	atmosphere
measuring	area	barometer
voltmeter	beats	pressure

Figure 6 illustrates how to play with the vocabulary to learn how to read, say, understand, recall, and write it.

3.4.3. Coding Words

Using a pencil as he reads is an excellent way for a dyslexic student to grow confident with the building blocks of literacy; the puzzle-solving element makes it fun. The reader can for example:

Mark off syllables	dys/lex/ic
Note short vowels, long vowels, and regular final syllables	mănūfac|ture|
Turn **c** /s/ into an **s**; **c** /k/ into a **k**	aksept
Turn **g** /j/ into a **j**	rēġent
Write "sh" above "ti" and "ci" when each is before a vowel	ini*ti*al
	pre*ci*ous

Unlocking the code makes for confidence and enjoyment—both rare and precious experiences for the dyslexic student.

3.4.4. Saying Words Aloud

The less confident dyslexic people feel about their control over words, the fewer times they speak. The less they speak, the weaker their control over words. This cycle is nowhere more apparent than when they learn foreign languages. Probably the most useful and simplest multisensory self-help is for the speaker to keep speaking the words aloud, no matter how reluctant and embarrassed he feels. Subvocalizing is a good compromise. H classroom policy for saying new or difficult words aloud will raise everyone's standards of literacy.

3.4.5. Enough Time for Words

Research into the speed of language processing of dyslexic subjects (Tallal, 1997) demonstrates two things: (1) milliseconds make a difference; and (2) training can improve the speed and efficiency of language processing. If, therefore, a teacher speaks even fractionally faster than the dyslexic pupil can process, the lessons, however well presented, will prove disastrous for him. The gift of time is probably the most valuable support a classroom teacher can offer a dyslexic pupil, while specialist remediation can center on the increased speed of processing which proven neural plasticity implies.

3.5. Teaching Ideas for the Classroom: Organizing to Master Words

3.5.1. *Know the dyslexic student in your classroom:*

- Know his particular difficulty with words.
- Know his preferred channel for words: listening, looking, speaking, writing.
- Give him time to ask and respond in class.

3.5.2. *Introduce the vocabulary before the topic:*

- Teach the words: students should see, hear, say, and write them.
- Teach mnemonics and symbols; use color and games; make up memory pegs and stories.
- Give semantic clues; affixes, derivations, associated words.

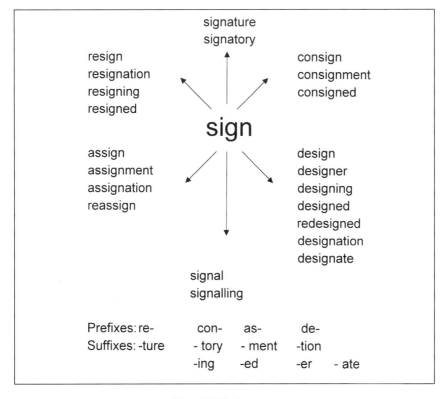

Figure 5. Word patterns.

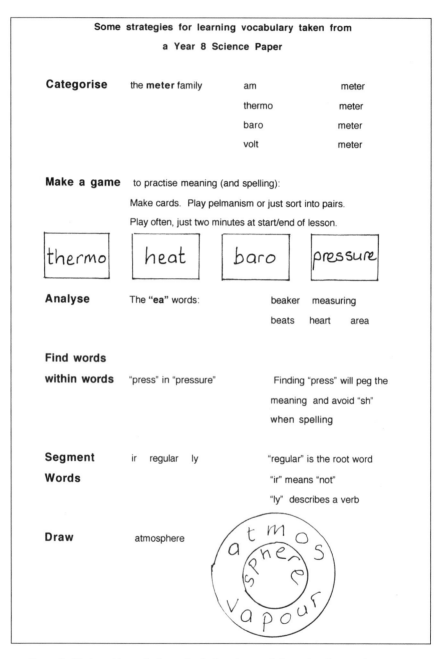

Figure 6. Playing with words. Strategies for learning vocabulary taken from a science paper.

3.5.3. See if the student can use the vocabulary he needs for each topic:

- Can he give a verbal account?
- Can he recall and spell the technical words he needs?
- Check his notes for word facility and spelling.

3.5.4. Find ways of easing the load:

- Encourage and facilitate word processing.
- Put crucial text on tapes.
- Make textbooks available at all times for dyslexic students to consult; their own notes may be far from adequate.
- Encourage alternative modes of learning and expression, particularly using visualizing.
- Use alternative strategies yourself; example is by far the most influential teaching method.

4. THE ORGANIZATION OF WRITING

4.1. The Problem

Writing is hard on the subskills that underpin literacy. It requires the writer to keep both the overall picture and the immediate detail, technical and intellectual, simultaneously in mind from start to finish. The overload on unautomatic skills when dyslexic students attempt to write causes problems: They may write too little or too much; their arguments may be muddled and repetitive; they may omit vital points; their conclusion may contradict their introduction; their spelling may be exasperating; and their handwriting may be illegible. The dyslexic writer knows this will happen, so he dreads writing and develops a writing block.

4.2. In the Classroom

Yet writing is a daily classroom activity as is homework, course work, and exams. To confuse the issue further, the dyslexic student, whose written work is so unsatisfactory, may make excellent verbal contributions in class and show talent for the subject. This contradiction bewilders and disappoints all concerned: student, teacher, and parent.

4.3. Organizing Solutions

The way to manage the problem of overload on writing skills is to break the task into steps and deal with each separately. The first step must be to assess the writing task. Is it to copy or take notes? Is it to write a story or an essay? Will its greatest demands be on speedy writing, summarizing information, balancing arguments, or an imaginative style? Who is the audience? What is the time scale? The selection of writing strategies is affected by the answers to these questions.

4.4. Copying from the Board

Teachers commonly assume that all children can copy, thus it is well worth the dyslexic student organizing himself to do it effectively, despite possible weaknesses in perception, short term memory, spatial and hand–eye coordination. He can support his weakness by subvocalizing when he focuses on the board, repeating the words to write as he looks down at his page. He can guide his writing, using the index finger of his free hand. If his copying is inaccurate or too slow, he should persuade his teachers to give him a handout to annotate.

A laptop computer is the ideal solution to the problem of unsatisfactory copying skills in the classroom. Touch typing is essential for this, and frees the dyslexic student to keep his eyes on the board while his fingers type. Not having to remember words or look from board to book or form legible letters, releases him to take an interest in the work he is copying. This alone could revolutionize the standard of his work.

4.5. Notetaking

This classroom skill is sometimes not taught, checked, nor supported with a textbook. It is usually assumed at a certain stage in education that a student can now make full, accurate, legible notes of his lessons. As with other writing tasks, the dyslexic student needs to survey his problems and select an appropriate strategy, choosing the style of note-taking which best suits the combination of his strengths and the topic's requirements.

If the dyslexic student word processes in class, he is likely to be able to keep up, get guidance from his teacher's body language, and make a legible record of the lesson to edit and revise later. In addition, he may have time to ask questions, note details which make the material live, and even remember afterwards what the lesson was about.

Whether handwriting or typing, the dyslexic student should feel able to select from a range of note-taking styles: perhaps using the Cornell note system (see Section 5.3.3.) for history, mind-mapping electric currents from his physics textbook, or laying out ideas for an essay under de Bono's plus/minus/interesting (PMI) headings. He may rely on a combination of keywords in class and discussion with a friend later. He could note coursework references on to tape or listen to his set book while annotating the text. The type of task will prompt the best choice of note-taking strategy, if the student is made aware in the first place that he is in a position to choose.

4.6. Writing Essays

Dyslexic students characteristically approach an essay question from unexpected angles and express themselves in an idiosyncratic style. This creative advantage is usually offset by poor mechanical and organizational output, particularly if they are writing against the clock. Their frequent complaints are: "I don't know how to begin," "I can't finish in time," and most frequent of all, "I never seem to answer the question." Knowing that restricted short term memory and lack of automatic literacy skills underlie these complaints, dyslexic students must organize their essay writing into manageable components, starting with an analysis of the essay question. Figure 7 presents a scheme for "questioning the question." It breaks a question down into categories: topic area, limiting words and key verbs.

Essays are a tool for thinking. A dyslexic student's essay rarely emerges as a coherent and focused product, unless the thinking was done before the writing began. It is therefore unwise for the student to start thinking about the essay question by writing the "introduction." Instead, the writer should take a step by step approach, first brainstorming the topic, then, with an eye on the question, mind-mapping the essay structure. These thinking steps allow for the central idea to change and the direction and conclusion to become clear. It may next be possible to start straight into writing the "meat" of the essay, reserving the writing of a brief introduction to the very end, thus minimizing the problem of how to begin.

Finally the step dreaded by all dyslexic students—checking. Again, the step by step approach will help. Apart from basic spell checking (an electronic dictionary is an excellent friend here), the dyslexic student ought to look out for his "favorite" mistakes; leaving "ed" off a verb, crossing l as well as t, for example. Reading his essay out loud will alert him to any non-sense he has written. The natural pauses he makes during his reading aloud will indicate the need for punctuation. For obvious reasons, checking and editing are infinitely more rewarding if the essay is word processed.

4.7. Teaching Ideas for the Classroom: Organizing to Write

4.7.1. Copying:

- Don't expect listening and understanding at the same time as copying.
- Either allow enough time for copying or give the dyslexic student a handout.
- Write lines of text on the board in different colors.

Question the Question

1.   Highlight the words or phrases which indicate the **TOPIC AREA**
      to be covered.

2.   Note the **LIMITING WORDS**.   These control the slant required
      on the topic area.

3.   Circle the **KEY VERBS**.   These indicate the structure into which
      the answer must fit, for example:

describe	offer a detailed account
trace	note turning points and stages
summarize	isolate key ideas, present concisely
discuss	consider all sides of the argument
compare	emphasize similarities, mention differences
contrast	show differences between

A student might question a history question like this:

"Why was the United Nations Organization unable to
prevent wars and international tension between 1945
and 1987? Explain your answer carefully."

1.   **TOPIC AREA**   the United Nations

2.   **LIMITING WORDS**   1945 – 1987

                              prevent wars and international tension

3.   **KEY VERB**   explain

Figure 7. Questioning the question.

4.7.2. Note-taking:

- Ask yourself what purpose this note-taking serves.
- Teach note-taking skills, e.g. abbreviations, keywords, highlighting, color coding, layout, word processing, filing.
- Keep a check on the dyslexic student's note-taking and filing.

4.7.3. Essay writing:

- Teach and insist on question analysis as first step.
- Encourage mind-mapping.
- Encourage word processing.
- Give feedback. Expect dyslexic student to follow it. Point out improvement.

5. MEMORY: PUTTING IT IN

5.1. Introduction

People with dyslexia usually have short term memory difficulties. Whether the weakness is in the auditory or the visual channel, the problem will be critical in schoolwork unless it is recognized and accommodated.

This section on memory is divided into three parts: 'Putting It In', which is the most important part of the memory process, 'Keeping It In', and 'Pulling It Out'—the stage which is often neglected. The subheadings within the sections will deal with memory in the context of typical school activities or tasks.

5.2. Reading to Remember

Comprehension and memory are affected by the same underlying problems which hinder dyslexic students from learning to read, and later from decoding unfamiliar words quickly and reading familiar ones accurately.

The student can get overloaded when he holds the parts of a sentence in his mind while getting at the meaning, particularly if the text contains difficult words and subsidiary clauses. This sort of overload prevents fluency, enjoyment, and interest. Without these the student is unlikely to remember what he has read.

To get beyond decoding and reach the meaning, the dyslexic student must make sure that input is multisensory. He must process the information that he is reading himself if there is to be any hope of him understanding and remembering it. The words on the page must become pictures and sounds, smells, tastes and feelings.

5.2.1. Visualizing

Training dyslexic students to visualize while reading text is one of the most constructive ways to help their memory. Poor readers can be taught to visualize what they are reading by teaching them to break the task into smaller steps and follow the procedures used by Oakhill and Yuill (1991) in their research into improving comprehension. They used a simple story for their experiment, but their method is applicable to any school topic. A group of poor readers were asked to:

- Read through a story to decode the words and get an overview.
- Read it again and choose events or images that they could visualize.
- Draw cartoon pictures of their chosen sequence.
- Decide on the main event and draw that.

The selection of what has to be remembered, where the characters in the story had come from, where were they going and why, what happened and why, should all be reflected in the pictures. The cartoon of the "main event" should be the key picture.

Oakhill and Yuill carried their research into a second phase. They got the students to think of the pictures and discuss and describe them to their teachers. In the third phase, the children simply read and thought of the pictures themselves. This research showed clearly that the exercise improved poor comprehension.

This technique is invaluable too, for memory, particularly for dyslexic students. Teach the student to stop and visualize, stop and visualize, while he is reading, so that he trains himself to see the landscape and action to such an extent that he can describe it to you. He'll be able to answer such questions as "What was he wearing?" "Where was the oak tree?" "Was it morning or evening?" Readers who struggle with comprehension and the nuts and bolts of reading often need help in developing these higher level skills.

5.2.2. Mind-mapping

Mind-mapping a book, play, or chapter is an effective way of making the reader visualize and, later, remember what he has read. Asking him to cover his map and revisualize and describe the map afterwards will treble the likelihood of his remembering the material. He will integrate both sides of the brain by processing the information, visualizing, turning words into pictures, seeing the sequence of events spatially, and turning his pictures back into his own words.

The main branches on a mind-map of a set text might be

- The main characters
- The most striking images from each chapter—and linking them to a quotation or chapter heading

We had left Liverpool and were on our way to Cornwall for our summer holidays. It was raining and hailing, and we were stuck in a traffic jam. We three children were hot and tired in the back of the car, and we started squabbling.

The portable phone rang. As Mum reached for it she spilled the thermos of soup all over the sandwiches. It was our neighbor calling to tell us that when she had been to feed our cat she'd found that Pushkin had had two kittens.

Our mood changed at once. We decided to turn round and go home and see the kittens (we couldn't wait!), and delay our journey until the next day when the weather might be better and the roads quieter.

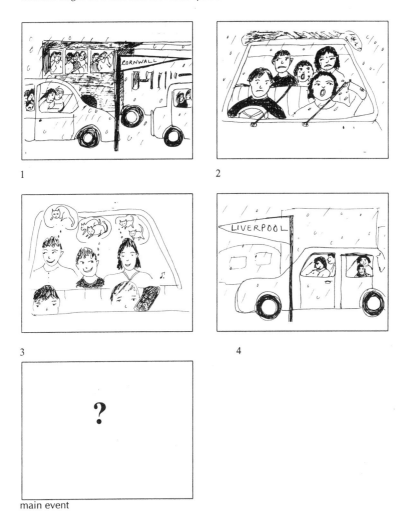

Figure 8. Selecting and drawing key elements in a story.

- Themes or imagery—linking a quotation
- Act by act

Figure 9 gives an example of a mind-map. It summarizes the first few chapters of Charles Dickens' *A Tale of Two Cities*.

5.2.3. Listening to Novels, Plays and Poetry on Tape

The main barriers to reading enjoyment are inaccuracy, slowness, limited memory, not noticing punctuation. These weaknesses cause poor comprehension, little interest, and poor motivation. Listening to literature on tape can solve all these problems at once. A professional reader can show the author's intention with the help of expression, emphasis, and character differentiation.

Texts in dialect, or with a lot of dialogue, are notorious for being difficult for the dyslexic student to read. For example,

> 'I see a light a-coming roun' de p'int, bymeby, so I wade' in en shove' a log ahead o'me, en swum mor'n half-way acrost de river, en got in 'mongst de drift-wood, en kep' my head down low, en kinder swum agin de current tell the raff come along. Den I swum to de stern uv it, en tuck aholt. It clouded up en 'uz pooty dark for a little while. So I clumb up en laid down on de planks.'
>
> Extract from *The Adventures of Huckleberry Finn*
> by Mark Twain, Chapter VIII

This would be immediately understood if the student listened to a tape while he looked at the text. The mind is free to visualize and therefore imprint images on the memory while listening rather than while reading words off the page. This skill can improve dramatically with training.

Most students find Shakespeare challenging but dyslexic students find him more so because of their poor short-term memory, sequencing, and slow and inaccurate reading. They may be the most *literary* people in the class, but it is their *literacy* skills which get in the way. Language problems inhibit their understanding of plot and affect their appreciation of the poetry on first reading. Meter is a problem, and so is stress. Reading around the class is not good for everyone: handling the play at a slow rate, lesson by lesson, with weekends to break up the flow, means that details can be forgotten and momentum lost.

Shakespeare's plays become more accessible if the student listens to the tape of the play as he reads the text. He then becomes familiar with the layout of the verse and the pronunciation of unfamiliar words and names. He can see who is speaking, and he can hear meter. He can see the punctuation and how it affects the phrasing. His understanding of character and motivation become clear as he is helped by tone of voice and timing.

Visualizing, listening, and seeing the words on the page make the experience multisensory and therefore memorable. Watching a video of a play is also helpful—

but for studying the language, it is better to have the combination of tape and text. The student's enjoyment of the play on stage or video later will be greatly enhanced.

5.3. Remembering Lessons

The student is largely at the teacher's mercy in the classroom. How multisensory the input is affects the amount the dyslexic pupil understands and remembers. The ideal learning experience will involve the student in listening, looking, drawing, talking, doing, and making the material his own in some way. However, many lessons involve a great deal of listening and perhaps looking, but not so much of the others. For the dyslexic student, note-writing can overload and prevent him from understanding and remembering the lesson at all.

What can the dyslexic student himself do about this?

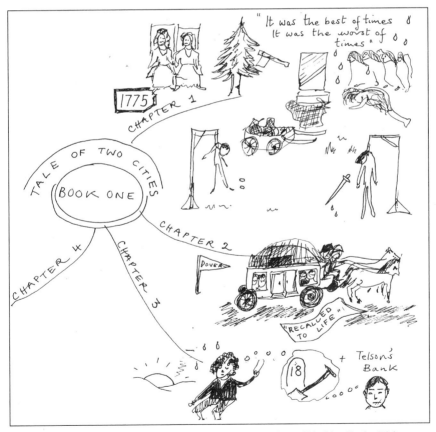

Figure 9. Mind map summary of first chapters of "A Tale of Two Cities" by Charles Dickens.

5.3.1. Make the Teacher Aware

The student should tell the teacher that his understanding depends on his being able to participate in the class and give full attention to explanations. Note-taking, although a good way for many students to process information, may not be effective for him. Can the teacher suggest alternative ways of keeping a record of the lesson? However well understood the lesson may be, there needs to be some record from which the student can later reinforce his memory. If the teacher can provide outline notes or substitute notes, then the student should make sure he involves himself in some activity that will make him process the information. If writing prevents him from understanding and remembering, then he must DO something to make sure he will remember the lesson:

- Draw.
- Mind-map.
- Participate.
- Add to summary notes.
- Make notes which invite further work.
- Illustrate.

5.3.2. Use a Laptop in the Classroom

If the student is a competent touch typist (perhaps typing at 35 words per minute (wpm), or maybe 50 wpm when he has used his laptop for a year), he will have plenty of time to listen, understand, and organize his notes as well as participate in class. A student whose writing speed when processing information is only 12 wpm is not going to benefit from the lesson because he is struggling to write, nor will he have a useful account of the lesson to revise from.

5.3.3. The Cornell Note System

The idea behind the Cornell system of note-taking is that a page of notes should invite further work. This system makes good sense for the dyslexic student who can't remember what he wrote in class. He needs to process its information, understand it, and transfer it to his long-term memory.

The note-taker should draw a wide margin on one side of his page before he begins to take notes. He takes notes in the normal way (see Section 5.1). The wide margin can be used later (either soon after the lesson, or for exam revision) for summary headings, questions on each paragraph, or pictures (see Section 7).

Figure 10 shows some notes on sources taken in a History class. The student had a slow handwriting speed and therefore always a used a word processor in his classes (history, biology, chemistry, and philosophy). You can see that he is able to include the amusing memorable bits as well as the rather dull bullet points. His Cornell layout has left room for picture symbols.

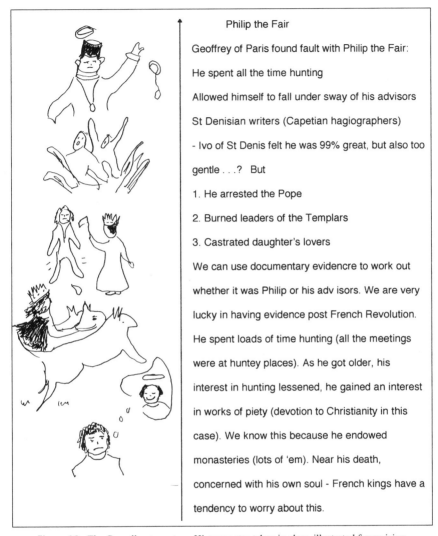

Philip the Fair

Geoffrey of Paris found fault with Philip the Fair:

He spent all the time hunting

Allowed himself to fall under sway of his advisors

St Denisian writers (Capetian hagiographers)

- Ivo of St Denis felt he was 99% great, but also too

gentle . . .? But

1. He arrested the Pope

2. Burned leaders of the Templars

3. Castrated daughter's lovers

We can use documentary evidencre to work out

whether it was Philip or his adv isors. We are very

lucky in having evidence post French Revolution.

He spent loads of time hunting (all the meetings

were at huntey places). As he got older, his

interest in hunting lessened, he gained an interest

in works of piety (devotion to Christianity in this

case). We know this because he endowed

monasteries (lots of 'em). Near his death,

concerned with his own soul - French kings have a

tendency to worry about this.

Figure 10. The Cornell note system. History notes taken in class, illustrated for revision.

5.3.4. Learning for a Test

The dyslexic student struggles to remember formulas, historical sequences, themes in a novel, points in a treaty, French vocabulary, or mathematical procedures. His short-term memory deficits *must* be counteracted by multisensory techniques if he is cope with school work and exams. Each dyslexic person has strengths and weaknesses he can learn to recognize and use. Whether the strengths are auditory or visual they will be improved with the multisensory approach, which supports the weakness with the strength.

5.4. Foreign Language Learning

All the problems that inhibit dyslexic students from learning reading, writing, and spelling in their own language manifest when they try to learn a foreign language.

It is important to think of multisensory learning with every memory task set. A dyslexic learner will have trouble learning vocabulary and grammar straight off the page. Therefore, he must:

- Say words aloud while looking at the writing.
- Write while looking at the written word and saying it.
- Listen while looking at the word.
- Remember sequences aurally as well as visually.
- Break up words into syllables while speaking.
- Visualize the object or action while saying the word.

5.4.1. Working with Pictures in Vocabulary Learning

Students should match labels to pictures, saying the word while looking at the picture. Then cover the labels and try to visualize the printed word—and say aloud again. Repeat. This is much easier in one-to-one teaching than in a class, but with a bank of pictures on an overhead, a whole class could do vocabulary building at the start of each lesson. For example, looking at the picture and saying the French word seems to be a much more direct link into memory than just translating a written English word into a written French word (see Figure 11).

5.4.2. Focus on the Gender

- Clearly say the definite or indefinite article.
- Link with an adjective: *le fromage blanc*
- Find some mnemonic link
- Visualize blue (for a boy) cheese.
- Highlight all the words in a list which follow a gender rule.

5.5. Formulas, Definitions, and Equations

Understanding scientific data is the key to remembering it. The dyslexic student may need extra strategies until the formulas, equations, and definitions are practiced enough to be stored in his long-term memory.

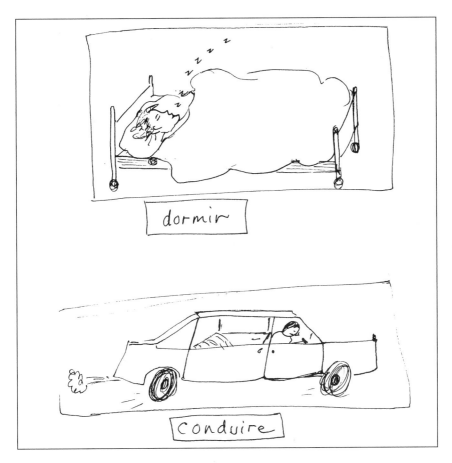

Figure 11. Using pictures and cards for vocabulary learning.

These strategies may help:

- Visualizing
- Saying aloud in a rhythm
- Putting on tape:

"Charge is measured in?"	(Pause)	"Coulombs."
"Q = ?"	(Pause)	"1 × t"
"What is osmosis?"	(Pause)	"Osmosis is the process by which . . ."

- A student could write a question on one side of a card and the answer on the other. If he carries the cards in his pocket and tests himself frequently (always saying the answer aloud and checking for accuracy), he will make the equation or definition and its terminology part of his expressive vocabulary, as well as remembering it aurally (see Figure 12).

5.6. Sequential Information

Lists of information can be very easily remembered by using a *peg system*. The "one bun, two shoe, etc." pegs are probably the most well known: Once the pegs are learned (and because each item rhymes with the number it represents, this is easy), the student can attach or associate each symbol with the information he wants to remember (see Figure 13).

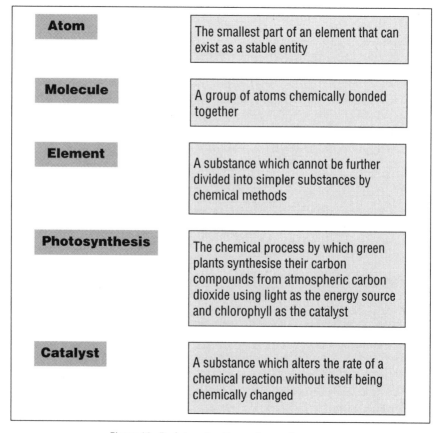

Figure 12. Pocket cards with questions and answers.

WOODROW WILSON'S FOURTEEN POINTS

1.	BUN	The end of secret diplomacy and secret treaties
2.	SHOE	Freedom of the seas in both peace and war
3.	TREE	International free trade
4.	DOOR	International disarmament
5.	HIVE	A fair consideration of all colonial claims
6.	STICKS	German troops evacuated from Russia
7.	HEAVEN	Belgian independence
8.	GATE	Alsace and Lorraine to be returned to France
9.	WINE	Italy's frontiers to be re-drawn on basis of nationality
10.	HEN	Peoples of Austro-Hungary to become self-governing
11.	CRICKET XI	
		Serbia, Montenegro, and Romania to be restored
12.	SHELVES	Turkey to become a nation rather than an empire and the subject peoples of the old Ottoman Empire to gain independence
13.	UNLUCKY	Poland to be given back her independence
14.	COURTING	A general association of nations to keep international peace to be created

---

Figure 13. Example of peg system being used for memory work.

The important thing to remember in this exercise is that the link should be visualized, not just described. Something visualized will be remembered much more effectively. Asking the student to close his eyes and describe what he sees is a good way of ensuring he is really visualizing (see Figure 13).

5.7. Teaching Ideas for the Classroom

- Check on notes, teach appropriate note-taking.
- Make sure your speed of delivery is not too fast.
- Actively support, praise, and protect the dyslexic pupil.
- Support word processing in the classroom and for homework.
- Encourage participation.
- Encourage mind-mapping.
- Make sure the lesson is multisensory.
- Listen to tape with the class and verify the school library has relevant tapes.

- Check textbooks are at correct reading level and suitable for the dyslexic student—if not, provide others.
- Supply slow readers with essay questions and themes to consider when they start reading, so they focus their ideas and immediately interact with the text. They may not have time to read the book twice.

6. MEMORY: KEEPING IT IN

A dyslexic schoolchild needs to learn how to transfer material that he wants to remember from his short-term to his long-term memory. This important skill is a problem for all students—especially when the reading matter, data, or foreign vocabulary bores them—but it affects almost every aspect of a dyslexic student's school work.

We have looked at some multisensory methods of putting information into the memory. The ways of keeping it there by multisensory reviewing are just as important.

6.1. The Forgetting Curve

Most students would agree that if a list of foreign vocabulary, a chapter on the Russian Revolution, or the definitions for osmosis and photosynthesis are learned once, then only 20 percent of this will remain in the memory for the end of term exam (or the rest of life). "If that," is their frequent rejoinder. Of course, if the first learning was multisensory, with much processing of the material, then the percentage of retention would be higher.

Good teaching does, of course, build in the concept of the forgetting curve: lesson, discussion, homework, test. But students often do not understand the value of these procedures—why they are doing them and how they could turn the forgetting curve to good account in their own work and revision. Each student should be able to draw the forgetting curve himself and by looking at the diagram, be able to link it to the work he is trying to remember (see Figure 14).

The time to introduce students to the forgetting curve is when they have an approaching test or final exam—something they want to do well on. Let the students deal with just one task in this way so that the effectiveness can be measured against other less successful learning techniques (or no techniques at all).

6.2. Learning Foreign Vocabulary Using the Forgetting Curve

1. Put the vocabulary on tape:

English word   (pause)   Foreign word

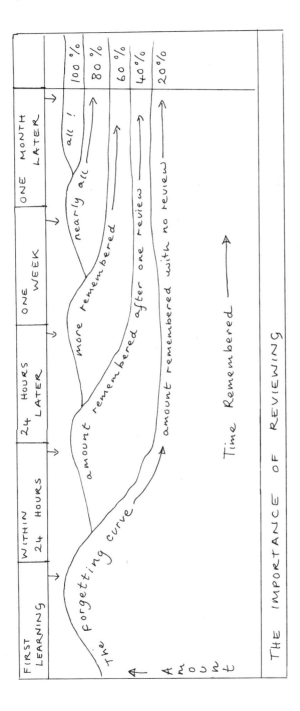

Figure 14. The forgetting curve.

2. Play the tape back, looking at the list of vocabulary and saying each word aloud.
3. Play the tape again but don't look at the list. The student should find his ear and tongue will anticipate the foreign word, which hangs in the pause. Do this several times.
4. When he knows them orally, he should try to *write* them in the pause.
5. Repeat.

These activities should be spaced out, covering about a week.

When the student tests himself, or when he is being tested, he should always look at the English word but cover the foreign word. In that way, he makes the *foreign* word the one he has to search his memory for, visualize, and say aloud, thereby using the memory in his ear, tongue and eye. To say the *English* word aloud wastes effective memory routes.

6.3. Question Technique with Notes or Text Book

After reading a paragraph from notes or a text book, the reader should ask himself "What questions are answered here?," and write them down. There may be one, two, or more. The questions should prompt a full and thoughtful answer so that the student has to rephrase the material he has read. Whatever has been read has to be well understood and digested for him to do this. It makes for very active reading. At the end of the chapter, or notes, he has a list of questions. He should run quickly through them to make sure he knows the answers. Otherwise, his reading may have been a waste of time! He should keep this list with the book so he can test himself before the test, lesson, or exam. He can get a family member or friend to test him, using this list. Some students put the questions on tape and leave a pause after each question so that when it is replayed they have a chance to answer the question before the voice on the tape answers it for them.

Some students like to write out the answer as well as the questions—but this encourages rote learning of the answers. It may be too laborious for the dyslexic student and can discourage him from using the technique at all. The questions must, however be kept with the notes or textbook, for future use (see Figures 15a and b).

6.4. Teaching Ideas for the Classroom

- Teach forgetting curve.
- Ask children to review during the last five minutes of the lesson and during the first five minutes of the next lesson.
- Gear lessons, homework and tests to the forgetting curve.
- Clearly guide students through what they should know for exams. and make sure dyslexic students have good enough notes.

7. MEMORY: PULLING IT OUT

Much memory work in the form of data to be learned for homework or revised for exams is receptive rather than expressive. The dyslexic student should not merely recognize what he knows (by looking at his notes or textbook), he should be able to express it twice: (1) in his own words so that it is truly his own, and (2) in writing, because this is usually the way he will be examined (and is also the mode in which dyslexic students need most practice). Students who have had an eye on this stage of the memory process will have committed their reading or learning work to memory in such a way that they can effectively test themselves.

VOLCANIC HAZARDS

Primary Effects – are the volcano's immediate effects when it erupts, and can cause damage in a short time.

1. Lava Flows – hot molten rock (magma) from Earth's upper mantle, emitted through the crater.

2. Pyroclastic Flows – a mixture rocks, ash and lava, fuelled by a cushion of extremely hot gas.

3. Ash Falls – fragments of magma from explosions.

4. Volcanic Gases – H_2O, CO, CO_2, SO_2, H, Helium.

Secondary Effects – these take longer to develop and thus occur longer after the start of the eruption, and often last longer than some of the Primary Effects.

1. Lahars – large avalanches of debris and material travelling up to 22m/s.

2. Landslides – occur after a violent eruption or slope deformation.

3. Tsunamis – giant waves, simply the intense energy from the eruption transmitted through the   water.

The most dangerous hazard of the primary effects is *undoubtedly* pyroclastic flows. This enormously hot mixture (700C) of rocks, ash and lava is lethal purely due to the fact that it travels so fast – up to 100mph. There is little friction because the solid materials ride on a "cushion" of hot gas, which allows them to tear down the mountainside. A pyroclastic flow would incinerate everything in its path: trees, animals, buildings.

Figure 15a. Example of word-processed geography class notes.

7.1. Notes

"I'll read through my notes," is the way most students answer "How are you going to revise?" It is probably the least effective method for a dyslexic learner.

Students who have made questions from their textbook can "pull out" their knowledge by answering the questions, either verbally or in writing. The virtue in this method is that the student uses his own words, rather than producing a pat answer.

7.2. Mind-Maps

The student should look at his original mind-map, and talk his way around it adding as much information as he can. If there are gaps in his memory, he should

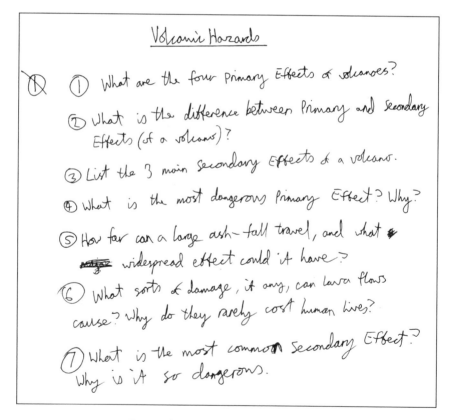

Figure 15b. Questions made from class notes.

look up the necessary information and put something on the mind-map to remind him of it. Next, he should turn the map over and revisualize it, describing the symbols and where the information is on the map. He should do this several times over a period of time so that it will be easy to conjure up on his "mental clipboard" during the exam or whenever he needs the information.

7.3. Sociable Revision

Both of the previous methods of "pulling it out" lend themselves to sociable revision: students revising together after preparing questions, mind-maps, or diagrams. The presence of another person encourages the student to express himself aloud. The tester, in his turn, learns while he asks the questions; he sees their relevance, anticipates their answers and then hears them.

7.4. Planning and Timing for Maximum Recall

Stress is the enemy of memory. The act of "pulling out" information during an exam is one that is often bedeviled by stress. Many answers are spoiled because a student is not calm enough to focus well on the question (see Figure 7), and realize its implications, marshall the facts he knows, and write a balanced answer.

A dyslexic student, who easily becomes overloaded, should split up a task into stages. This process will help him when he has to do too many language functions at the same time: remember, argue, plan, write, spell, and punctuate while he is sequencing fluent sentences. A student will usually say that he "didn't have time" to plan his answer in an exam, and so he should practice the procedure, timing each stage (see Figure 16). For example, a one-hour question might be split

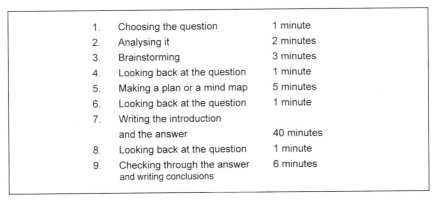

1.	Choosing the question	1 minute
2.	Analysing it	2 minutes
3.	Brainstorming	3 minutes
4.	Looking back at the question	1 minute
5.	Making a plan or a mind map	5 minutes
6.	Looking back at the question	1 minute
7.	Writing the introduction and the answer	40 minutes
8.	Looking back at the question	1 minute
9.	Checking through the answer and writing conclusions	6 minutes

Figure 16. Organizing time in an hour exam.

up in this way: By breaking the task into steps, the student can avoid overload, by timing the stages you can show the dyslexic student how little time planning actually takes. He then learns how steadying this process is, enabling him to focus on the question and pull out relevant information.

7.5. Word Processing

A word processor is an enormous help for a dyslexic learner. "Pulling out" information from memory in good fluent prose is often impeded by the act of writing itself. Handwriting, spelling, and punctuating are less automatic for a dyslexic writer and can take so much available memory that arguments and the way they are expressed and sequenced often suffer. A word processor can solve these lower-order language skills and leave the mind free for ideas and their expression.

7.6. Suggestions for Classroom Teachers

- Explain the difference between expressive and receptive learning.
- Arrange "timed" questions.
- Make sure slow workers get enough practice (especially in mathematics).
- See that dyslexic students have adequate notes to revise from.
- Give dyslexic students more rehearsals than others.
- Insist on the "small steps" procedure.
- If a student is going to use a word processor during an exam, he should practice timed questions and mock exams on it first. In that way, any possible snags (layout, ink, printing, plugs, saving, disabling spell checks, cleaning hard disc of relevant files) can be overcome before the exam itself.

8. METACOGNITION

8.1. What Is Metacognition?

Dyslexic students learn best if they understand how their brain works. This understanding, called metacognition, is the explicit awareness in an individual person of his own unique mental processes. The essence of metacognition is self-knowledge. To be metacognitive is to think about thinking, usually not to solve a problem, but to work out *how* to solve it and then how to generalize from it to a similar problem. So a student in school, faced with some physics to learn or an essay to write, would articulate the task, plan its solution, monitor, and adapt the process, evaluate its success and bridge from the final solution to other learning or writing tasks. Since it confers the power to control, a capacity for metacognition will enhance any student's learning, but for those with learning difficulties, and for their teachers, it is essential.

8.2. Why Is Metacognition Necessary to Dyslexic Learners?

More often than not, dyslexic students learn in a different way from the way their teachers teach and the way their peers learn. If a dyslexic student understands his own learning style, he is in a position to control the material a teacher offers him. If, for example, a teacher writes "metacognition" on the board, the rest of the class may learn to spell it simply by looking. The dyslexic learner may need to break the word up, saying each syllable and recognising "meta" as a prefix and "tion" as a regular final syllable, before he too can use the word. He need not rely on his weak visual memory, which will fail him, provided he knows the method which suits him best: He needs to know his own mind. It helps immeasurably, of course, if his teacher knows it too.

8.3. How Else Can Metacognition Help Dyslexic Learners?

8.3.1. Creativity

There is a line of thought which relates learning difficulties to the creative process: "Especially with respect to the modes of thought now associated with visual processing in the right hemisphere (of the brain)" (West, 1991). To illustrate this connection between creativity and learning difficulties, West quotes Einstein's description of his personal experience of "playing with images": "The words or the language, as they are written or spoken, do not seem to play any role in my mechanism of thought." Later in the same passage, West quotes Einstein: "Conventional words or other signs have to be sought for laboriously only in a secondary stage, when the mentioned associative play is sufficiently established and can be reproduced at will." (West, 1991, p26)

Most of the school curriculum, especially in secondary school, is taught through the medium of words. Teachers themselves have learned their trade through verbal channels. They naturally teach through those channels and most of their students learn fine that way. In every class, however, there are a few students who learn via a "different configuration in the brain" (Hales, 1998). Their modes of thinking are fundamentally different and less stable. They may be seeing ideas, which are presented in words, as images. They may understand a concept, not sequentially in time, but holistically in space, as a picture or a diagram—possibly in three dimensions—which they can then rotate and manipulate. They may find, as Einstein seems to have done, that words are not their natural medium for thinking and that any work they process through words is slow, laborious, and disappointing.

Metacognition can help the unconventional thinker (in this case, the dyslexic thinker) in three ways: (1) It will first help him recognize how his mind works differently. (2) It will prompt him to resist accepting his unconventional way of learning as a disadvantage. (3) It may give him the self confidence and courage to develop his own unique thinking mode as a strength and thereby open the way for his creativity to flourish.

8.3.2. Staying Power

In the context of classroom, homework, exam results, qualifications and curriculum constraints, dyslexic characteristics are noted chiefly for their exasperating drawbacks. Poor time-keeping, random sequencing, inattention, lost possessions, social ineptitude, unfinished work; these are the negative aspects of dyslexia that dominate in school, where order, system and smooth progress are the goals. Can the dyslexic student learn to recognize and mobilize his strengths, tipping them into the balance against his undeniable weaknesses? If so, he is likely to develop the motivation to enjoy and keep going at his work, reversing the familiar downward spiral of failure, discouragement, and dislike for the subject he is trying so hard to study.

8.4. Learning to Think about Thinking

Dyslexic students need to tease apart and learn distinctive skills in thinking, many of which, because of underlying difficulties, may not be automatic for them as they are for others. There is for example the fundamental skill of developing thought through listening. This may be extremely difficult for the dyslexic student who has weak auditory perception and a restricted sequential memory. The difficulty will be intensified if he is longing to join in the discussion. He may miss points made by others, then burst in, out of turn, with his own and be marked down as stupid and disruptive. It is easy to see what a vicious circle of inappropriate behavior and stunted thinking class discussion could set up for this type of dyslexic student, unless he learns how to sort out and manage the skills involved. Fortunately, thinking skills can be taught and learned, both in daily subject lessons and through formal programs.

8.4.1. Matthew Lipman's Philosophy for Children

The Philosophy for Children program gives equal time and an equal rôle to each child in the group. It encourages a disposition and the courage to think. It is centered in the belief that people best learn how to learn in a social context. Thus its format is described as a "community of enquiry." The group explores a topic with the aim of enlarging each member's perception of it. Inspired by the model of socratic dialogue, it obliges children to operate excellent structures for thinking and learning, such as comparing, analyzing, categorizing, deducing, questioning, summarizing, and evaluating. It teaches respect for other people's views, and emphasizes a rigorous standard of precise and appropriate language.

Such a constructive and explicit framework allows the dyslexic student to recognize the separate skills involved in listening, thinking, and communicating, and it encourages him to analyze his own levels of skill. Over a period of time, the program is expected both to curb impulsivity and to win the most diffident student to take risks in these fundamental areas of learning.

8.4.2. Cognitive Acceleration through Science Education

The Cognitive Acceleration through Science Education (CASE) program, like the Philosophy for Children program, sees talking in a group as the most effective environment in which to learn how to learn. The course teaches general thinking skills through the specific medium of science. It uses a method of "cognitive conflict" to modify and develop a concept in Science by means of successive challenges; each added level of difficulty proves the child's current model of the problem to be inadequate and he is obliged to formulate a new model which allows for the added variant.

The main reasoning patterns developed by this method are visualization, prediction, probability, proportionality, classification, and the control of variables. These reasoning patterns are of obvious value to dyslexic children whose learning flourishes in a multisensory, step by step procedure and whose lateral minded style may depend upon rethinking from whole to part and from part to whole to keep it on track.

8.4.3. Instrumental Enrichment

The Instrumental Enrichment training program sprang from Reuven Feuerstein's researches into measuring intelligence. Feuerstein defined the components by which intelligence is usually measured. He then looked at the underlying cognitive processes and asked some important questions: Is intelligence fixed? If it is not fixed, can it be trained—and how?

Feuerstein's work is relevant for the dyslexic learner because Feuerstein assumed that intelligence was *dynamic,* that weak cognitive functions could be trained. He believed that once children understood their own strengths and weaknesses, they would become empowered to learn more effectively.

His training program is based on the common deficits he observed in the children he tested who were not succeeding in education. These children were impulsive and disorganized. They lacked either the ability to categorize or the ability to deal with data. In addition, they could neither analyze a problem nor focus on the main issues.

Instrumental Enrichment, when implemented as a school policy, is a training course in its own right. It has been shown to enhance learning across the disciplines when teachers dedicate their time to this program.

For those who help dyslexic students at home, school, or in individual lessons, they will find Feuerstein's philosophy of teaching has features which are of great value:

- The principle of the teacher following a structured and cumulative program
- Helping the learner to recognize his own cognitive strengths and weaknesses and the importance of these skills in relation to thinking effectively
- Mediating the learning experience by discussing the mental processes involved in doing a particular exercise and then
- Helping the learner to generalize from one learning experience to another by bridging from the exercises or "instruments" to subject-specific material.

8.4.4. Neurolinguistic Programming

The term *Neurolinguistic Programming* (NLP) was coined to reflect three aspects of Richard Bandler and John Grinder's theory. They believe any form of human excellence can be modeled, replicated, and taught. Thus, they chose: (1) *neuro* because our senses and nervous system are the source of all our experience; (2) *linguistic* because experience is stored, coded, organized, and transformed through language; and (3) *programming* because organizing the components of a system (sensory representation) achieves a specific outcome.

The dyslexic learner often comes to special education feeling discouraged and demoralized because orthodox learning methods have failed with him. Therefore NLP has a particular appeal to those who teach dyslexic students. It focuses on the relationship between the teacher and student, the cognitive profile of the learner, and the morale and motivation of the student. The main tenets of NLP programs are:

- The attitude of the learner must be appropriate. If the student is in a low state of morale or motivation, he will not learn effectively. His attitude must be worked on first.
- The success of any communication is in the response of the learner. However "good" the lesson or lecture, it can only be judged by the response of the learner. The teacher must observe how the student learns and be prepared to adapt his teaching style accordingly.
- People learn according to patterns they have developed. Teachers must help them to see other choices.

- Body language rather than verbal language is a better indicator of how the student is feeling. The teacher should always be aware of this.
- It is important to be the student's ally and to see problems from his point of view.
- The teacher must study how his student learns (visually, auditorily, or kinesthetically) by observing his behavior, studying his language, and monitoring his success.

NLP theories marry well with two successful strategies for teaching dyslexic students: (1) the multisensory approach and (2) the emphasis given to the morale of the student.

8.5. From Skills to Strategies—A Whole School Policy

When students are trained to be aware of their own thinking skills, they acquire a greater flexibility and control in the strategies they apply to their school tasks. All students benefit, not just the dyslexic ones, if they are able to survey a range of reading techniques and select one that suits a particular reading task: previewing the subheadings in a geography textbook to find a particular topic, listening to *The Mayor of Casterbridge* on tape while following the text, mind mapping a question while studying a teacher's handout on electric currents.

However, it is difficult for any student to develop independent learning strategies if his teachers are not accustomed to using a metacognitive approach. Hence the ideal school is one where teachers habitually ask "How will you do this? What skills do you need and how will you monitor their use?"

8.6. Independent Learning Lightens the Burden of Dyslexia

Teachers and their dyslexic students need to work in a metacognitive partnership so that dyslexic students can eventually take independent charge of their own learning. Both teacher and student need knowledge of dyslexia in general to combine with precise information about the student's profile of strengths and weaknesses. A subject teacher should articulate and teach the skills on which the subject discipline relies, while her dyslexic student must know how those subject skills relate to the way his particular mind works. The dyslexic student can build his learning confidently on this foundation, monitoring and adapting his performance and relying on his teachers to act as allies and facilitators for his progress. This partnership of mutual awareness can start at any age, but, in principle, the earlier it starts the better for the student.

Figure 17 is a secondary school illustration of the partnership between a dyslexic student doing GCSE English and his English teacher. It is in the form of a ladder where each rung represents either mutual or independent markers on the

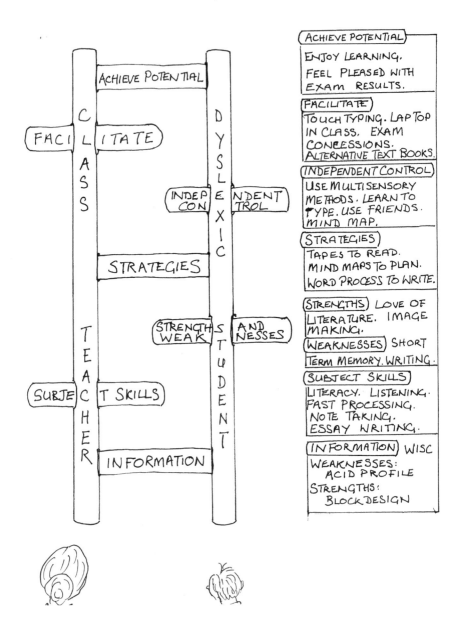

Figure 17. Metacognition ladder.

climb to the top, where the dyslexic student can achieve his potential—and enjoy his work.

People with dyslexia should not have to pass their days in the state of bewildered frustration which is so often "the burden of dyslexia" (Hales, 1997). Metacognition is the means by which they can ease this burden and gain control over their lives. Metacognition is a habit of mind, an attitude to life which serves everyone well, but which dyslexic people *must* have. Where better to learn it or use it than in school?

REFERENCES

Bandler, R., & Grinder, J. (1979). *Frogs into Princes.* Real People Press.

Ellis, N. (1991). Dyslexia Integrating Theory and Practice. Paper presented at the Second International Conference of the British Dyslexia Association, "Meeting the Challenge," held in Oxford, England. London: Whurr Publishers.

Feuerstein, R. (1980). *Instrumental Enrichment: An Intervention Program for Cognitive Modifiability.* Baltimore: University Park Press.

Galaburda, A. (1991). *Proceedings of the National Academy of Sciences* quoted in *The New York Times,* September 15, 1991.

Hales, G. (1997). Dyslexia Institute PGDip. Psychology Lecture.

Lipman, Matthew. For further details, contact Roger Sutcliffe at 106 High Street, Bletchingly, Surrey RH1 4PA.

Oakhill, J., & Yuill, N. (1991). The Remediation of Reading Comprehension Difficulties. Paper presented at the Second International Conference of the BDA "Meeting the Challenge," Oxford, 1991.

Tallal, P. (1997). Language Learning Impairments: Integrating Basic Science, Technology and Remediation. Keynote lecture at BDA 25th Anniversary Conference, York, April 1997.

West, T. (1991). *In the Mind's Eye.* New York: Prometheus Books.

10

Students, Dyslexia, and Mathematics

Pauline Clayton

1. INTRODUCTION

Teachers who work with dyslexic students are aware of their students' literacy problems. Such teachers may be less intune with the problems that arise for many of these students, and others, when faced with mathematics. There is a growing awareness of those students who experience difficulties in mathematics yet have little or no literacy issues. These students are often labeled as dyscalculic. Increasing research in this area backs up previous anecdotal evidence. For example, Varda Gross-Tsur et al. suggests that as many students are affected by dyscalculia as are affected by dyslexia and attention deficit hyperactivity disorder (ADHD).

We must not, however, assume that all dyslexic students have difficulties in mathematics. For some, their main issue is language. Their understanding of concepts and mastering of arithmetic may cause few problems. Opinions, from experienced practitioners, as to the number of dyslexic students experiencing difficulties in mathematics varies: Joffe (1983) suggests about 60 percent of dyslexic students experience substantial difficulties in mathematics; Miles and Miles (1992) believes the percentage is higher, and that even good mathematicians will have some difficulties with mathematics but they can better compensate for their weak areas. Dyslexic students who experience few problems with mathematics tend to show strengths in applied mathematics, e.g., engineering and architecture. Pure mathematics is often more difficult for them.

Pauline Clayton, Furzewood Bungalow, East Street, Turners Hill, Crawley, Sussex RH10 4QQ, United Kingdom

2. PROBLEMS FOR DYSLEXIC STUDENTS

Because mathematics is the only subject in which students can consistently obtain no grades, confidence and self-esteem play a vital part in its mastery—especially for adults. Essays can usually be started, and some attempt can be made to answer the question. With mathematics it is possible to read a question and not be able to start to answer it in any way. Continual failure, when others are succeeding, often can cause disillusionment, lack of confidence, poor self-esteem and, therefore, lack of motivation and an increase in avoidance tactics.

To improve our understanding of the issues these students, especially those who are dyslexic, face in mathematics we need to first discuss their weaknesses and strengths. Next, we should examine how problems in managing verbal codes affect not just literacy but mathematics as well.

A student with poor reading skills (i.e., decoding skills) will not be able to read many specific mathematical words. The complexity of the mathematical words needed by the average 13-year-old appalls many dyslexic students. Consider, for example, words such as isosceles, rhombus, permutation, dodecahedron, etc.

Mathematics uses English in a specific way. Students who struggle with literacy will also struggle to interpret words in their mathematical context. Such students, because they tend to read less than their peers thus use what they consider to be safe language are not exposed to the secondary meanings of many words. The meaning of words in their mathematical context has to be taught; for example, students confuse terms such as "divided by" and "divided into"; they interpret words such as "leaves" as being "*things on trees*," and "integration" is something that relates to minorities, and not calculus (Durkin and Shire, 1991).

Sharma suggests that when we learn a new subject, we first relate it to something known (Sharma, 1990). It is more efficient to use an "existing mental file" rather than open a new one. However, if the wrong file is opened, then the student becomes confused. Teachers must ensure they use language that is understood in its mathematical sense.

One area of weakness, which many teachers associate with dyslexia, is working, and short-term, memory. This affects a person's ability to create automatic links in basic skills, from the immediate recall of number bonds in the primary school student to the physics student who does not know his seven times table. Poor working memory also means numbers may be remembered incorrectly, either when copying from a question or when entering in and reading from a calculator display. These problems lead to memory overload, inaccuracy in complex tasks and frustration—especially in the more able student whose grasp of concepts and understanding of the language in its mathematical context is high.

Sequencing and logic skills are often weak. This, in turn, affects the student's ability to recognize patterns and follow procedures. Much of mathematics is taught sequentially. Although the British National Curriculum allows for change, many older students are still taught in school to "show all of your work," and to follow the method taught. It is important, but it may not be the easiest approach for the dyslexic student.

Much of mathematics is taught at the abstract level and requires a high level of abstract thinking. Even the basic mathematics taught early in primary school involves abstract thinking. Of the primary school students who can correctly give the sum of two numbers, how many are really working at an abstract level? Or are they giving an answer they picture, using concrete apparatus, or that they learned by rote and know will give them the necessary approval for the correct answer?

Students who have a slow "speed of information processing" on an educational psychologist's report may get left behind in lessons. This, combined with their lack of automaticity, means that many dyslexic students, who need more practice and reinforcement than their nondyslexic peers, do, in fact get less. For example, in the classroom, a dyslexic student may have trouble keeping pace with the lesson. Group teaching may progress too fast for the student to assimilate. Furthermore, all mathematics is reinforced by practice. Often, toward the end of a lesson, the teacher assigns a worksheet, or a group of examples from a textbook to complete before the bell rings. While his or her peers may complete the task, the dyslexic student will complete perhaps three-fourths, thus getting less, not more, reinforcement. This leads to inadequate learning and a lowering of the student's confidence in his ability to complete a set task.

Speed of information processing also affects the time spent on homework and projects. Mathematics is perhaps the easiest subject in which to predict the time a task should take a student who understands it. If you are processing information more slowly than your peers, then you will take longer to do your assignments. Added to which, the effort of concentrating during the day at school will make a student more tired so homework becomes harder and takes longer. Perhaps setting aside time before school, rather than after, could be a possibility for some students?

A percentage of dyslexic students may have perception skills that are weak, or different from those of their teacher. Thus these students do not interpret diagrams in the same way as their teacher. Dyslexic students who show strengths in mathematics will have no trouble with perception and therefore they will find the interpretation and drawing of diagrams to be easy. They will also be good at visualization, hence they will have a propensity to succeed in the areas of applied mathematics. Those dyslexic students with difficulties may find that they cannot interpret a two-dimensional drawing as a representation of a three-dimensional object. However many ways a diagram is colored or shaded it may remain for them "just lines and colors." For example, a diagram of a tetrahedron from the side, may appear as an envelope or a kite.

There is a small percentage of dyslexic males who are also color blind. The advent of color printers and the use of colored pens on a white board, rather than the reliance of a board and chalk, hinders their progress in the classroom. Dyslexic students now find that as paper has become whiter and print blacker, the contrast is harder to read. This does not always indicate the need for screening for the use of colored overlays, but it can be comparable to reading in the sun, when the glare from the paper becomes a problem. This is obviously not just a problem in mathematics, as perception affects all subjects, but it is a problem in biology and geography, where color is used extensively in diagrams.

There are three components necessary to master any idea in mathematics: language, concepts, and arithmetic-procedure (Sharma, 1990). A dyslexic student may struggle with one, two, or even all of these areas. The difficulties in language have already been discussed. The concepts must be mastered for mathematical competence. A student may know his five times table, which is the arithmatic element, but may not understand what multiplication is, which is the concept. Without an understanding and knowledge of the concepts the student will approach all elements of mathematics individually. Mathematics reduces memory load and the number of possible "files" to be accessed mentally through its strenth in interlinking both horizontally and vertically. Without the concepts the interlinking "wall" of mathematics cannot be built, and knowledge that was learned in one area cannot be used in another. For example, instead of algebra being a logical extension of arithmetic, it becomes a new subject that brings out a sense of insecurity in the dyslexic student.

Much has been made of the learning style with which a student approaches mathematics. The different learning styles have been given a variety of names including: "inchworm and grasshopper," from Dr. Steve Chinn, principal of Mark College (Chinn and Ashcroft, 1998), which is perhaps, the most descriptive; "sequential" and "holistic," which are the terms often used in higher education; and "quantitative" and "qualitative," from Sharma (Sharma, 1989).

Examples

Simple case: 29×6

Inchworm Approach

$$\begin{array}{r} 29 \\ \times\,6 \\ \hline 17\underset{5}{4} \end{array}$$ completed "following the rule"

Grasshopper Approach

$$30 \times 6 = 180$$
$$29 \times 6 = 180 - 6$$
$$= 174$$

Higher level: Integrate $\sin^5 x \cos x$ with respect to x.

Sequential, by the rule, if you can remember it!	Holistic
Let $\sin x = u$	When I differentiate, I reduce
$\dfrac{du}{dx} = \cos x$, etc.	the power; when I integrate,
	I increase the power.
	Guess $\sin^6 x$ and test.

A dyslexic, *inchworm*, student with reasonable memory skills will attempt to rely on rote learning of procedures to master mathematics. This may work through primary school, but will break down at some stage, as the memory load soon becomes too great, by which time there is a great deal of work to explain and understand.

Some dyslexic students achieve good, even excellent, grades in mathematics. But as they progress in mathematics, they may go from a teaching style that is largely inductive to one that is deductive. This change means some students will be unable to cope. This is often not understood by teachers. Such students may, however, show strengths in various areas of applied mathematics.

3. TESTING AND ASSESSMENT

Before dyslexic students can be helped in mathematics, they must be tested and assessed. There is, at present, no simple test available to assess dyslexia-related problems in mathematics. It is not sufficient to test solely for mathematical attainment. Doing so will not show how a child's dyslexic problems are affecting his or her performance in mathematics. Consideration must be given to the skill areas previously discussed, including particularly:

- Understanding and mastery of the *language of mathematics*
- *Short-Term* (or working) *memory*
- Understanding of *concepts* versus the knowledge of *facts*
- *Preferred learning style* of the child. There may be no strong preference, but if a child does express a strong preference for one style then the teacher must be aware of this.
- *Speed of information processing.*

Perception and visualisation skills are less easy for a teacher to assess.

Ideally a child should be assessed by an educational psychologist prior to receiving any mathematical assessment (see Chapter 4). The psychologist's report should indicate the child's strengths and weaknesses. Although the main area of concern is often literacy, yet all reports should contain some form of information on performance relating to mathematics.

For example, there is, although now under discussion, generally thought to be a strong correlation between the results on the Raven's Matrices Tests (NFER Nelson), or Matrix Analogies Test (MAT), (Psychological Corporation) and problem solving abilities in mathematics.

The following are all skill areas that will be tested by an educational psychologist. All will affect the student's mathematical ability to a greater or lesser extent:

- Short-term memory (tested using Differential Ability Scales (DAS), a closed test available to educational psychologists only) problems will apply to all areas.
- Speed of information processing (tested using DAS) affects mathematical learning and performance in the classroom.
- Sequencing and pattern recognition (DAS test of sequential and quantitative reasoning) are vital in mathematics.
- Reading and comprehension are also necessary in mathematics.

Results of these tests and others can be interpreted with a view to teaching the student mathematics.

Further useful information can be found by using the "One Minute Addition and One Minute Subtraction Test" (Westwood et al., 1974) which not only tests knowledge of very basic number bonds but also shows speed of recalling information. Some dyslexic students have a marked discrepancy between their addition and the subtraction scores.

Most published tests will prove useful when used diagnostically. This must involve the teacher or tutor in:

1. Talking to the child
2. Offering a different language if the student doesn't understand first presentation
3. Asking how a question was done
4. Finding out why a question cannot be answered, should that be the case.

The tests below are a selection of the many available.

- The Gillham and Hesse Basic Number Screening Test (ages 7–12, approximately) is a good basic test, although the format is rather dated. It takes about 20 minutes upwards to administer (Gillham and Hesse, 1976). Its main advantage is its lack of language or instructions on the test sheets. Therefore the tester has to play an active part and can gain useful information about the student's understanding of mathematics.

- The Maths Links Tests of Mastery (NARE/NASEN) covers many areas, although its presentation is not ideal. It is available at two levels covering ages 7–12+. It is comprehensive and designed to indicate specific problem areas. It is a purely diagnostic test and will not give a "mathematical age" (Turnbull, 1986).
- The Wide Range Achievement Test (WRAT, available from the Dyslexia Institute) is thought by many to be useful. It is a timed test. Its advantage is that its results for reading, spelling, and mathematics are normed from the same extensive population so it should provide a good comparison in performance between these three skills (Jastak and Jastak, 1984).
- A useful Diagnostic Test Protocol is included in *Dyslexia and Maths: A Teaching Handbook* (Chinn and Ashcroft, 1998). This test is designed primarily for students between nine and 13. The aim is to measure the student's present level of achievement and highlight the areas of difficulty.

  Many other tests are available, providing the level of the test is suitable for the student most tests can be used successfully. The following test is recommended for assessing learning style:
- *Diagnostic Inventory of Basic Skills and Learning Styles in Mathematics* (Chinn, 1998).

The way a test is administered is more important than the actual test chosen. No student should be handed a test then left to "get on with it." Some tests are not timed so that during the test, the tester can ask the student what they are doing, how they obtained an answer. For older students doing a timed test (e.g., WRAT) the discussion can take place afterwards. An indication of the speed of information processing can be seen from the number of questions answered in the allocated time. Discussion is vital. The test should be seen as a diagnostic tool, and the opportunity must be taken to use the language of mathematics, both on the part of the teacher and the student.

A calculator is not allowed to be used on a test. However, it can be relevant to ask an older student to to take the test twice, the second time using a calculator and different colored pen. This will show how much the student relies on a calculator, how efficient the student is at using one, and the extent, if any, to which the student estimates and checks to ensure he or she gets the correct answer.

In the event of an educational psychologist's report not being available do *not* assess the student's mathematical competence only. It is important that a teacher is aware of the child's innate ability.

The following tests can be used successfully by teachers:

- British Picture Vocabulary Scale Second Edition (BPVS) (Dunn et al., 1997)
- *Raven's Matrices* (Raven & Court, 1993). This is available at three levels colored for children below 7, standard for students 7–14 and advanced for students of 14+ and adults.
- MAT (Naglieri 1995) for nonverbal ability.
- Digit Span Test (Newton & Thomson, 1982) is a screening test to indicate possible dyslexia for short-term memory. This can be found in the Aston Index (Newton and Thomson, 1982).
- The One Minute Addition and One Minute Subtraction Test (Westwood et al., 1974) will indicate both the student's grasp of basic addition and subtraction facts and the speed at which they are recalled.

4. HOW CAN WE HELP?

As teachers, parents, and administrators, the type of support we offer must relate to the student's needs. School-age students will see their priority as coping in the classroom and passing tests and examinations. Students in high school will either see mathematics as a skill necessary for their chosen subjects or as a skill necessary for life.

For such students support involves: improving basic skills; suggesting efficient strategies to encourage independent work; providing support for the higher level work experienced by the student within the classroom.

It is vital to use concrete apparatus where possible. The majority of dyslexic students have strong spatial skills and the use of concrete apparatus makes mathematics practical for them. Cuisenaire rods or Deines apparatus are examples of suitable materials for the holistic thinker. A pegboard with pegs and a number line are suitable for the sequential thinker. Both types of apparatus can help make the most of a student's strengths while supporting his or her weaker approach.

Dyslexic students improve in mathematics when it is done as a means to an end and not as an exercise in itself. For example, an older student who has an interest in motor bikes would be more motivated if work was structured around that topic.

Unlike literacy, mathematics has rules that cannot be broken. There are no choices in mathematics, but there are choices in reading. For example, "lead" has two pronunciations and several meanings, and "rain," "rein," and "reign" all have the same pronunciation. In addition, all reading and spelling begins at the top of a page, on the left and moves consistently from left to right down the page. This is not so in mathematics. A thorough knowledge of the rules of mathematics is vital for all students.

Often the computer is invaluable. Many dyslexic students are computer literate and prefer using the computer to using pen and paper. The superb graphics in many programs allow three-dimensional objects to be represented realistically, and simulations can clearly illustrate theory. However, few programs successfully teach mathematics, the majority providing only practice and reinforcement. Both are important.

The importance of talking has already been discussed, but again, it must be stressed that students must be allowed to talk through procedures. This uses mathematical language and enables the teacher to see whether students understand what they are being taught. The language used should be precise and repeated so students get consistent aural reinforcement. Talk in the support lessons should be equally divided between the teacher and the students.

Teachers should follow the guideline of being prepared to teach, teach, and teach again for learning to take place. The first time, information will largely be forgotten. The second time, it should be recognized. The third time, it will be remembered—we hope!

Remember that dyslexic students need to make more links to learn than their nondyslexic peers, so they will need more practice to master procedures. It is difficult to allocate time for this in the classroom. Students will feel it is unfair to be expected to finish work during breaks at school or at home. Each teacher, knowing the teaching setup, must decide how best to tackle this sometimes insurmountable problem.

Some students seem to understand or absorb mathematics by a process of osmosis! Dyslexic students do not "pick up" skills; they have to be taught. We must not assume knowledge that they may not have. Because topics are revisited and built on each year, they will be familiar to most students, but recognizing is not the same as remembering.

Students should be encouraged to produce their own key cards for every topic. The aim is understanding. Mathematics is *not* primarily a memory exercise. Strategies should be found wherever possible to reduce a student's memory load.

It is often suggested that teachers should give copies of overhead projector sheets and notes. It may be better to offer outline notes so students will know what is important, but will still have to take their own notes. However, it must be remembered that dyslexic students cannot easily carry out multiple tasks. Taking notes while listening is difficult for them. Unless note-taking is taught to *all* students, there will be many—including those with dyslexia—who will struggle.

Remember, most dyslexic students need extra time to copy from an overhead projector sheet and from a board. Dividing a white board into four quadrants with a permanent marker helps students find their place when copying. Also, many dyslexic students find reading cursive handwriting noticeably more difficult than reading printed script. Although students should be encouraged to use a cursive style for writing it is advisable for the teacher to have reading material printed in lowercase.

There is a move, especially in secondary schools, to teach study skills to all students. This must include study skills for mathematics. Improving question analysis, organization, time management, revision and exam techniques are vital. Revising for, and taking examinations in mathematics require skills different from those required in the humanities. These skills must be taught, and the student must practice them. Whereas the holistic thinker (grasshopper) can jump from one topic to another, the sequential thinker (inchworm) finds it difficult to move from one question type to another. This makes examinations difficult for the sequential thinker because each question is on a different topic. Teachers must monitor time management and offer ongoing support to help students organize, plan, and complete projects.

Often a list of instructions is given to students which may prove too many for a dyslexic student. It is better to give two or three instructions at a time, rather than four or five, and then ask the student to repeat those instructions.

Team teaching is being used in some colleges and schools. This style of teaching can often reduce the problems arising from different teaching and learning styles.

Many support tutors are literacy specialists; more tutors who understand *both* mathematics and dyslexia are needed. Many colleges now offer dyslexia support but this is often only for literacy and literacy-based study skills.

Last, a heartfelt plea from many students, not just those who are dyslexic. There is a tendency for classroom teachers to give homework right at the end of a lesson, sometimes after the bell has rung. Dyslexic students need time to write down their homework. They will not remember later!

5. WHAT CAN PARENTS DO?

Parents often ask teachers how they can help their child. Mathematics at home should be fun. Much can be learned by playing games, cooking, etc. Younger children can learn to count from the games with which we are all familiar, such as Ludo, Chutes and Ladders, etc. For older children, games like RummiKub may provide sequencing and counting practice. In addition, card games offer endless possibilities for older students. Even just scoring is good practice. Many dyslexic students are good at chess. All games help improve concentration. Darts, snooker, and ball games (such as tennis and badminton) all provide the opportunity to count and practice memory skills.

A potential difficulty may arise if parents attempt to explain homework to their child. It is important that they implement the same methods and procedures being used at school. Also, parents often work on showing the procedure necessary to complete a task rather than on teaching the child how to understand it. This is because many parents are so familiar with the simpler areas of mathematics that they no longer have to think about the concepts involved.

Parents tend to become over anxious about multiplication tables, especially if the school shows concern. When the student tries to learn the times tables, the teacher should help by suggesting multisensory learning strategies. However, by the time many students receive support for mathematics, they have become disillusioned about learning the times tables. Provided students understand the concepts involved in multiplication, they should be offered strategies to cope until they are ready to try again. These coping strategies could include, for example, a multiplication square. It may be necessary to reassure the student that the use of such aids is not cheating.

6. CONCLUSION

Supporting and teaching a dyslexic student in mathematics involves three specific areas: (1) an understanding of the difficulties a dyslexic student may bring to the subject of mathematics; (2) an assessment of an individual's range of difficulties and strengths; and (3) an awareness of how to teach mathematics using a structured, cumulative, multisensory approach. The last of these areas is a long term learning experience. Mathematics is a vast subject that is taught to our students for at least eleven years. Teachers with expertise in teaching literacy skills to dyslexic students can bring that knowledge to the subject of mathematics. One of the greatest barriers is that of teachers' confidence, not competence. Working with dyslexic students in the subject of mathematics and appreciating the difficulties they have can be a rewarding experience.

REFERENCES

Ashlock, R., Johnson, M., Wilson, J., & Jones, W. (1983). *Guiding Each Child's Learning of Mathematics.* Columbus, OH: Merrill.

Chinn, S. (1998). *Diagnostic Inventory of Basic Skills and Learning Styles in Mathematics.* London: The Psychological Corporation.

Chinn, S., & Ashcroft, J.R. (1998). *Mathematics for Dyslexics: A Teaching Handbook,* second edition. London: Whurr.

DeBono, E. (1970). *Lateral Thinking: A Textbook of Creativity.* London: Ward Lock Educational.

Department for Education & Employment (1995). *The National Curriculum,* London: Her Majesty's Stationary Office.

Dunn, L.M., Dunn, L.M., Whetton, C., & Pintille, D. (1982). *British Picture Vocabulary Scales.* Windsor: NFER-NELSON.

Durkin, K., & Shire, B. (1991). Primary school children's interpretations of lexical ambiguity in mathematical descriptions. *Journal of Research in Reading, 14(1),* 46–55.

Fawcett, A.J., & Nicolson, R.I. (eds.). (1994). *Dyslexia in Children: Multidisciplinary perspectives.* London: Harvester Wheatsheaf.

Gillham, W.E. & Hesse K.A. (1976). *Basic Number Screening Test.* Sevenoaks: Hodder & Stoughton Educational.

Henderson, A. (1989). *Maths and Dyslexia.* Llandudno: St. David's College.

Henderson, A. (1998). *Maths for the Dyslexic: A Practical Guide.* London David Fulton.

Hopkins, D. (1985). *A Teacher's Guide to Classroom Research.* Milton Keynes: Open University Press.

Hornsby, B. (1984). *Overcoming Dyslexia.* London: Dunitz.

Jastak, S.J., & Jastak, G.S. (1984). *Wide Range Achievement Tests,* third edition. Wilmington, Delaware: Wide Range Inc.

Joffe, L. (1983). School mathematics and dyslexia . . . a matter of verbal labelling, generalisation, horses and carts. *Cambridge Journal of Education, 13 (3):* 22–27.

Miles, T.R., & Miles, E. (eds.) (1992). *Dyslexia and Mathematics.* London: Routledge.

Naglieri, J.A. (1985). Matrix Analogies Test-Short Form. Columbus: Charles E. Merrill Publishing Co.

Newton, M., & Thomson, M. (1982). *The Aston Index.* Cambridge: LDA.

Raven, J.C., Court J.H., and Raven, J. (1998). *Crichton Vocabulary Scale.* Oxford: Oxford Psychologists Press.

Raven, J.C., Court J.H., and Raven, J. (1998). *Mill Hill Vocabulary Scale.* Oxford: Oxford Psychologists Press.

Raven, J.C., Court J.H., and Raven, J. (1993). *Standard Progressive Matrices.* Oxford: Oxford Psychologists Press.

Sharma, M.C. (1988). Levels of knowing mathematics. *Math Notebook,* Vol. 6, Nos. 1, 2.

Sharma, M.C. (1989). Mathematics learning personality. *Math Notebook,* Vol. 7, nos. 1,2.

Sharma, M.C. (1983). Visualisation: Its Applications to Mathematics Learning. *Math Notebook,* Vol. 3, nos 1 & 2.

Turnbull, J. (1986). *Maths Links Tests of Mastery.* Tamworth: NASEN.

Varda Gross-Tsur et al. (1996) Developmental dyscalculia: Prevalence and demographic features. *Developmental Medicine and Child Neurology, 38,* 25–33

Westwood, P., Harris-Hughes, M., Lucas, G., Nolan, J., Scrymgeour, K. (1974). One Minute Addition Test–One Minute Subtraction Test. *Remedial Education, 9(2).*

11

Information and Communication Technology and Dyslexia

Margaret Rooms

1. INTRODUCTION

This chapter will be out of date by the time this book is published. Computer technology is advancing at a rapid pace. Thus, discussion will be confined to general trends and skills development rather than to specific software or hardware considerations. Information and Communication Technology (ICT) considered here is limited to the technology commonly found in schools, colleges, and homes.

When viewed as a tool to enhance learning and to make learning and writing easier, ICT, and its interactive nature, becomes apparent and compelling. It is how dyslexic people can interact with computer technology that is of interest to us here. Is it the pathway to a golden age of dyslexia-free literacy and learning, or are there hidden obstacles that will trap our dyslexic learners, yet again, as they try to overcome their difficulties?

This chapter will show that there are many advantages for the dyslexic learner to use ICT. These advantages need to be taught before students can utilize ICT, and, inevitably, the dyslexic student will encounter *specific* obstacles. Ultimately, dyslexic learners will have to assess their own needs as to how ICT can assist

Margaret Rooms, The Dyslexia Institute, 2 Grosvenor Gardens, London SW1W ODH, United Kingdom

them, balanced against their individual obstacles. A knowledgeable teacher, by guiding these students, can save much time, frustration, and disappointment of unrealistic expectations.

2. ADVANTAGES OF INFORMATION AND COMMUNICATION TECHNOLOGY

2.1. General

Many of the advantages of ICT apply equally to the dyslexic learner as to everyone else. These include

- Most children enjoy using computers, and most are motivated to use them.
- ICT enables students to learn at their own pace.
- Computers are more patient than teachers.

2.2. Advantages for the Dyslexic Learner

- Multimedia computers enable multisensory (oral, aural, kinesthetic, visual) elements to be incorporated into the natural education process.
- Overlearning is easily accessible as computers do not tire.
- Work printed out from the computer is neater than handwritten work.
- A spell checker can provide spelling assistance.
- All of the above are available without the dyslexic learner being singled out and made to feel "different."

3. HARDWARE

3.1. Desktop Computers

Most personal computers are either IBM compatible (PCs) or Apple Macintosh. Additionally, in the British education market only, there are Acorn computers. The difference between them is defined by the operating system. In recent years the windows operating system developed for PCs has mirrored the Apple system. Apple computers have a dedicated following, but PCs have the lion's share of the market.

Unfortunately software is not yet compatible across the three systems so that a user is essentially locked in to whichever computer he, or the school, has purchased. The further development of Java as the standard for software composition should permit cross platform software in the future.

3.2. Laptop Computers—sometimes known as notebooks

Laptop computers are portable computers that mirror the functions of desktop computers. Their portable function makes them more expensive than desktop computers, therefore the security factor alone in carrying them around a school puts their use at risk.

3.3. Palmtops

There are smaller, lighter computers called palmtops, so called because they can fit into the palm of the hand. These are more likely to find a considerable market in schools due to their lower purchase price and ease of portability. Potentially, they are as powerful as any other computer although not everyone is comfortable using such a small keyboard.

4. HARDWARE AND SOFTWARE

4.1. Word Processors

There are still a number of dedicated word processors being produced. Because they only do word processing, they are cheaper than PCs and often easier to use. It is also possible to get dedicated word processors in the notebook size, which are often given to dyslexic students to use in school.

4.2. Spell Checkers

Hand held spell checkers are a relatively simple way of providing a computer function without incurring the expense of a computer. A child using a hand held spell checker in the classroom has direct IT assistance even with handwritten work.

5. SOFTWARE

5.1. Word Processing

Word processing is still the most widely used computer function. It is, after all, essentially writing. For the dyslexic learner, word processing is particularly valuable. The main advantages of word processing for a dyslexic learner are:

- Presentation—Neat work, always.
- Spell checker—Aids the dyslexic person in spelling words.

- "Cut and paste" facility—Eliminates the need to rewrite by allowing work to be rearranged.
- Delete—Surely the single most valuable function on the software. No erasers. No crossing out. Just remove the error and write over.
- Layers—Content, spelling, punctuation, layout can all be worked on as separate discrete tasks rather than simultaneously as is required with handwritten work.
- "Labor"—Handwriting labor is eliminated.
- Copy and paste facility—This allows difficult words to be typed in only once and then copied as needed.

Although I am in favor of teaching dyslexic people how to use a word processor, I feel honor bound to list some drawbacks to word processing.

- Word processing skills take time to develop like anything else. Competence does not happen instantly.
- Facility to waste time—almost boundless for the determined student. It can be compelling to "fiddle" with text when so many tools are available.
- Poor keyboard skills can be a painful experience for teacher and student. Word processing cannot be executed efficiently and timely unless the student has good keyboard awareness.
- Spell checkers can be frustrating for poor readers who cannot recognize the correct word from those listed. Spell checking can also be time consuming.
- Accidentally deleting work or not saving at the end of a lesson. Not all word processors have an "undo" function.

Although these drawbacks could apply equally well to anyone, for the dyslexic learner they can have serious consequences. The dyslexic person may approach word processing with high expectations. He may have been led to believe that this is the answer to his written language difficulties. Any difficulties he encounters during word processing can disillusion him and reinforce any feelings of inadequacy or frustration. Skilled guidance and systematic teaching can help to prepare these students.

5.2. Speech Technology

There are two forms of speech used in software: synthesized and digitized. Synthesized speech is inexpensive. and is the one that sounds like a robot. This is the speech that is normally incorporated into a word processor. It can make mistakes when reading text, however there is usually a function to alter mispronunciations.

Digitized speech is a real voice that has been recorded digitally. Its quality and accuracy are excellent. The disadvantage is that the words have to be pre-recorded which limits the vocabulary and therefore subsequent use. They also use a lot of hard drive space. Digitized speech is used in many literacy programs but not normally with a word processor.

5.3. Text to Speech

Since word processing became widely available there have been many developments to enhance its capabilities. One of the most useful to the dyslexic learner is text to speech. This software literally speaks the text that is on the screen. It enables the dyslexic learner to hear the words he has typed as well as see them. Many children do not catch the errors they have made until they have heard them.

The text to speech facility may be comforting for the dyslexic person in that it can be programmed to fit his needs. It can be set to read single words, sentences, or paragraphs according to the level of need, or it can be turned on or off as he wishes. In this way the level of auditory "interference" can be regulated to the individual.

5.4. Word Prediction and Word Completion

A word predictor attempts to predict the next word the writer wants to use by analyzing the sentence under construction then drawing from the writer's own vocabulary, as previously used with this program. The writer reads the list of predicted words (or uses a speech engine to read them to him) and selects the word he wants. Thus the more someone uses the software, the more accurate the program's prediction will be.

Word completion works in a similar fashion but operates once the first letter of a word has been written. Again a menu of words appears from which the writer makes his selection.

This type of software was originally designed for the physically handi-capped user to reduce the number of keystrokes they used when writing. Dyslexic people tend to love these functions when they are first introduced, but often drop their use when composing. The prediction and completion functions can distract and interfere with the dyslexic student's focus on the writing content. Instead of concentrating on the flow of ideas and the sequence of words required, the student is constantly referred to lists of unrelated words that can interrupt his concentration and sequencing. The student may also be the tempted to select one of the words because they are being offered rather than to persevere with the word he originally intended. For a reluctant writer, however, this software could give sufficient support to encourage his writing where previously there had been none! A teacher's careful guidance when demonstrating the functions and following up on their use would be advisable.

5.5. Spell Checker Designed for the Dyslexic Student

A number of spell checkers have been designed specifically to help the dyslexic student. Their attempt to understand every "bizarre" spelling leads to extensive analysis which generates numerous suggestions. The correct spelling may well be included in the choices, but the program demands the student persevere to reach the correct choice. In my experience, unless the correct spelling is offered in the first menu option list, most dyslexic students are not interested in pursuing it further. They may also find it a time-consuming task—which can be difficult to justify when the correct spelling is not reached. This is not to say there isn't a need for a better spell checker; for it to be useful at the school level, it needs to be more user-friendly than those currently on the market.

5.6. Voice Activated Software

Speak to the computer and the text appears on the screen! The possibilities of voice activated software (VAS) are awe-inspiring. This is the future for all people who have good verbal skills. Although the technology still has room for improvement, it presents issues that need to be resolved before being considering for the dyslexic student. They are described in the following sections.

5.6.1 High Specification of Hardware Needed to Run Voice Activated Software

The high level of hardware specifications needed to run VAS means that some potential users will be excluded even though they have relatively current hardware. The paradox is that software costs have come down, but hardware costs have had to go up to accommodate the higher specification needed.

5.6.2. Time Needed to "Train" the Computer

The amount of time needed to "train" the computer to recognize the user's voice varies with the different systems, but the process is usually reported to be onerous. Assistance should be given by someone who is familiar with the system, and can make the process easier.

5.6.3. Reading Complexity of the Training Material

The complexity of the training material required for the dyslexic user to read remains an issue. Again, help may be needed at this stage. This is particularly off-putting for the adult who is looking to this system to make his residual difficulties with literacy less apparent. When it appears to highlight his problems, it may induce his feelings of frustration and inadequacy.

5.6.4. Continuous Speech and Discrete Speech Systems

Continuous speech systems allow the user to speak at a normal pace without having to pause between words. The words appear on the screen *after* the user speaks and thus do not give immediate visual feedback, allowing the speaker to check for accuracy. With discrete speech systems the user has to pause slightly between words but the text appears on the screen right away. The choice of either discrete or continuous has to be made according to the needs of the individual student. Some students prefer to check their work as they go (discrete) and others prefer to concentrate on the content first and do their checking all together. BECTA (British Educational Communications Technology Agency) is currently carrying out research with its "SEN Speech Recognition Project" into the use of this technology with students with a variety of special needs.

5.6.5 Synthesized Speech Feedback

Some software combines VAS with text to speech. By so doing, it creates synthesized speech feedback on the accuracy of the input.

6. KEYBOARD SKILLS

6.1. Introduction

Central to word processing is *keyboard awareness*. Unless the learner knows where to find the appropriate keys on the keyboard then he cannot achieve much writing. The interruption of finding keys when sequencing words and sentences places a burden on the writer.

There are many keyboard awareness programs and touch typing programs available to resolve this problem. Which of these is most appropriate for a dyslexic student will depend on individual circumstances. Inevitably, students use the one the school has bought!

Touch typing originated when manual typewriters were the norm and were confined to offices. There was a need for fast typing from the typist or secretary. The typist was not composing the text as she typed; her skill was to quickly copy, using the typewriter, text that was already composed. Keyboard awareness skills are adequate for people when they are *composing* as they are writing. Pausing to think as you write slows the whole process down anyway. Typing speed needs to be as fast as handwriting speed for it to be a useful tool.

For the dyslexic typist there is an added advantage in looking at the keys while typing. It may be easier to *recognize* the needed letter rather than having to conjure up the shape from visual memory.

6.2. Keyboard Awareness

Keyboard awareness promotes just that: knowing where the keys are so they can be accessed quickly. Students can look at the screen or at the keyboard and they can use as many or as few fingers as they wish. Note that I do not call this "hunt and peck"; there is no hunting and very little pecking because they are aware of the keyboard layout.

6.3. Touch Typing

Touch typists develop a kinesthetic *feel* for the keyboard that turns typing into an automatic skill. This could be compared to the action many people use when they key their personal identification number into a cash machine: They may not be able to recall the number but they can remember the pattern of key strokes. Touch typing is not an easily acquired skill for some dyslexic people. Motivation is a key element: A student will practice until he is fast enough for his individual needs.

6.4. Literacy Skills Practice

There are many programs which practice and develop literacy skills: spelling, phonological awareness, rhyme, word recognition. Reading practice programs tend to incorporate text to speech so students "hear" the words as they are read. This is the largest group of special needs software, and offers much to choose from. Children are usually enthusiastic about using such programs, and motivating them to spell cannot be a bad thing! Care must be taken, when using such programs, that they are part of a *structured* language lesson and are not used on an ad hoc basis.

7. CORE TEACHING PROGRAMS

7.1. Integrated Learning Systems

There are an increasing number of programs that aim to teach core literacy skills.

Integrated Learning Systems (ILS) contain teaching material plus an elaborate management system that tests the student, grades the test, guides the student to material, grades that work, and then selects the next task according to the results. Theoretically, the student is always given material at his correct learning level. The student works independently at the computer.

7.2. Open Integrated Learning Systems

Open Integrated Learning Systems (OILS) follow the same concept as ILS except a teacher can overrule the program and place the student herself when necessary. This flexibility enables the teacher to adjust the program to fit the needs of the individual.

Whether such systems would benefit the dyslexic student would depend on the student's individual profile. The program's independent learning element is excellent for building a student's confidence and self-esteem, plus the overlearning potential is high. Programmed learning tends to be cumulative, and a multimedia computer would provide the multisensory element. Commercial programs aimed at all students might not be sufficiently structured to meet a dyslexic learner's needs especially if his literacy level is low. Such programs are more useful after the primary literacy problem has been overcome.

8. INTERNET

8.1. Introduction

For some years, word processing has been acknowledged as the single most useful IT function for dyslexic people and probably for everyone. The Internet is now threatening to dominate IT in school and at home. The power of the Internet will have an impact on the lives of everyone who uses a computer. The British government is committed to giving Internet access to every school in the country and aims for every student to have his or her own e-mail address. But what will be the specific issues for the dyslexic learner?

8.2. Electronic Mail

Electronic mail (e-mail) involves reading, writing, and spelling. Thus it does not immediately lend itself to being particularly dyslexia friendly as the optimal choice as a means of communicating. However, e-mail protocol encourages an informal style of writing where even spelling mistakes are attributed to *typing errors* because the assumption is that e-mails are quickly composed. Many of the aids described earlier for use with word processors can also be used in e-mail and for World Wide Web (www) access.

The precise nature of e-mail addresses will cause some problems for dyslexic users, (as they do for everyone else,) but the advantage is that they only have to be typed in once and thereafter can be copied directly.

8.3. Access to Information

As search engines for the Internet become more sophisticated in their *hunting* techniques and less specific in their demands for information, then accessing the Internet for information will become more dyslexia friendly (i.e., less exact information will be needed). Dyslexic people should not be disadvantaged when they use it. What people do with these vast quantities of information is a separate question with infinite answers! Again, the potential for time wasting is enormous.

9. CONCLUSION

9.1. The Crystal Ball

Is ICT the great leveler that allows dyslexic people to compete on equal terms with their non-dyslexic peers? The facilities are there in the software already, although not everyone has access to them. Neither do they all have the skills needed to maximize their usefulness.

Children now entering the school system are going to be using computers at a much earlier age than their teachers did. Increasingly they will use ICT across the curriculum and for long stretches of time throughout the week. Home computer use is growing at such a rate that some familes already own two or three computers.

This growth in the user base for computers will have a greater impact on education because it will become a major vehicle for learning. For the dyslexic person, this means *everyone* will be using computers, and he or she will not be singled out for special treatment with ICT.

9.2. Strengths

It must be remembered that the dyslexic person has many strengths as well as weaknesses. Many dyslexic people will find these strengths will have an outlet in ICT. Computers are the means of expressing creativity as well as being useful for crunching data. The language of programming, being totally logical, *can* be easier for a dyslexic person to handle than the English language. *In the Mind's Eye* West (1977) highlighted the many creative achievements of dyslexic people. ICT offers another vehicle for such successes while, as always, requiring effort, perseverance, and skilled guidance from the beginning.

REFERENCES

textHELP! textHELP systems Ltd., Enkalon Business Centre, 25 Randalstown Road, Antrim, N. Ireland BT41 4LJ.
KeySpell. Keyspell Ltd., 9 Military Road, Newcastle upon Tyne, NE15 OBQ.
West, Thomas (1997). In the Mind's Eye, Prometheus Books.

12

The Challenge of
Dyslexia in Adults

Jenny Lee

Dyslexia's a cloak over your intelligence.

This comment, made by a 19-year-old dyslexic undergraduate, sums up, not only the personal frustrations but also the misconceptions that others can have of a dyslexic adult.

1. INTRODUCTION

This chapter will discuss some of the difficulties common to dyslexic adults, how they relate to some theories of dyslexia and the impact they can have on a dyslexic adult's life. It will examine and evaluate a selection of screening and assessment tools for specialist teachers. It will also explore some of the issues that need to be addressed when negotiating learning programmes and during teaching. Some examples of learning programmes will be used to illustrate this and a range of practical teaching methods will be suggested. Ways for both the dyslexic student and teacher to monitor progress will be discussed.

By the time the dyslexic individual has reached adulthood, his or her dyslexic difficulties can be complex and diverse. They will almost inevitably be overlaid with problems of self esteem and confidence. Dyslexia affects adults, not only in their personal lives, but also at work and study. Thus this chapter will suggest

Jenny Lee, Adult Basic Education Coordinator, Education Department, Durham
County Council, LEAP Adult Education Centre, Barnard Castle, Co. Durham DL12 8BG, England.

some ways of supporting adults in these two specific areas by developing part-nerships between specialist teachers, universities and businesses. It must be ap-preciated however that no one approach will succeed for all.

This chapter will offer a selection of approaches and techniques from which the specialist teacher and the dyslexic student can choose. How effective these ap-proaches are will depend upon a number of factors, including the depth of the as-sessment, the commitment of the dyslexic adult and the skill of the teacher.

2. SOME POSSIBLE CAUSES AND CONSEQUENCES

Much exciting research continues to be carried out in an attempt to establish the core deficit or deficits in dyslexia.

Figure 1 attempts to relate some of the current ideas to the primary and sec-ondary indicators of dyslexia most commonly seen in adults.

It is generally agreed that the underlying cause of dyslexia is likely to be ge-netic and will be located primarily in the language area of the brain. This leads to a core phonological deficit; see for example Hulme & Snowling (1991), Rack and Snowling (1985), DeFries et al. (1996), Hynd et al. (1995), Galaburda (1993), Galaburda and Geshwind (1989), Goswami and Bryant (1990). Paulesu et al. (1996) suggested that a break in the bridge or insula, between the part of the brain that recognizes words visually (Wernicke's Area) and the part that segments them auditorily (Broca's Area) reduces the dyslexic adult's ability to activate these ar-eas in concert.

Dyslexia seems to affect more than just language. New theories are attempt-ing to relate the diverse difficulties to abnormalities in the cerebellum. Nicolson and Fawcett (1995) propose that cerebellar abnormalities can affect motor control, the development of automaticity and organizational skills as well as phonology and language. At this stage in the research, the links are still speculative.

Lovegrove (1990), Livingstone et al. (1991), and Cornelissen et al. (1995) have attempted to correlate deficits found in the dyslexic's visual processing sys-tem with learning to read. Again, although an association between the two has been established, the precise nature of the link is not yet clear.

These theories may eventually help to explain some of the more puzzling symptoms that teachers observe, which seem to be unrelated to phonological deficits. For summaries of these studies see Hulme and Snowling (1997), Faw-cett and Nicolson (1994), and Snowling (1985).

As Figure 1 shows, brain abnormalities can result in deficits in the cognitive area and thus, without remediation can lead to both primary and secondary be-havioral indications in adults. Ideally it would be useful to be able to correct some of the problems in these biological and cognitive areas, and this in turn, would have an impact on the behavioral signs. However, at present it seems that

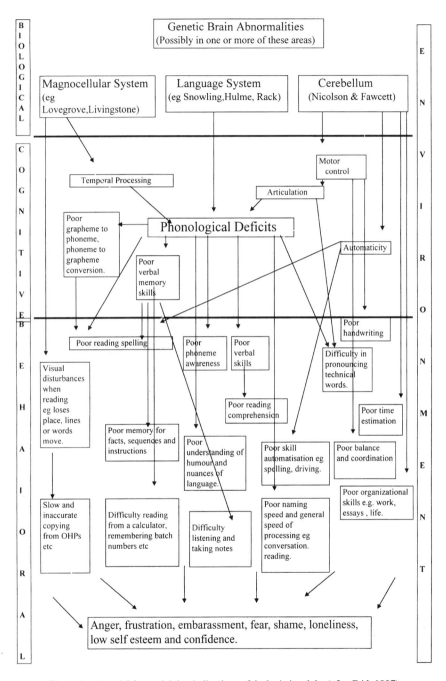

Figure 1. A model for explaining indications of dyslexia in adults (after Frith 1997).

the majority of our efforts are concentrated on dealing with the primary behavioral problems. Remediation in this area does seem to have *some* positive impact on the cognitive area, but despite striking improvements in reading and spelling, many underlying cognitive deficits remain surprisingly intractable in adults. Underlying skills such as short term memory, phonological awareness and automaticity often show only slight improvement, indicating that the dyslexia as such has not been "cured" but strategies have been found to remediate the presenting problems. Specialist teaching, which improves basic skills, undoubtedly ameliorates some of the secondary features of dyslexia such as anger, low self esteem, embarassment and lack of self confidence.

3. THE EFFECT DYSLEXIA CAN HAVE ON THE ADULT

Abnormalities in the brain structure leading to deficits in some of the cognitive skills can often result in a wide range of problems for the dyslexic adult.

3.1. Reading & Writing

Reading problems can persist into adult years but spelling and general written expression seem to remain the most stubborn problems.

The following are some comments made by dyslexic adults who describe the problems they have experienced because of their weak reading and spelling skills:

"When you write, things never come out as they're meant to, but you compensate with other skills."

"If you're asked to fill in a form, you feel like your head's going to burst and you feel physically sick."

"You feel inadequate in society because society's mode of communication is written."

"Going to restaurants; you end up eating what you can read."

"Reading is intense work."

"You dread letting other people see what you've written."

"When I read a story to my 3 year old son, my wife tells me the way I read is incomprehensible, but my son doesn't complain."

"At home, it's so upsetting when your kids can read and write better than you."

"At work you have to get other people to get things out of the stores, then they think you're lazy."

"I've still not got my sick pay because I couldn't fill in the six page form."

"There is so much I would like to write but I'm limited to basic words that a seven-year-old could do. Frustrated? YES."

"I was offered promotion but I left my job rather than explain that I couldn't read or write well enough to cope."

3.2. Problems with Short-Term Memory, Verbal Naming and General Language Processing

Short term memory, verbal naming and general language processing problems can result in unexpected difficulties for an adult.

"It's hard to make myself understood, especially when someone is annoying me."

"You can't keep up with a conversation between four or five friends."

"I lose track in team briefs and forget instructions."

"My husband says I'm stupid because I can't "get" jokes."

"I'm always being pulled up because I've recorded batch numbers wrongly."

"If I do a crossword I have to constantly look at the clue and keep reading it while I'm trying to think of the answer. Then I forget what the clue was again."

"Being dyslexic caused a lot of friction in my second marriage. If he saw any writing of mine, he used to laugh and say I was thick which used to upset me. It caused arguments which I wasn't very good at because I couldn't think of the words to argue back, so I felt worse than ever."

3.3. Problems With Organizational Skills

Deficits here can result in missed appointments, exams not completed, essays muddled, poor awareness of time at work and difficulties in organizing paperwork.

"I find it hard to think of more than one thing at a time."

3.4. The Emotional Impact

The overall impact of dyslexic problems in adults cannot be overstated, although it may take some time before they feel secure enough to share their feelings. Here are some writings from dyslexic adults, where they describe the pain and isolation that can be felt before help and understanding was given:

"Dyslexia—
The boy must be thick
Yes that's it
The boy's thick
It's the only thing
Small words won't go in
Your son is way behind
He's what we call word blind
There's no white stick
The boy's thick
From outside he looks just fine
We'll never ask more from his mind
Put him down there with all the rest
Believe me it's for the best.

I'm here
Can you not see me?
I'm speaking
Can you not hear?
I'm trying
God know I'm trying

Can you not help?
Inside I'm crying
Can you not feel?
Hope is dying
Doors slam shut
Life stands still

Voices tell me
"This is it"
Only myself
To blame
A life sentence
My heart sobs
At the news
I am a prisoner
For a crime

I have not committed
Will I never be a free man?"

"You don't expect to be valued."

"The real killer isn't the dyslexia itself, it's the guilt and lack of confidence it brings."

"There is a process in metal work called 'work hardening'. This is when you get a soft bit of metal, you beat the metal with a hammer until it gets hard and unyielding, this is called 'work hardened'. The attitudes of my teachers and parents had the same effect on me, I became disillusioned with the whole process and rebelled. I hardened my attitude to everything and became skeptical and mistrusting; I would take no more of their education. Now, I try to keep my mind dormant. In this way I don't get too disappointed and get on with my lot."

4. IDENTIFYING DYSLEXIA IN ADULTS

"Before being tested, I was frightened. I was scared that everybody would be right—that I really was stupid."

"I was relieved, but my dad's old fashioned—he wouldn't like it—it's hereditary, isn't it?"

It is clear from these comments that there is more to testing adults for dyslexia than just collecting and interpreting the results. However, the key to solving some of the problems discussed in this chapter's previous sections must lie in identification and assessment.

4.1. Screening

A good screening test should be quick, easy to administer and provide the necessary data to tell whether a full assessment is necessary. The term "screening" is perhaps a misnomer as related to adults, because it is usually carried out only on request in industry or university. It is not felt to be right or economically sensible to screen everyone in an organization for dyslexia.

There are two adult screening tests which can be useful, the Michael Vinegrad Adult Dyslexia Checklist published by the Adult Dyslexia Organisation and the Fawcett & Nicolson Dyslexia Adult Screening Test (DAST).

The Adult Dyslexia Checklist comprises a set of 20 questions requiring a "yes" or "no" response. It is very quick to administer and could be completed by the dyslexic adult alone provided his or her reading skills were adequate. "Yes" answers to certain specific questions suggest a strong indication of dyslexia. Nine or more "yes's" overall indicate dyslexia. The test is clear and user friendly but if the scoring was purely numercial, it could be difficult to distinguish between dyslexic adults and other adults with basic skills problems. This caveat is, however, noted on the test instructions.

The Fawcett & Nicolson Dyslexia Adult Screening Test is an extremely reliable instrument both for screening and remediation. The whole test takes about 35 minutes to complete and is made up of a series of 11 sub-tests which are designed to tap some of the cognitive and behavioral areas that are typically dyslexia sensitive, for example, speed of information processing, verbal memory, phonological awareness, balance, reading and spelling. It also includes tests in which some dyslexic adults tend to do well, for example, nonverbal reasoning and semantic fluency.

Scoring is very straightforward and indicates both graphically and numerically whether an adult is "at risk" of being dyslexic. Information provided by the individual sub tests is also valuable when planning a teaching program.

4.2. Diagnostic Assessment

4.2.1. Psychologists' Tests

Once a decision has been made to obtain a full assessment, an assessor must be found, preferably one who specializes in adult dyslexic problems.

A first choice would be an educational psychologist, but often they can be too expensive for adults on a limited income. A psychologist can do a battery of tests, usually the Wechsler Adult Intelligence Scale (WAIS). These can be used to produce a detailed cognitive profile to identify precise areas of strengths and weaknesses.

For a readable and detailed analysis of psychologist's tests, see Turner (1997) and also McLoughlin, Fitzgibbon, and Young (1993).

4.2.2. Specialist Teachers' Tests

A good assessment, carried out by a specialist teacher, trained to post-graduate level, can provide a reliable analysis of an adult's difficulties as well as detailed recommendations for teaching.

4.2.2.1. Choosing Tests   The norm-referenced tests chosen should be well standardized with recently obtained norms, established across the full age range. It is difficult to find tests that are both normed and appropriate for adults; the age ceiling on many excellent tests is often around 13.5 to 15.5 years. Both norm-referenced and criterion-referenced tests must be chosen carefully so that the assessor is sure they are testing what they claim to be testing. For instance, if a student is asked to identify the "odd one out for sound" from "bad" "cad", "pan", "sad", is this a test of phonological awareness or working memory or both?

It is important when choosing tests to be sure to read the 'fine print' and check when and how a test was standardised. For instance, many practitioners, myself included, are unhappy about the most recent standardization procedure for adult norms of the Raven's Matrices. However, this test is still useful for estimating nonverbal reasoning skills. The Kaufman Brief Intelligence Test (see Turner) has a reliable nonverbal component but the verbal test may cause some problems in the UK because of differences in spelling.

4.2.3. Principles of Assessing for Dyslexia

What general principles should a specialist teacher consider when assessing an adult? In broad terms, the tests chosen should answer three central questions.

1. *Is the adult underachieving?*
    Is there a discrepancy between achievement and potential?
2. *Why?*
    To find this out, it is necessary to establish a profile across a range of cognitive skills.
3. *What are we going to do about it?*
    What specific action can be taken to remediate the problems? This will include detailed recommendations for teaching based on individual needs, strengths, weaknesses and learning styles. Recommendations for extra support or for further investigations may also be needed.

It is important to supply the adult with a realistic estimation of how long the assessment will last before beginning testing as it can take up to three hours! A rough outline of the test procedure should be given. It can be unnerving to be asked to write something if you have not written much more than your name and address for years. Explain that a break can be taken at any time during the assessment; that the results will be discussed and a written report will be given. Stress that all information obtained is highly confidential and will not be passed on to any one without the student's express permission.

A good first step in assessment is to use a structured interview format as a basis for initial discussion. Klein's (1993) interview form (Diagnosing Dyslexia) is useful in establishing important background information, for example present needs and difficulties, educational history, relevant medical information, early eyesight, hearing, motor, speech problems, familial incidence and students' own perceptions of their problems. This first stage may take some time, but it is extremely useful, not only to establish any other possible reasons for the difficulties, but also to develop a rapport. Initial observations regarding general test behaviour, for example, speech and language abilities, nervousness etc, can be made.

4.2.4. Is the Adult Underachieving?

A comparison of scores can be made between tests of verbal and nonverbal intellectual ability and tests of basic skills. Verbal and nonverbal tests which are standardized for adults include Raven's Standard or Advanced Matrices, Kaufman Brief Intelligence Test, Mill Hill Vocabulary Test. The BPVS Test is standardized up to 15.8 years. Basic skills (eg single word reading/spelling and arithmetic) can be tested using the Wide Range Achievement Test, WRAT 3 or Woodcock Reading Mastery Tests, WRMT.R (see Turner, 1997).

A more detailed analysis of single word reading can be gained by examining word attack skills and decoding skills using tests of irregular words and non-words, e.g., tests adapted from Nelson and Snowling (see Klein, 1993).

Prose reading will need to be assessed using the miscue analysis technique (see Klein, 1993). It is also valuable to obtain knowledge of reading speed and comprehension. This can be evaluated informally by having the student read one of the higher levels from the Neale Analysis of Reading, or if necessary simpler passages (see Klein 1993) or if appropriate the student's own college texts. Adult reading rate (with reasonable comprehension) should be at about 90–100 words per minute when reading aloud, and more when reading silently.

Spelling errors can be analyzed using spellings either obtained from the WRAT or from dictated passages, e.g., Margaret Peters' diagnostic dictations. This spelling error analysis (Klein 1993) is very useful because it determines what type of spelling instruction is necessary. It also helps to answer our second major question, "why." Certain types of spelling errors can suggest deficits in specific skills, for instance, phonological awareness, verbal or visual memory.

A range of writing skills such as handwriting, sentence construction, use of punctuation, organization, use of vocabulary, speed etc can be assessed by giving a 10 minute free writing task. Thinking time should be offered before timing begins.

Writing speed can also be assessed by giving a 1 minute copying task, such as that in the Dyslexia Adult Screening Test, DAST, (Fawcett & Nicolson 1998). Speed for free writing and copying should be around 20–25 words per minute for an adult.

4.2.5. Why?

To establish a possible cause for the problems the teacher needs to consider any background information and examine a range of cognitive skills. Verbal memory skills can be tested diagnostically by using either the Bangor Dyslexia Test (Digit Span) or, if a rough percentile score is required, the Backwards Span Test in the DAST, (Fawcett and Nicholson, 1998). Informal indications of short term memory abilities can be gained from checking an adult's knowledge of alphabetical order, times tables, months of the year, etc.

Phonological awareness (or the ability to identify, segment and manipulate sounds in words) can be easily evaluated using tests such as the Rosner Test of

Auditory Analysis Skills (Rosner, 1993). This test is normed for children, but it may be used diagnostically for adults. The Perin Spoonerism Test which is derived from a piece of research and is not a published test, can provide useful information about higher level phonological processing skills. Phonemic segmentation is also tested on the DAST (Fawcett and Nicolson 1998).

Visual recall is tricky to evaluate. This is because most tests of "visual memory" inevitably involve people recoding visually presented material by "rehearsing" items in their heads using a speech code. Dyslexic people however, do not always automatically do this and therefore it is still helpful to see how well they can integrate these two modalities. If a more in depth assessment of visual perceptual skills is needed, use the Gardner Test of Visual Perceptual Skills (1990). The scores are standardized up to 17 years, but the test manual suggests that the 17 year norms would hold well for adults.

For the majority of adults, the assessment process can be a positive experience. Many adults who come for testing hope that dyslexia will provide an explanation for the problems they experience, so careful handling will be required if there seems to be no evidence of dyslexia. I find it best to discuss this possibility before assessment and to point out that whatever the results, something positive can be done to sort out whatever problems are identified. An assessment report must explain succinctly all the relevant information gathered from the discussion and the test results. It should cite examples of the student's performance and give details of the tests used. An interpretation and analysis of the evidence should then be given. This must be followed by clear recommendations for a teaching program and any support that may be required at work or college.

The most common reaction, if dyslexia *is* proposed to be the problem (and remember, that as teachers we can only give our opinion on this and not a diagnosis) is relief. As one adult memorably said:

> "It's like finding out you've only got one leg and thinking, 'Good . . . that's why I can't walk.'"

I like the "good"!

5. NEGOTIATING LEARNING PROGRAMS

By the time a dyslexic individual has reached adulthood he or she has often experienced a great deal of failure in the basic skills. The job of the specialist teacher is to demonstrate that, using multisensory methods, an adult *can* learn effectively. The first step is to negotiate a learning program that describes specific, relevant and measurable targets which can be reviewed at a later date. Before setting learning plans, it is useful to have the following information, in addition to the results of the formal assessment:

- The student's needs and goals as regards work, study, home;
- Barriers to learning;
- The student's preferred learning styles;
- The time the student has available (contact time and private study time);
- The student's degree of commitment (e.g., does he/she work full time; have many other commitments? Is he/she a shift worker?);
- What materials, resources are available;
- What are the student's priorities and how urgent might they be;
- What expertise is available from teachers;
- Whether the student is interested in certification as a way of accrediting learning;

Learning programs should be stated in terms of:

- Measurable goals;
- The skills and knowledge needed and/or the steps required to achieve these goals;
- The time scale for achieving these goals;
- The priorities;
- The materials needed to achieve the goals.

Most students with severe dyslexia-related reading and spelling problems will need, as part of their learning program, a highly structured multisensory language program such as the Dyslexia Institute's Literacy Programme (DILP 1993), or Cathy Diggle's "Write/Right to Read" (Cornwall LEA). They will also need to address pressing needs such as learning how to spell the words they need for work or college. Word processing, organizational and memory skills, report writing, form filling, essay writing and reading for meaning, may also need to be included in a learning program.

Figures 2–4 show examples of learning plans for dyslexic adults in different situations. Notice how each general aim in Section 1 is translated into specific measurable objectives in Section 3.

When negotiating learning plans it is important to bear in mind both the general learning styles of dyslexic adults (see Fig. 5) and any particular learning styles the individual might prefer.

6. TEACHING DYSLEXIC ADULTS

> *"I've failed and failed and failed at this all my life. I'm scared I'll fail again*—a dyslexic student, sitting down to his first teaching session."

Learning Plan

Name: Jane   **From** September 9th   **To:** December 17th

A   What do I need/want to learn?

1   Start work on the structured language programme, with the long term goal of achieving an open college structured language programme certificate.
2   Develop multisensory strategies for spelling priority words.
3   Learn how to extract meaning from reading;
4   Develop short term memory and sound awareness skills.
5   Improve punctuation and form filling.
6   Organise life!
7   Develop word processing skills.

B   How much can I do already in these areas?

- I know names of letters of the alphabet, apart from G & J.
- Can spell name and most of address.
- Can read slowly and sound out regular unfamiliar words.
- Can remember 4 digits in same order.
- Can write most letters as capital but not J & G.

C   What skills and knowledge do I need; what steps do I need to take to achieve these goals?

1.1 Reach end of Module 2 in Write/Right to Read Programme.
1.2 Know sounds, names and shapes of 13 letters & blends.
1.3 Know basic language terminology, ie open and closed syllables, definition of a suffix, a vowel and a consonant, long and short vowel sounds, voiced and unvoiced consonants.

2   Spell 10 priority words, by experimenting with a range of multisensory strategies.

3   Extract meaning by experimenting with inference, cloze strategies, imagery, dual code techniques.
4.1 Extend auditory memory skills to 5 digits by chunking and picturing.
4.2 Segment words into syllables, using one syllable pattern, vc/cv.
5.1 Use full stops and capital letters correctly.
5.2 Practise name and address on forms, using block capitals. Find out the meaning of and be able to read terminology of forms eg "marital status" etc.
6   Organise correspondence at home using a filing system.
7   Know main parts of computer and be able to input text.

D   What are the priorities?

Spelling words for form filling.

E   What about materials?

Right/Write to Read, (Diggle) Reading & Thinking, (Evans) The Punctuation Book.
Sample and real forms, Left to Right (Brown & Brown), filing cards.
The Multisensory Spelling Programme for Priority Words, MUSP, (Lee)

F   We'll review your work after about a term and a half.
Would you prefer to review more often?   Yes, termly.

Everyone involved at this Centre will be respected and appreciated irrespective of gender, race, culture or disability.
Signed: *(tutor)*   **Signed** :*(student)*

Figure 2. Sample learning plan (general literacy skills).

Learning Plan

Name: John   **Date:** From September 19   **To:** July 17

A   **What do I need/want to learn?**

1   Memory techniques for recording batch numbers.
2   Multisensory strategies for spelling priority words for reports.
3   Reading skills for reading & understanding SOPs (Standard Operating
      Procedures).
4   Improve maths for internal tests (Numerical Estimation)
5   Follow instructions accurately.

B   **How much can I do already in these areas?**

- I can record 5 digit numbers well.
- I can spell the words that I use a great deal.
- I can read SOPs very slowly.
- I can add and subtract without carrying; I can use a calculator.
- I am quite good at visualising things.

C   **What skills and knowledge do I need; what steps do I need to take to achieve these goals?**

1   Learn how to chunk numbers, picture, then subvocalise and proofread.

2   Use multisensory strategies, particularly the 'Mind's Eye' spelling
      technique for learning 30 priority words for report writing.

3.1   SOPs: scanning skills to gain overview of document;
3.2   chunking long words, eg base word & suffix, syllables;
3.3   sightreading (flash cards for difficult irregular words;
3.4   using imagery to picture the procedures when reading;
3.5   creating diagrams from text.

4.1   Understand basic maths concepts - place value, decomposition, method of
      subtraction, decimals, percentages, using concrete operations ;
4.2   once understood, learn short cuts.

5.1   Learn assertiveness skills - *"can you repeat that/write it down/check I
      can do it please."*
5.2   Use 'rehearsal' skills to carry out instructions.
5.3   Make diagrammatic notes of instructions.

D   **What are the priorities?**

      Reading and understanding SOPs.

E   **What about materials?**

      The Multisensory Spelling Program MUSP (Lee).
      Worksheets for practising, recording batch numbers.
      ALBSU (BSA) Numeracy Pack, Deines Rods, 'Maths The Basic Skills (Greer)
      Worksheets for practising numerical estimation.

F   **We'll review your work after about a term and a half.**
      Would you prefer more often?   No

**Everyone involved at this Adult Basic Education Centre will be respected and appreciated,
irrespective of gender, race, culture or disability.**

Signed: (*tutor*)   **Signed** (*Student*)

Figure 3. Sample learning plan (for an employee in industry).

Learning Plan

Name: Ann   **Date:** From October 1st   **To:** June 12

A   What do I need/want to learn?

1   Improve general spelling ability.
2   Be able to spell confidently the words I use most commonly on my course.
3   Develop effective study skills - research reading.
4   Be able to write a good essay.
5   Become more organised at university.

B   How much can I do already in these areas?

- Can spell most regular simple words.
- Can read all but the most difficult words accurately.
- Know what I want to say in an essay.
- Can find my way to lectures, can write out a timetable.

C   What skills and knowledge do I need; what steps do I need to take to achieve these goals?

1.1 Know how to identify and use the 3 main syllable patterns ie: vccv, vcv and vv - be able to identify and spell vowel and consonant suffixes.
1.2 Be able to work out, using logic and rules, how to add these suffixes to base words.

2   Be able to spell confidently 30 words for study using multisensory spelling strategies.

3.1 Try out and evaluate the effectiveness of 3 research reading techniques
3.2 Use imagery.
3.3 Highlight keywords using colours for different categories, eg causes, main points etc.
3.4 Create mind maps from text.

4   Essay writing - analyse the question, selective reading, planning, organising ideas, drafting, proof reading.

5.1 Organisation; using colour/highlighting on timetable.
5.2 Developing an effective diary system.
5.3 Creating an assignment/essay timetable.

D   What are the priorities?

Essay writing.

E   What about materials?

DILP worksheets, Exercise Your Spelling (Elizabeth Wood), Use Your Head (Buzan), 'Get Sussed' Study Skills, Sunderland University, MUSP (Lee)

F   We'll review your work after about a term and a half.
Would you prefer more often?   No

Everyone involved at this Adult Basic Education Centre will be respected and appreciated, irrespective of gender, race, culture or disability.

Signed: *(tutor)*   **Signed:** *(Student)*

Figure 4. Sample learning plan (for a university undergraduate).

Teaching dyslexic adults requires:

- A good understanding of the nature of dyslexia; adult students need to know that you understand and can explain their difficulties to them;
- The ability to interpret psychologists' and specialist teachers' assessments, both to explain them to students and to use them for developing learning plans;
- The ability to design, deliver and evaluate a teaching program which takes into account all the adult's learning needs;
- An in-depth knowledge of spelling rules, reading strategies and also an ability to teach them in a multisensory way using a structured language program;
- An understanding of how vulnerable the dyslexic adult feels and an ability to balance listening with teaching;
- A sense of humor, delicately used, to help students come to terms with their difficulties;
- An understanding of the importance of over learning, no matter *how long it takes;* half-learned spellings will be half forgotten;
- The ability to explain repeatedly *why* a student has to learn in a multisensory way and that "saying it in your head" does not work. (This takes some doing!) "Selling the product" requires knowledge, confidence and persistence but learning *must* be multisensory or the adult will fail yet again.
- Enthusiasm for the teaching and respect for the learner.

6.1. Options for Teaching

If time is limited, it may be necessary to use what I would call the "bandaid approach". This would embrace teaching the adult how to use spell checks, voice activated computers, tape recorders, as well as readers and writers for exams.

I prefer to use a combination of both the "bandaid approach" and the "antibiotic approach": directly teaching students how to spell, read and study by using multisensory learning techniques. This usually results in greater independence in the long run.

7. TEACHING SPELLING

Teacher:	*"I'm sorry but I'm going to nag, until you practice that spelling in a multisensory way."*
Student:	*"It's great; I wish they'd nagged like this at school. I was put at the back of the class and told to 'color in'".*
Teacher:	*"Oh!"*

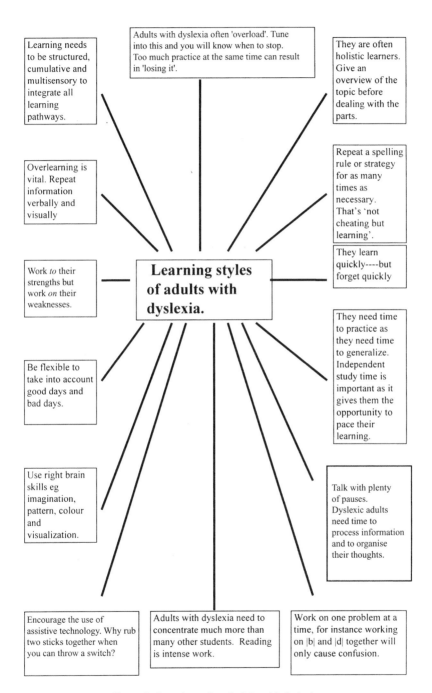

Learning needs to be structured, cumulative and multisensory to integrate all learning pathways.

Adults with dyslexia often 'overload'. Tune into this and you will know when to stop. Too much practice at the same time can result in 'losing it'.

They are often holistic learners. Give an overview of the topic before dealing with the parts.

Overlearning is vital. Repeat information verbally and visually

Repeat a spelling rule or strategy for as many times as necessary. That's 'not cheating but learning'.

Work *to* their strengths but work *on* their weaknesses.

Learning styles of adults with dyslexia.

They learn quickly----but forget quickly

Be flexible to take into account good days and bad days.

They need time to practice as they need time to generalize. Independent study time is important as it gives them the opportunity to pace their learning.

Use right brain skills eg imagination, pattern, colour and visualization.

Talk with plenty of pauses. Dyslexic adults need time to process information and to organise their thoughts.

Encourage the use of assistive technology. Why rub two sticks together when you can throw a switch?

Adults with dyslexia need to concentrate much more than many other students. Reading is intense work.

Work on one problem at a time, for instance working on |b| and |d| together will only cause confusion.

Figure 5. Learning styles of adults with dyslexia.

It is often difficult for the inexperienced adult dyslexia teacher, when faced with a highly articulate and intelligent but extremely dyslexic adult, to teach to the level of the *dyslexia* whilst, at the same time, acknowledging the level of *intelligence*.

7.1. Structured Programs

For a severely dyslexic student, use one of the structured multisensory language programs for example DILP (Walker 1993) or Write/Right to Read (Diggle Cornwall LEA) as a major element of each lesson.

However profuse apologies and explanations should accompany the giving of sentences to read and spell in the early stages of these programs. For example giving the sentence, "Pip sits in tins" can lead on to a discussion of Pip's mental faculties and his bizarre and worrying personal habits, once the sentence has been read, spelled and punctuated.

The reading and spelling cards routines which are an integral part of these programs will be accepted eventually;. . . . *"You want me to do what?!"*, ...if their value in developing *automaticity* is explained.

Careful and thorough explanations of syllable patterns need to be given if you as a teacher are not to be held personally responsible for the irregular vc/v syllable pattern (I have encountered many a reproachful glance when I have apologetically introduced *that* particular pattern.)

Structured multisensory programs are highly effective with adults, but it is vital to insist on a *full* multisensory approach and to build in work on phonological awareness. Remember to explain the theory at regular intervals or dyslexic students will forget.

7.2. Dealing with Priority Words

Although the structured programs are invaluable, they are rarely sufficient for the needs of an adult. There needs to be another systematic way to teach the words they need to spell most urgently. The spelling method described below (MUSP, Lee) has been found to be highly effective. When the method is used *exactly* as suggested, an 85% to 97% success rate on a long term basis can be achieved.

Appendix 1 sets out MUSP, the Multisensory Spelling Program for Priority Words in detail. It should be used as a *4 week* program, longer if necessary, but not shorter.

Some important points to bear in mind when using the MUSP spelling program:

- It is important to insist on adhering to *every* step so the student benefits fully from the multisensory techniques. For instance, emphasise

the reasons for always saying the *word* followed by the *strategy;* Students, when writing at work, will find the word comes into their heads and, if this process is used, the strategy will automatically "click in."
- The second stage in the Look Say; *Cover, Picture, Say;* Write Say; Check procedure is *extremely* important. Once the word and strategy have been *covered,* a student is usually anxious to write the word "before I forget it." By covering the word and strategy whilst working on them phonologically and visually they commit them to both auditory and visual memory. They also integrate the two modalities.
- Proof reading, using the strategy encourages students to check what they have written by "rehearsing" the strategy. They also gain a visual sense of "rightness" for the whole word.
- The systematic overlearning of lists is built into the program. It is crucial to retain old lists because they should always be learned using the same strategy.

Almost all our students report this program is the most effective way they have ever found of learning and retaining the miscellaneous priority words they need for everyday life. They find too, that with only a little practice, they can use this system independently.

7.3. Choosing Multisensory Spelling Strategies

As the examples in Appendix 1 show, it is important to use right brain skills to enhance the left brain skills when devising spelling strategies. Pattern, rhythm, pictures, imagination, images all help the automatization process. Students soon begin to identify their own best learning style and so develop metacognitive awareness.

Mind's Eye Spelling Technique

Visual learners often love to use this Mind's Eye Spelling Technique which I have adapted to learn words on the MUSP spelling lists. It should be used at the *Cover, Picture, Say* stage of the procedure.

Write out the word as a whole word and in chunks, e.g., **cirrhosis ci rr hosis**. Ask the student to study the chunked word, say the whole word then say all the letters or chunks, (depending on the length of the word). The student then looks away and makes a mental image of the chunked word in his or her "mind's eye" by saying the word a bit at a time and building up a mind picture of the word. For example *"ci ... double r .... hosis"*

Next, ask detailed questions about what he/she "sees" in the "mind's eye". For example, "what letter comes before the 'h'? ....'"; "what comes after the first 's'," etc. Do this for some time until both student and teacher are sure that the image is secure, then ask the student to spell it by "reading it off" from his mind's eye, both forward and backwards (it is usually surprisingly easy for visual learners to do this!). Finally ask the student to write the word (saying the letter names or chunks *as he/she writes them*) and then check against the original.

7.4. Some Other Approaches to Spelling

Adults whose dyslexic problems are not so severe may need a less structured spelling program. The LEAP Fast Track Spelling Program, Fig. 6, is one possible alternative. Despite its name, this program should never to be taken *too* fast. Work sheets and spelling exercises from a variety of sources can be used within this structure, and further spelling rules can be added as required.

Appendix 2 is an example of a spelling logic summary worksheet that can be used with adults. *Much* practice would be done with every stage, although it is helpful to give the student a holistic view, so that he can see the whole picture before working on each part. This logical approach can empower adults, enabling them to work out how to spell many words from first principles.

8. TEACHING READING

8.1. Word attack skills

Word attack skills can be taught using some of the logic described in Appendix 2. Students need to be able to break down the jumble of letters into recognizable chunks. They should, for instance, be able to spot the prefix or suffix at 40 paces!

8.2. Comprehension

8.2.1. Inference

Reading "comprehension" is sometimes misunderstood when it is taught.

For instance, having read this sentence *"The plund fell onto the gesbink"* you would have no difficulty in answering the question: *"Who fell onto the gesbink?"*, but would have no clear idea of what the sentence was about.

Take a sentence such as this, *"He put on his scarf and turned up his collar"*. A correct answer to the question, *"What did he do to his collar?"* may not necessarily show true comprehension, whereas a reasonable answer to this question; *"What do you think the weather was like?"* . . . would show a much deeper understanding of the text.

THE LEAP FAST TRACK SPELLING PROGRAMME
SOME SPELLING TERMINOLOGY, LOGIC & RULES

1 Terminology -
- 1a   Consonants, voiced and unvoiced & vowels
- 1b   Long and short vowel sounds
- 1c   Syllables, open & closed
- 1d   Base words
- 1e   Prefixes and suffixes
- 1f   Parts of speech (optional)

2 Vowel/consonant patterns -
- 2a   vc, eg hat
- 2b   vowel consonant vowel pattern (double vowel power) vcv eg hate

3 Syllable division - (link to double vowel power logic):
- 3a   Short vowel pattern - vc/cv - eg rabbit
- 3b   Long vowel pattern - v/cv - eg lupin
- 3c   Discrimination between long and short vowel pattern
- 3d   v/v eg diet

4 Suffixes (part 1)-
- 4a   Consonant suffixes
- 4b   Vowel suffixes - (i)   the doubling rule eg shopping
      (ii)   drop the 'e' rule eg hoping
      (iii)   ed saying (id), (t) or (d)

5 Useful Rules & Logic -
- 5a   One syllable words with short vowels ending in the sounds (l) (f) or (s) - 'floss' words
- 5b   The rules for the hard (k) sound -
      (i) 'c' or 'k' for the (k) sound at the beginning of words
      (ii) 'c' saying (k) at the end of 2 syllable words
      (iii) one syllabled words with short vowels ending in the (k) sound and spelled 'ck'
      (iv) 'c', 'k' or 'ck' inside words eg broken, locket, crocus
- 5c   vc/v (irregular) "robin" words
- 5d   words ending in 've', and the (j) sound

6 Suffixes (part 2)
- 6a   Suffixes with words ending in 'y'

7 Useful Rules & Logic
(part 2)
- 7a   'c' & 'g' rules - (i)   Soft 'c' & 'g' rule
      (ii) Adding suffixes to words ending in soft 'c' & 'g'
      (iii) 'd' as a wall to keep the vowel short eg hedge
- 7b   '-tch' eg match

8 Prefixes
- 8a   Prefixes
- 8b   Prefixes and suffixes - word segmentation
- 8c   Difficult prefixes

9 Useful Rules & Logic -
(Part 3)
- 9a   The 'wa' rule saying (wŏ) (link to 'qua' 'squa')
- 9b   Regular, final syllables - eg -ble, -tle, -cle, -dle etc (double vowel power logic again)
     -tion, -sion, -cian, saying (sh'n)
     -ture saying (chu)
- 9c   silent letters eg lamb, comb

10 Useful homophones
      eg to, too, two etc

Lee J

Figure 6. The LEAP Fast Track Spelling Programme. Spelling terminology, logic & rules.

Teaching these 'inference' skills where the answers have to be inferred from the text using keywords is a much better use of time than giving the type of 'comprehension' question which can be answered using innate grammatical knowledge.

8.2.2. Using a Dual Code and Imagery

Pat Lindamood (1997) suggests that the sensory system can be taught to use a "dual code" if students are encouraged to visualize and verbalize what they have read. Students start by visualizing and verbalizing a picture, then a given noun. They are next shown how to image a sentence and then a paragraph by reading it and visualizing it. They then place a colored square on the table as an "anchor" for the image, saying as they do so *"here I see . . . "*, describing what they see in their mind's eye. When they have finished reading they can recall the whole text by picking up each colored square in turn and saying *"Here I saw . . ."* this time translating from visual to verbal code. The text's main idea can then be retrieved by "seeing" what most of the colored squares are about. This technique develops skills such as inferring, summarizing, predicting and evaluating.

8.2.3. Keywords

Identifying and highlighting key words in a passage is a useful technique but it can be made much more effective if students are shown how to colour code, for example, red for names, green for evidence, yellow for examples and so on. Students can then read the key words to help them pull back the information they want to learn.

There are many other techniques that can be taught to aid comprehension. Some of these include using cloze passages; prediction exercises; learning new vocabulary; skimming and scanning; using "signal words" e.g., "in conclusion". They can also work with a friend, by reading and discussing alternate paragraphs; reading onto tape then playing back the tape and highlighting the text. They can use the SQ3R (Survey, Question, Read, Recall, Review) technique, they can prepare text before hand, by highlighting punctuation and phrases, they can work on difficult words and create mind maps from text (Buzan 1986)

9. A WORD ABOUT NUMBER

If teaching mathematics is a priority, a careful assessment will be needed to understand how adults are thinking and which concepts they do not fully understand. Teaching should always start with concrete operations which use language in a precise way so that, as Kibel says in *Dyslexia and Mathematics* (Miles, 1992)

"Language and manipulation work together in a mutually supportive way. . . . This is verbal labelling."

Dienes Rods (which come in ones, tens, hundreds and thousands, and seem to be acceptable to most adults) are one of the best tools to explore grouping, place value, addition with carrying and the decomposition method of subtraction. The precise language which is used while manipulating the rods, e.g., "I exchange 1 ten for 10 units and put them in the units column" is then transferred fairly effortlessly to the algorithm.

It is important, unless time is at a premium, to teach concepts and estimation skills before giving quick or trick ways of computation (mental arithmetic). This way the student feels in charge and should be more able to explore new ideas independently. Calculator skills should always be taught alongside and used for self checking.

10. FUNCTIONAL LITERACY

"I came here as a last resort; my business is growing and I have to get the wife to write all the checks."

"He (her husband) *tried to commit suicide. He thought he'd never have to read and write as a shepherd but then the Ministry gave him some forms to fill in. He pretended he'd lost his glasses and brought the forms straight home but he's terrified they'll find out."*

It is clearly of utmost importance that part of the teaching session should be used to address everyday needs.

A task analysis can be carried out for each problem area so the component skills and knowledge can be taught in a multisensory way.

For instance, writing a check involves:

- Understanding the layout of a check;
- Being able to write a signature consistently;
- A knowledge of the order of months of the year and their relationship to numbers or abbreviations;
- Knowing how to write numbers, as words and symbols (place value);
- Knowing words for checks, e.g., "only", and useful names;

All the spelling required for checks could be learned using MUSP (Lee J). Sequencing months and numbers can be taught using sequencing games and flip cards. Each flip card has a month on one side and the number on the other with a strategy if necessary. For example, the "O" in October could relate to the "0" in 10 and the "A" in April looks a bit like the "4" for the fourth month

April	4		October	10
front	back		front	back

The cards are then placed at random. The student reads aloud what is on one side and predicts what is on the other. Because the goal is to achieve automaticity the student is told to look on the other side immediately, if at all unsure.

Priorities for university students often include spelling, punctuation, multi-sensory revision techniques, presentation skills, essay writing, reading, notetaking, time management, exam techniques, and learning new vocabulary.

Appendix 3 shows a procedure for learning meanings, pronunciation and spellings of new vocabulary in a multisensory way. A phonological and visual representation of the word is created and linked to meaning. Motor memory for the word is then developed. This facilitates storage in long term memory.

11. MONITORING PROGRESS

Progress will need to be monitored accurately, so that both student and teacher can be convinced that, at last "it's working". Most adults need to know at regular intervals exactly where they are in a program and what skills they now possess. Ongoing progress can be monitored through discussion, tests, observation and assignments. Progress can be recorded in the appropriate section on the lesson plan during lessons. Always tell students what you are writing (see Fig. 7).

Reviews and Summative Assessments

Reviews and summative assessments should take place at intervals agreed with the student. They need to relate precisely to the targets set out in original learning plan. For example

September Learning target: to understand and be able to use the three main syllable patterns by March;

March Review of that target: I understand the three main syllable patterns. I can use them when I concentrate, but still forget when writing reports; (more practice needed).

September Learning target: to spell 20 priority words with confidence by May, using multisensory strategies (MUSP).

May Review of that target: I never forget how to spell 18 words, even when writing quickly (effective strategy is saying it as it's

Lesson Plan

AIMS:

1 To enhance short term memory.
2 To introduce letters 'a', 'd' & 'h' and the concept of open and closed syllables.
3 To develop multisensory spelling strategies for a new list of priority words.
4 Develop reading for meaning techniques using skimming, scanning & imagery.

Plan	Material	Comments/Action
1 Alphabet and sequencing work. Use alphabet arc to develop memory skills. Try 6 letters. Use chunking, semantic links & picturing. Use same system for tel numbers	1 Alphabet cards. Telephone directory	1 Found remembering 6 letters easy if they are chunked into 2 x 3. Tried same method with local numbers & it worked (6 again next week)
2 Practice reading & spelling packs	2 R & Sp packs	2 becoming automatic now.
3 give 'a', 'd' & 'h' reading & spelling cards with words and sentences to read & spell using these new letters.	3 New R & Sp cards 'a', 'd' & 'h' Worksheets for Module 2 (Right/Write to Read)	3 'a', 'd' & 'h' given (worksheet for homework)
4 Remind definition of syllable. Introduce idea of open & closed syllables. Play open & closed syllable pairs game. Give open & closed syllable to read and identify.	4 Open & closed syllable pelmanism game	4 Open & closed syllables understood, but will need more practice
5 Start MUSP list B–devise strategies for the words student. brings	5 Multisensory Spelling Program notes (MUSP)	5 Needed to be reminded of the full Look, Say, Cover, Picture, Say, Write & Say, Check process—left out 'cover, picture, say' bit (Check next week)
6 Show how to initially scan text for titles, headings key words—what's it about. Skim 1st para—what is it saying. Read each para, Stu to say what it is about & to create image in head. Use squares to anchor image then retell using squares.	6 Student's text. Coloured squares–dual code method	6 Found skimming very hard– needs to read every word. Loved imagery technique. Try again next week.
7 Review lesson		7 Quick recap on open & closed syllables.

Figure 7. An example of part of a lesson plan for a dyslexic adult.

spelled). I still occasionally get "business and sincerely" wrong.

12. A MODEL FOR DEVELOPING A DYSLEXIA POLICY IN INDUSTRY

It has been realized for some time that industry annually loses a great deal of money through some employees having difficulties with literacy and mathematical skills (CBI Conference London 1995). The issue of dyslexia in industry, however, is a separate one and requires more detailed attention than this chapter will allow. The benefits of addressing this issue can be immense both for the employer and the employee.

The key factor in creating a successful dyslexia policy in industry is the ability to development of a strong partnership between the company and the dyslexia specialists.

12.1. Awareness

A series of one day and half day dyslexia awareness seminars, run by the dyslexia specialists will enable team mangers and training coordinators to:

1. Understand the nature of dyslexia, become aware of some of its indications and see what it could feel like to be dyslexic at work.
2. Be able to identify people in their departments who maybe dyslexic;
3. Be able to approach these people in a nonthreatening and supportive manner.

12.2. Assessment

Assessment is a sensitive issue for the members of staff involved, and it must be undertaken by either an educational psychologist or a qualified specialist teacher. The assessment report should include:

1. A clear description of the extent and nature of the difficulties;
2. Detailed recommendations for a suitable learning program in relation to the nature of the work being done by the employee and the support required from the manager;
3. A statement as to who will have access to the report (issues of confidentiality must be discussed and agreed).

After assessment, and if the employee agrees, a specialist education program can be planned.

12.3. Information and Publicity

It is important, once key staff have taken part in dyslexia awareness training, to raise awareness amongst all employees. This is difficult in a large firm and needs to be seen as an ongoing task. One effective method is to hold regular, high profile "Enrolment Days" during which employees can meet the specialist teachers and key staff from the business informally to discuss general work-based literacy and arithmetic problems. These days provide a good platform for helping staff to become aware of the specific nature of, and difficulties related to, dyslexia.

12.4. Flexibility

It is very important that both partners in a dyslexia project are willing and able to respond to needs as they arise. Funding should be available to allow a dyslexia team to respond quickly to any need.

12.5. Outcomes

Team managers notice positive differences, both in the attitudes and skills of their dyslexic staff.

As awareness of dyslexia spreads, this allows more people in the workplace to understand and appreciate both the problems and the strengths of their dyslexic colleagues.

13. SOME SUGGESTIONS FOR A DYSLEXIA POLICY AT A UNIVERSITY

As with industry, three main threads combine to develop a successful dyslexia policy in university—staff awareness, identification, and teaching.

13.1. Staff Awareness

Staff awareness should be encouraged across all departments. If staff awareness courses are built into the university's annual staff development program and are available to all staff—lecturers, administrators, library staff, etc., this will gradually develop an awareness of the dyslexic student's problems and needs.

13.2. Identification

A screening, assessment, and counselling service should be available on site; ideally it should be funded by the university.

13.3. Teaching

Specialist tuition can be in the form of:

1. Group learning support sessions where topics such as essay writing, spelling note taking etc. are worked on;
2. One on one sessions with specialist teachers;
3. A dyslexia module. We have recently piloted this in the University of Sunderland in the UK. Students who were diagnosed as being dyslexic have the option of choosing dyslexia as one of their degree modules. The module we have developed is credited with 20 credit points for 150 hours of study. It is assessed by the specialist teachers on the presentation by the dyslexic student of a portfolio built up over 1 semester. Portfolio evidence includes an academic knowledge of dyslexia, the ability to plan learning, their development of essay writing skills, their ability to plan, deliver and evaluate a presentation, and their ability to use spelling strategies and multisensory learning skills for study. Lectures are given on the above topics as well as on dyslexia assessment, reading strategies, spelling, time management, exam techniques, punctuation and using technology.

It seems to be an exciting idea which may prove to be an effective way of developing the potential of dyslexic students at university.

14. CONCLUSION

This chapter explored some ways in which dyslexia can affect adults. It discussed only a small selection of the many teaching approaches and techniques which are available. Many dyslexic adults have experienced failure in the basic skills for years, so our job as teachers must be to create an environment where intellectual risks can be taken and success assured.

I will leave the last word to one of my talented dyslexia teachers who is herself dyslexic.

> *"I don't remember much about Infants and Juniors—mainly flashes. I can remember the initial excitement, the eagerness to learn—a clear memory of straying into Juniors, seeing maps on the wall and feeling excited that one day I'd be learning all about them.*
>
> *After that the feeling of dread creeps in—and the dreadful stomach pains, I ended up in hospital with suspected appendicitis eventually, but it wasn't that, I assume it was psychosomatic—I took little blue pills and they started saying I was "sensitive".*

I can remember insisting that the letters do move—and a teacher telling me it was nonsense, and I can remember how bewildered I felt when it dawned on me that it did make sense to the rest, and how frightened I was that they might find out.

The last memory of Juniors was sitting on the school steps the day my year took the 11 Plus—just two of us had been excluded. The other girl played in the sun; I stayed on the steps—out of sight.

Strange, I never cried then, never, but I can now."

REFERENCES

Journals

Cornelissen, P., Richardson, A., Mason, A., Fowler, S., & Stain, J. (1995). *Contract sensitivity and coherent motion detection measured at photopic luminance levels in dyslexics and controls.* Vision Research 35, 1483–1494.

DeFries, J.C., & Light, J.G. (1996). *Twin studies of reading disability.* In J.H. Beitchman, H. Cohen, M.M. Konstantareas & R. Tannock (Eds.) *Language, Learning and Behavior Disorders.* New York: Cambridge University Press.

Galaburda, A. (1989). *Ordinary and extraordinary brain development: Anatomical variation in developmental dyslexia.* Annals of Dyslexia 39, 67–79. Baltimore Orton Dyslexia Society.

Hulme, C. and Snowling, M., (1991). *Phonological deficits in dyslexia: A 'sound' reappraisal of the verbal deficit hypothesis?* In N. Singh & I. Beale (eds.), *Progress in Learning Disabilities.* Berlin: Springer-Verlag.

Lindamood, P., Bell, N., and Lindamood, P. (1997). *Sensory Cognitive Factors in the Controversy over Reading Instruction.* Journal of Developmental and Learning Disorders 1, No. 1.

Livingstone, M., Rosen, G.D., Drislane. F. & Galaburda. A., (1991). *Physiological evidence for a magnocellular defect in developmental dyslexia.* Proceedings of the National Academy of Sciences, 88, 7943–7947

Lovegrove, W.J., Garzia, R.P., & Nicholson, S.B. (1990). *Experiential evidence of a transient system deficit in reading disability.* Journal of the American Optometric Association 61 137–146.

Nicolson, R.I. & Fawcett, A.J., (1995). *Dyslexia is more than a phonological disability.* Dyslexia: An International Journal of Research and Practice 1, 19–37.

Paulesu. E., Frith. U., Snowling. M., Gallagher. A., Morton. J., Frackowiak. R., Frith. C., (1996). *Is Developmental Dyslexia a Disconnection Syndrome? Evidence from PET Scanning.* Brain (1996). 119. 143–157.

Rack, J.P., & Snowling, M.J. (1985). *Verbal Deficits in Dyslexia: A Review.* In M.J. Snowling (ed.), *Children's Written Language Difficulties Assessment and Management.* Windsor: NFER-Nelson.

BOOKS AND TESTS

Burt, A., (1983). *A Guide to Better Punctuation.* Cheltenham. Hodder & Stoughton.

Buzan, T., (1986) *Use Your Memory.* London. BBC.

Diggle, Cathy (1996). *Write/Right to Read,* 4th Edition. St Austell Cornwall. Link into Learning.

Dunn, L., Dunn, L., Whetton, C., Burley, J., (1997). *The British Picture Vocabulary Scale.* Windsor. NFER Nelson.

Evans, A. J., (1987). *Reading & Thinking.* Wolverhampton. Learning Materials Ltd.

Fawcett, A.J., & Nicolson, R I., *Dyslexia Adult Screening Test* London. The Psychological Corporation.

Fawcett, A J., & Nicolson, R.I., (1994) *Dyslexia in Children, Multidisciplinary Perspectives.* London. Harvester Wheatsheaf.

Gardner, M.F. (1992) *TVPS-UL Test of Visual, Perceptual Skills* U.S.A. Psychological & Educational Publications Inc.

Goswami, U., & Bryant, P., (1990). *Phonological Skills and Learning to Read.* Hove: Laurence Erlbaum.

Hulme, C., & Snowling, M., (1997). *Dyslexia, Biology Cognition and Intervention.* London. Whurr Publishers Ltd.

Klein, C., (1993). *Diagnosing Dyslexia.* London. ALBSU (now the Basic Skills Agency)

Lindamood, P. and Lindamood, P. *LiPs Trainer's Manual.* Gander Publishing.

Llewellyn, S., & Greer, A., (1983). *Mathematics, the Basic Skills.* Cheltenham. Stanley Thornes Ltd.

McLoughlin, Fitzgibbon & Young, (1994). *Adult Dyslexia Assessment, Counselling & Training.* London. Whurr Publishing Ltd

Miles, T. R. (1982). *Bangor Dyslexia Test.* University College of North Wales, Bangor. LDA Duke Street Wisbech Cambs England

Miles, T.R., & Miles, E., *Dyslexia and Mathematics.* Routledge (1992)

Neale, M. D. (1989). *Neale Analysis of Reading Ability.* Windsor Berkshire England. NFER Nelson.

Raven, J.C., Court, J.H., & Raven, J. (1994) *Raven's Progressive Matrices* Oxford England. Oxford Psychological Press.

Raven, J.C., Court, J.H., & Raven, J. (1980) *Mill Hill Vocabulary Scale* Oxford England. Oxford Psychological Press.

Rosner, J. (1993) *Helping Children Overcome Learning Difficulties* - 3rd edition. New York. Walker & Company

Snowling, M.J., (1985) *Children's Written Language Difficulties* Windsor Berkshire England. NFER-Nelson

Turner, M. (1997). *Psychological Assessment of Dyslexia.* London. Whurr Publishers Ltd.

Vinegrad. *Adult Dyslexia Checklist.* London. Adult Dyslexia Organisation.

Walker, J., Brooks, L., (1993). *The Dyslexia Institute Literacy Program (DILP)* London. London, James & James Ltd.

Wilkinson, G., (1993) *Wide Range Achievement Test* (WRAT) Wide Range Inc. Wilkington, Delaware.

Wood, E., (1982). *Exercise Your Spelling.* Sevenoaks. Hodder & Stoughton.

APPENDIX 1

MUSP

THE MULTISENSORY SPELLING PROGRAMME

FOR PRIORITY WORDS

How to learn the words **YOU** need in a systematic way, so that they are retained in your longterm memory.

In other words, you can **always** remember how to spell them.

WHAT TO DO

WEEK 1

1   Choose a list of 5 to 15 words that **you** need to spell, eg words for work, forms, letters, study etc.

2   Call that list '**A**' and date it.

3   Write the words on the left hand side of the page, as <u>whole</u> words in joined up writing.
On the right hand side of the page, print the word showing the <u>strategy</u> you've chosen.

   Note   (i)   Strategies must be multisensory - seeing, hearing and feeling.
          (ii)   They must address the bits of the word you have got wrong, for instance:

permanent	perma frost at Nent Head
necessary	1 collar & 2 socks (1c & 2s's)
architect	arch i tect
	(visual clue & you say it as it's spelt)
solicitor	sol ICI tor
	(see a symmetrical pattern)
opportunity	op port unity
	(split up double consonants auditorily & visually & find hidden words)
queue	q ue ue (say it in rhythm)
specific	spec if ic
always	al ways one flag

....get the idea?

Fiddle about with a few strategies until you find one that clicks for <u>you.</u>

Important - once you've decided on a strategy, **stick to it.**
Your teacher will probably have to suggest strategies to start with, but gradually
you'll take over because **you** know which ones work best for **you.**

4   Now use the 'LOOK, SAY, ...COVER PICTURE SAY,.... WRITE, SAY,...
CHECK' method to practise.

(i)   LOOK at the word and study the strategy;
SAY the word then say the strategy;
(ii)   COVER the word and the strategy;
SAY the word, then say the strategy; PICTURE the strategy;
(iii)   WRITE the word as a <u>whole</u> word, in joined up writing.....but....
SAY the strategy <u>as</u> you write it - <u>tell</u> your hand what to write.
(iv)   CHECK - letter by letter to see if it's right.

(Don't leave out any stage)
Always practice writing the word as a whole, using
joined up writing - it develops your motor (muscle) memory.

**   <u>During the week</u> - Practise at least a couple of times using the 'Look, Say,...
Cover Picture Say,..... Write, Say,.... Check' method.

WEEK 2

1   Go over each word and <u>relearn</u> the strategies with your teacher (Always use the
above method.)

2   Let your teacher test you like this: she/he says the word, you <u>repeat</u> the word,
then say the strategy. Write the word, saying the strategy <u>as you write it.</u>

Don't write it until you can think of the strategy. If you've forgotten,
look and say - that's "not cheating but learning".

3   Afterwards **you** look at your test (<u>without</u> the original) and <u>proofread</u> it for errors.
Look at the word, say the strategy; have you written what the strategy says?

4   Then look at the original and mark it.

<u>During the week</u> - Yes, you've guessed it - practise using the above LS, CPS,
WS, C method.

(Week 2 can be repeated as often as necessary if you haven't had time to practise at
home.)

WEEK 3

Ask your teacher to test you 'cold' without looking first at the list . Remember-**You** proofread first, then check with original.

<u>During the week</u> - practise using the same LS, CPS, WS, C method.

WEEK 4

1   Your teacher will dictate the words you've learnt by putting them into sentences - she says the sentence, you repeat it, write it and proofread it.

2   Start List B - choose new words that have cropped up at work or college and add any words that you're not quite sure of, from list '**A**'. Use *exactly* the same system for learning this new list.

Remember

*   Both you and your teacher need to keep a copy of each list and the strategies used. Also keep a record of which list you're working on and what week of the list, eg:

    7 Oct   start List '**A**'

    14 Oct   List '**A**' (Week 2)

    28 Oct   List '**A**' (Week 3)

    4 Nov   Dictate List '**A**' - Start List '**B**'

*   After about 2-3 months, whilst learning a new list thoroughly, you should relearn an earlier list and be tested on both. (Keep a record of which lists have been relearnt and when.)

<u>All</u> old lists need to be systematically relearnt, about 2-3 months after they were first learnt.

This method really *works*. You'll find you can spell the words **you** need surprisingly quickly - **<u>and you won't forget them</u>**!

Lee J

APPENDIX 2

DOUBLE VOWEL POWER & SUFFIXING LOGIC

There is a lovely logic to these ideas that helps **us** to feel in charge of spelling, rather than **spelling** being in charge of **us**.

These are the vowels:

> a   e   i   o   u   and sometimes   y

Vowels can be long:

eg:	$\bar{a}$	$\bar{e}$	$\bar{i}$	$\bar{o}$	$\bar{u}$
as in	plate	these	kite	hope	cute

or short:

eg:	ă	ĕ	ĭ	ŏ	ŭ
as in	hat	pet	pip	hop	cut

y   acts like a vowel if it sounds like a vowel

eg:	happy	($\bar{e}$) or (ĭ)
	cry	($\bar{i}$)

All the other letters are consonants.

Double Vowel Power

Look at this word and listen: $n\bar{o}$

The vowel is **long** because there's no consonant wall, so the vowel can go on for as long as you've got breath to say it.

now look at listen to this word: nŏt

The vowel is **short** because the consonant is acting like a wall and blocking it from going on and on: nŏt

If you want to say **"note"** you need a way of lengthening the vowel, whilst still keeping the (t) sound at the end of the word, so we use:

Double Vowel Power
note double vowel power in action!

> note

Here the 'e' in **"note"** is giving the 'o' extra power to break down the consonant wall and become long.

However double vowel power only works if there's just **one** consonant wall between the vowels.

eg: **lōcal**   (double vowel power in action)

     cŏtton   (double vowel power can't work)

This idea works quite well in many words, but there **are** exceptions, it must be admitted:

eg: in **rŏbin**   there should by rights 2 consonant walls...

but......it works like a dream when adding suffixes...............watch...........

A Suffix

is a letter, or group of letters, added to a base word.

You can get 2 kinds of suffixes:

1   **Consonant Suffixes:** start with a consonant

eg:	**ly**	**less**	**ful**	**s**
	ness	**ment**	**some**	

2   **Vowel Suffixes:** start with a vowel

eg:	**ing**	**ed**	**able**	**age**	**er**

ALL suffixes come, I like to imagine, in packages and you can't alter them, eg:

    (ly) is always spelt **ly**, there's never an 'e' in it.

        '**ful**' is always spelt with one '**l**'

        and '**ness**' with **2** 'ss'

Do *not* disturb a suffix!

Let's look at suffixing logic

Consonant suffixes

We'll deal with **consonant** suffixes first because they're so easy.

All you have to do with consonant suffixes is **just**...

add them on to the end of a base word (the original word)

If you **know** how to spell the word & you **know** how to spell the suffix....

it's **easy** - eg: **love** + **ly** = **lovely**

hope	+	ful	=	hopeful
faith	+	ful + ly =		faithfully
manage	+	ment	=	management

There is only **one** exception and that's when the base word ends in **'y'**, but that's

another story!

Vowel suffixes

But with **vowel** suffixes, you can use the **double vowel power** logic.

Look at this word   hŏp

Now add the vowel suffix   **'ing'** - hop + ing

If we just add the: **'ing'** we'd get 'hōping' -

we'd get double vowel power working - hōping has a long (ō) sound.

So we must have **2 consonant walls** to keep the vowel short, eg:

$$hop + p + ing = hŏpping$$

So that double vowel power can't work

Now look at **'bite'** and think about adding the vowel suffix **'ing'**

bīte + ing

What is the **'e's** job in the base word **'bīte'** ?

Yes - double vowel power -

it's lengthening the **'i'** and without it, you'd have **'bĭt'**; a short (ĭ).

But we've already got a **vowel** that will do the job just as well in the vowel suffix

'ing'.

You never need **triple** vowel power so:

you must drop the **'e'** :   bīt e + ing

and add the vowel suffix <u>bīting</u> and *double vowel power*

keeps the **'i'** long. Here are some more:

$$wāke +   ing   =   wāking$$

make + ing = māking

bike + ing = bīking

Try some yourself :   *it works!*

Take suffixing a step further - look at and listen to the 'c' & 'g' in these words:

cat, cup, certain, circle, cycle, gone, guess, general, gist, gypsy

You can hear that if a 'c' or a 'g' is followed by an 'e', 'i' or 'y' they sound soft **(s)** and **(j).**

In **'manage'** the 'e's job is to soften the 'g' and in **'notice'** the 'e' softens the 'c'.

If you want to add a suffix to these words, and the suffix <u>**starts**</u> with an 'e', 'i' or 'y', you won't need to keep the 'e' at the end of the base word.

However, if the suffix <u>doesn't</u> start with an 'e', 'i' or 'y' you must keep the 'e' to keep the 'c' or 'g' soft.

Look: **manage   +   ing   =   managing**

manage   +   able   =   manageable

manage   +   ment   =   management

notice   +   ing   =   noticing

notice   +   able   =   noticeable

Try some more, easy, isn't it?..........well, <u>quite</u> easy!

APPENDIX 3

Multisensory Meanings

This exercise is a good way for dyslexic students to learn quickly the meanings, pronunciations and spellings of the new words that crop up at university.

1   Divide your page lengthways into 3 columns. Label the columns.

2   In column 1, write the whole word;

In column 2, write the word, split up into chunks, so that it's easy to say (pictures help);

In column 3, write the meaning (look it up or ask!) Work on about 5 - 10 words at a time.

eg:

It looks like this:	It sounds like this:	It means this:
litigation	(shun) lit iga tion	"to go to law"

3   (i)   Now LOOK at the word in column 1

(ii)   then LOOK at the word in column 2 and SAY it slowly, then quickly.

(iii)   SAY the definition in column 3.

(iv)   COVER the whole line, PICTURE it, SAY the word and the

definition out loud.

(v)   WRITE the word as a whole word but SAY it in chunks as you write;

(your mouth tells your hand what to write).

(vi)   CHECK letter by letter to see if you've got it right.

* Do this exercise with each word about twice a week until you are confident you know both spelling and meaning.

13

The Dyslexic Child at School and Home

Wendy Goldup and Christine Ostler

1. THE DYSLEXIC CHILD IN SCHOOL

1.1. Introduction

The dyslexic child must be *at the heart* of the classroom action. Too often he feels he is an outsider in his own classroom and his peer group, alienated and marginalized.

He will have known before anyone else does that he is "different." He feels clever but is not always able to show it. He has inconsistencies in his behavior that he finds puzzling. He feels bright in some areas and mystified in others. Language (instructions and talk) rushes by too fast and has pieces missing. Often he has a good grasp of the concept—frequently ahead of his peers—but his ability to produce a verbal response is patchy. His writing attempts are often disastrous; neither verbal nor written responses ever match what is inside his head.

He feels embarrassed that he cannot remember a simple sequence of instructions. He's bothered that he answers with the wrong words, that he cannot look and listen, or listen and write at the same time. He is bewildered and wonders "Why is this happening to me?"

The majority of his peers might consider him "dopey" because he can't get the rules of a game or talk about things in the same way as they do. They might

Wendy Goldup, The Dyslexia Institute, 32 Avebury Avenue, Tonbridge, Kent TN9 1UA, United Kingdom   Christine Ostler, The Garden Flat, Cobham Hall, Cobham, Kent DA12 3BL, United Kingdom

delight in his spoonerisms, encourage his acting up, and deify his anarchic be-havior. But at the end of the day, they will choose to pair up or play with someone who thinks more like they do.

His teacher will be puzzled by the erratic nature of his behavior and output, his good days and bad days. She will be irritated to find a word spelled correctly one day misspelled the next, let alone in the same piece of work. She might feel anxious that she doesn't know how to deal with a dyslexic student, that she hasn't had appropriate training. She might be willing to try some interventions at Stage one of the Code of Practice (1994) (See Appendix 1), but when the child moves to Stage two or three, she may feel that he has now become the province of the spe-cial needs team, special educational needs coordinator (SENCO), a special edu-cation teacher, or a learning support assistant (LSA) and may lessen her interactions. She may even expect him not to listen in class because she believes the support person will do it for him. When addressing the whole class she may not expect the child and support person to stop and listen too. This adds to the child's feeling that he is outside the action, marginalized, that the party is happen-ing elsewhere.

The learning support assistant might have little or no training and find her-self in support of someone she doesn't understand and can't follow. She may feel ill equipped to help. In a worst case scenario, she can find herself responsible for a large part of the dyslexic child's education. Even when well directed by the teacher she may often know what the child is to *do* but not what the child is to *learn,* causing empty experiences for the child. He will know inside himself that he hasn't improved, that he hasn't done it himself. He has a very thin grasp of what went on.

When the school works in partnership with parents and keeps them well in-formed, then failures that occurred during the day are carried home and the child has to suffer them again. Badly targeted homework can become a source of family friction, as can hesitant, labored reading, awful presentation, and paucity of output.

In school, in friendships, and even at home the dyslexic child can feel out of his depth, out of control and helpless.

Extrinsic rewards are often in evidence in the classroom: team points, mar-bles in a jar, stars, joyful letters sent home and so on. These have a limited life for most children—and particularly for the dyslexic child, who still feels different. He knows that, for him, it is not making an effort that counts but making the right kind of effort.

Reward and sanction systems may have been tried with the dyslexic child—more often than with anyone else, by different people for different reasons. These sanctions may result in *continuous* extrinsic motivation that reduces the child's be-lief of being in control of his own destiny. They may undermine the very thing teachers and parents want for children: intrinsic motivation, wanting to do well for its own sake, to manage one's own time and learning, and the good and positive self-esteem that comes with this success.

Other factors that undermine intrinsic motivation (Deci and Ryan, 1985) are:

- Negative feedback: "I can't read this," "Your spelling is awful," "Answer the question!"
- Unpredictable outcomes: *All* words on the spelling test graded, in red, as being wrong; or no words marked, but there is a single check on the paper, so that child is unsure whether or not "I got it right" or what parts he got correct. He will also be dealing with unpredictable outcomes in his own performance, good and bad days, fluctuating hearing ability, fluctuating perception of shapes and sounds, erratic mastery over his pen or pencil.
- Imposed deadlines: Things having to be done, or turned in to the teacher by a certain time when often the student needs more time. Room changes involving packing and repacking of bags, or selecting correct books and equipment will be hugely unsettling.
- Continuous surveillance of performance; the more he fails, the closer he is watched by his teacher, learning support assistant, or someone else. He may be moved closer and closer toward the teacher's desk, singled out as a problem.
- Mismatched and misgrouped (Moyles, 1997) with children who have other learning difficulties and do not match his intellectual level; these are children who are singled out as having "special needs."

The child who feels alienated for any of these reasons may attempt to gain respect from himself and his peers by making his behavior look intentional. His subconscious choice of self-preservation might be indifference, avoidance, non-cooperation, defiance, disruption, or withdrawal. He may very quickly "rise" through the school's behavior process to become the worst behaved boy in the class, group, or the ultimate accolade—school.

1.2. The Teacher's Role

The teacher's role begins with an understanding of the strengths and weaknesses of this erratic, disorganized character who is her dyslexic student. She must consider the underlying difficulty, the creation of a hospitable environment, physical and emotional, and finally the provision of teaching methods and strategies which will enable the child to become a successful learner in all areas of the curriculum.

Above all, the dyslexic child must be in the center of, *at the heart of,* the action. He must be fully included and fully integrated. He must be taught the curriculum by the teacher and have his work differentiated by her. He must be given discreet help from support personnel working in the classroom. This should be similar in amount and nature to support given to other children in the class for different reasons and general help given to any member of the class at any time for any reason.

In ideal circumstances the dyslexic child will participate in a specifically targeted literacy program delivered by a special education teacher. This should be tied in tightly to what is happening in the classroom, where he will spend the majority of his time, so that the class teacher knows what he has learned and what he is currently learning. In this way, she and the support staff help with reinforcement and overlearning to ensure maximum success and to convince the child that everyone is working together for him. Information should also flow from the class teacher to the special education teacher, so that the latter knows what topics, concepts, programs are being worked on at any particular time in class. She can then help the child with metacognitive and study strategies (see Chapter 9).

1.3. Organizing the Physical Environment

The dyslexic child should face the front of the room and have as few distractions as possible between him and the teacher. He should sit close enough to be able to gain information from facial expressions, lip shape, body gestures and language, but not so close that he feels under constant surveillance and "separate" from his peers. Thus the teacher should use the following strategies for gaining and sustaining the child's attention. These will be helpful for the whole class and be lifesavers for the dyslexic child.

1.3.1. Gaining Attention

To ensure all children are ready to listen and learn, wait for quiet and attentiveness from *all* the children in the group, including any child receiving help from another adult. The assisting adult can serve as a good model of watching and listening.

1.3.2. Ensuring Successful Input

Saying "Listen" rarely works because some children not only do not understand what is expected of them, but they do not know what listening means. Active listening strategies should be used in the classroom. Children should be taught the steps involved in listening. This could take the form of a visual aid that lists instructions something like:

- Sitting still
- Hands still
- Eyes watching
- Ears listening
- Brain waiting
- Brain thinking

Put the visual aid up high enough for the whole class or group to see. Walk over and touch it as you ask everyone to listen and then remind them of the steps involved. Tell the children that "brain waiting" means to be alert and attentive to what you are about to say while "brain thinking" means to run your words through their own brains, listening to them again and thinking about them. Using a well-paced talk or set of instructions with plenty of pauses will help this process.

Children for whom listening and attending is a particular problem might like to make their own "listening card" by writing down the previously given list and drawing their own illustrations to make it memorable. Or they might make a small card with the words "brain waiting" and add a suitable quirky illustration. When told to listen, they could actually pick up their card to signal the teacher "I am ready."

1.3.3. Structuring Input

The responsibility for obtaining and sustaining children's attention rests with the teacher, not the child. Three simple steps will preview, provide information, and then review the main points to ensure maximum success for the listener.

- Say what you are going to say.
- Say it.
- Say what you have said.

This will give children a preview of the main points they must listen out for. It will also help them become ready to receive the information and enable them to process their own understanding of it. Adding a further summary for the dyslexic child, using ten words or fewer, will help him secure the information or instruction (Sawyer, 1991). An outstanding way of ensuring the child has received the information correctly is to get him to say it back to you. Get him to summarize the information or repeat the instruction. Thus he will run the information around his own articulatory loop and have a much better chance of remembering it. Bear in mind that "in some circumstances such as verbal instructions, children almost inevitably appear to believe we mean everyone else in the room except them, so it is as well to ensure that for this, and other reasons, the children have opportunities to reiterate their perception of the task" (Kyriacou, 1997).

When you expect an answer from a dyslexic child you must increase the time you are prepared to wait so he may answer confidently and successfully. Sawyer (1991) tell us the average wait time for any child should be five seconds; the dyslexic child will need longer. Either tell the whole class in a relaxed and encouraging way, that you are prepared to wait for anyone to answer, or you can give the dyslexic child prior warning. For example: "Joe is going to tell us about places where we might find eagles, and then I want *you* to describe them to us."

1.3.4. Grouping

> It is best to avoid any situations where children's "academic" standing is made obvious to others as this can affect self image on both sides (Burns, 1982)

Does anyone seriously believe that calling groups "Green" and "Red," or "Hearts" and "Diamonds" masks who's who? It fools no one, not the children and definitely not the dyslexic children, whose senses in these matters are always sharp.

Many studies have shown the advantages of small group work. The dyslexic child can benefit fully from this type of situation if his class teacher makes sure he is not carried away by extraneous stimuli and lost in time, space, and purpose.

> Studies of small group work have indicated that its effectiveness is enhanced when the teacher shows skill in handling and understanding groups, gives a positive lead before the group work begins, and follows up the group work by pooling the discussion and giving feedback on the work produced. (Kyriacou, 1997)

The National Numeracy (1997 draft) and Literacy (DfEE, 1998) strategies are clearly founded on the same pattern: Teacher-led whole class work, differentiated group work and a plenary to draw ideas together.

Dyslexic children, like other children, need to be with children of mixed abilities and personalities so that group work can be dynamic. The children can bounce ideas about, making equal use of the good reader, the good logical thinker, the good recorder, the good ideas person, so that everyone gets a chance to shine and have their weaknesses supported by the group. Otherwise, why have groups?

The arrangement of classroom furniture needs to be flexible so that children are always focused on the teacher whether she is at the front of the room, or the center of their group. A routine should be established so that all children know where desks and chairs should be placed for any particular activity and can move them there quickly and sensibly.

The teacher will need to explain to the dyslexic child *what* is being investigated, *how* it is to be tackled, i.e., *what* stages to follow and in *what* order and finally *what* the expected outcome is. She should use the tactic previously described of requesting repetition of the instructions, not once but several times, from different members of the class or group, one of whom should be the dyslexic child. If the whole class knows the teacher is going to employ this strategy regularly, they will sharpen up their listening skills.

1.4. Organization in Time and Space

Make routines and regular activities visual wherever possible. An illustrated timetable for the week displayed prominently will help enormously, particularly if the teacher frequently talks the children through it. The children could also make one of their own, with their own illustrations and color coding. This could take the form of either a weekly plan or a daily plan and certainly a homework timetable (Figure 1), and would be much more meaningful to them.

Help to organize bag, books, folders, worksheets by using color coding, filing, storage systems, in–out trays for work, etc. will help to orient the dyslexic child spatially.

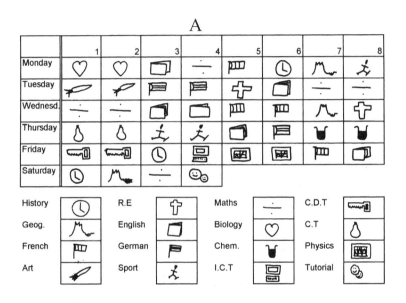

Figure 1A. Homework timetable; 1B Home-to-school timetable.

The teacher or LSA should have five sharp pencils about her at the start of every day. She can swiftly exchange a blunt or leadless pencil for a working one, and replace a missing one without much fuss or disruption.

1.5. Differentiating Input

Differentiation can be done in many ways. It does not mean having to make six different worksheets. It does not mean making the activity so transparent and easy that an amoeba could do it! It usually means changing something slightly, fine-tuning it, so that it can be thought about in a different way and grasped by someone who has not grasped it yet.

Much differentiation will have been done at the input stage if the advice of this chapter has been followed so far. Examples this chapter has given of differentiation include furnishing the dyslexic child with a listening card, summarizing information or instructions given to the dyslexic child as the task begins, increasing waiting time for response, etc. The teacher can also adjust her input to facilitate clearer reception by using different words, different examples, by modeling, by demonstrating, by pausing at intervals and rounding up comprehension, by giving children time and opportunity to reflect on their thoughts on the matter. Holt (1991) suggests that children should

> live with an idea or insight for a while, turn it around in some part of their minds, before they can . . . discover it, say "I see", take possession of the idea, and make it their own.

By so doing, children learn to make the experience greater than superficial "parrot learning" and learn how to assimilate and ultimately use this experience.

1.5.1. Multisensory Input

Truly multisensory experiences that maximize learning should be applied to every part of the child's education. Differentiated input, linked visually, auditorily, oral–kinesthetically, and manual–kinesthetically will then make information and instruction as secure as possible. Of course it is not always possible to have one, several or many children *physically* engaged at all times. However physical interaction can take place in the imagination.

Visualization is a technique that is useful in all areas of the curriculum: history, geography, biology, art, or English, and a vital one for mathematics and spelling. Have the children close their eyes and picture a scene. Tell them to imagine they are there, speaking and doing. Ask them to imagine what they might be feeling, to imagine what might happen next. Encourage children as often as possible to use this technique.

1.6. Help with Processing

1.6.1. Metacognition

The dyslexic child's disorganization is evident in his physical persona. It undermines his ability to keep track of books, pencils, and pieces of paper. It prevents him from keeping his book bag, his desk, or his room tidy. It lurks unseen and plays havoc with his thinking, planning, hypothezising, and testing, and even his storage and retrieval processes, all of which need help, through support and strategies, if he is to succeed.

Metacognitive strategies (based on Flavell, 1979), usually acquired from experience by nondyslexic students, will require specific teaching. For other students, these strategies tend to be implicit and internalized, but for the dyslexic child they have to be made explicit and externalized, that is, turned into language which can be spoken, listened to, and thought about.

Examples of this externalization in thinking and planning are:

- Establishing purpose
  What is the purpose of this activity?
  Why am I doing it?
  Am I reading for pleasure, information, or for a comprehension test?
- Determining outcome
  What will my work look like when I have finished?
- Marshaling relevant previous knowledge
  What do I already know?
  Have I seen anything like this before?
  Are these the Vikings we talked about last week?
- Determining an appropriate strategy
  How shall I tackle this?
  What works for me?
- Monitoring for success
  How did it go?
  Could I have done it differently/better?
- Ensuring further improvement
  How can I take this further?
  What have I learned that will help me next time?
- Transfer to other aspects of learning
  Can I do the same thing in math, history, etc?

At the "determining appropriate strategy" stage, children will need help to discover whether they learn better through auditory, visual, or kinesthetic channels.

Teachers can help them to find out by presenting information in the three different ways and discussing with the child which was most successful.

Teachers should know, and make use of, the child's preferred modality for learning, but at the same time teach the child how to translate from one to the other whenever he needs to. The child who learns best by watching, when given a verbal instruction needs to visualize, i.e., make pictures in his mind of that information. The child who learns best by listening, must learn to "talk himself through" visual information i.e. describe it silently to himself in words.

Most people learn best by actually doing, but this is not always possible. Therefore the child has to learn to "do in his mind." He needs to imagine himself in the situation, picture himself interacting, and then think about how he would feel and act.

At each of the previously described metacognitive stages, dyslexic children will need explicit help. They will need to think about each stage and pose their own questions. They will initially need to be helped to do this but ultimately they must learn to do it for themselves.

A cue card, made by the child, will help him keep these processes under review until he has assimilated them and no longer needs it (Figure 2).

Thinking–planning frameworks where the child can actually note his ideas are also useful (Figure 3). A framework can be made to fit any situation as part of the teacher's differentiation for the dyslexic child. It should be noted however that any framework given is *not* a worksheet; filling in the frame with thoughts and ideas is a beginning point for thinking and writing, not an end in itself.

Differentiated help to put thoughts and ideas into a framework can be given. This can range from full support from an adult, acting as scribe, to minimal

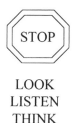

LOOK
LISTEN
THINK

What day is it?
Where am I going?
What do I need?
Where can I find it?
Who can help me?

Figure 2. Cue card used to support metacognitive strategies.

guidance, with a view to the student completing a framework by himself and eventually creating them for himself to fit a particular situation.

1.6.2. Help with Processing: Memory

The dyslexic child will need a great deal of help to gain control over this most slippery and elusive of functions. How well all children remember what they are taught in school depends on the following:

- How meaningful the information is to them
- How that information is laid down in the first place
- How the new information is linked to previous learning
- How often the learning is revisited

Structuring input and making learning real and relevant, as already discussed, together with metacognitive strategies will make a great deal of difference to the dyslexic child's understanding, retention, and retrieval of information.

Laying down information piece by piece, linking new information to existing information, e.g. "We were looking at which group of people last week?" "And they lived in . . . ?" "And obtained food by . . . ?" will provide hooks for the child to hang new information on rather than let it drift into oblivion.

Links between subjects will also be helpful. Many National Curriculum subjects are designed to overlap to facilitate this process (National Curriculum, 1995). Bear in mind that for the dyslexic child, those skills and rules, which for some are implicit, need to be made explicit. These children do not "pick up" links, rules, or generalizations. They need to learn them.

They need to be taught, for example, how often to review information to make it secure. Tony Buzan (1990) suggests revisions after 10 minutes, 24 hours, one week, one month and then three monthly, as a bare minimum, to prevent 80 percent of information being lost.

Helping children to plan a remembering timetable, like a revision timetable for exams later, will improve retention.

Conway and Gathercole's Translation Hypothesis (1990) states that

> When the brain moves from one modality to another, it is committing an act which is itself encoded in episodic memory.

Therefore retention and later retrieval of information will also be helped if the student is taught to transfer information from one modality to another and then another so he makes links between seeing, hearing, saying, feeling, and doing. One link reinforces another; a stronger channel supports a weaker one.

Many memory struggles occur when abstract concepts become involved. Abstract material can be made tangible by providing the students with concrete, manipulable aids such as: a wooden alphabet or an alphabet strip; visual timetable

What is the subject of my study?

Geography - Coasts

What main aspects of the subject should I consider?

Erosion

What do I already know?

I know it means wearing away of cliffs etc by water. I know it happens but I don't know how.

What should I research?

1 A clear definition of erosion/erode

2 Type of erosion and descriptions

3 Factors affecting erosion

What did I find out?

1 To eat into or wear away slowly
To cause to deteriorate or disapear
To produce or form by eroding.

2
Attrition.
boulders smash
together + break up

Corrasion
sand paper
effect

Corrosion
acidity in
water

Hydrlic action
movement of
water

3 Hardness of rock, weaknesses/faults, power of water, acidity of water.

Figure 3. Research framework.

for, say, historical events or other sequential material; multiplication square; number bonds visual aids; checking aids; lists of commonly used words; spellings of days of the week, months, etc. If these items are accessible to the whole class, they will help many. They do not have to be confined to one or several children. They can be placed in a small plastic basket and set on each table that any child can dip into without shame or fear of ridicule.

Metacognition and memory, key skills of information processing, are of crucial significance at a time when new information is replacing existing information moment by moment. Technological advances are making this information available to us as it happens. We cannot do better by a child than help him become master of his world; he can become dynamic rather than defeated.

1.7. Differentiating Output

There are many ways to "show what you know." Putting it down in writing is only one of these ways. You can speak into a tape recorder and write your words up later. You can tell your thoughts to a scribe who can write it down and then help you to transcribe later. You can use a word processor that has both spell and grammar check and then ask for help in editing. Alternatively, you can act out in drama. You can create a picture, diagram, flow chart, or a mind map. You can take photographs or make a film to demonstrate your understanding of a subject.

At some times in life, however, it is necessary to record in writing. It is helpful to have good cursive handwriting along with a system of decreasing support that uses frameworks or "scaffolds" (see Chapter 6).

The teacher can help further by showing understanding and by differentiating her standards of acceptable output. What is required from a piece of history? Is it knowledge of history or perfect secretarial skills?

The teacher's expectations of content and presentation should be high for *all* her students. Poor spelling should not undermine a piece of work that shows solidly good conceptual knowledge, but merely pinpoint for the teacher spelling and grammar issues which need to be worked on in later lessons. A positive comment at the end of every piece of work will encourage the struggler to keep going; he needs to know that what he has to say is worthwhile.

1.7.1. Grading

Grading should not crush feelings, with *every* mistake highlighted, nor absent, with nothing marked, so that the child is left wondering "Which parts did I get right?" Mistakes which the child can conceivably do something about are a good place to start. Offer meaningful directions. "This word is in the spelling family we learned last week, James," is helpful, whereas "Spelling!" is not.

A consistent set of markings will help the child to direct his thoughts for corrections, e.g., ^ for omissions, _____ for spellings, p for punctuation. Do no more than two or three per page. This should be school policy for maximum effectiveness.

1.8. Effective Use of Classroom Support

Many classes have a learning support assistant or paraprofessional allocated to them. Sometimes they serve as general classroom help and sometimes they are attached to the most needy children i.e., those at stage three or above in the Special Needs Audit (Code of Practice, 1994), sometimes at stage two. Some statemented children have a number of paraprofessional hours allocated specifically to them. This has not always been successful, and has been affected by the conditions required for intrinsic motivation. There has been a welcomed move in the UK toward hours allocated for special education teachers, although fewer per child, leaving paraprofessionals to do more general support.

Of all the "special needs" groups this move toward specialist intervention will be of maximum benefit to the dyslexic children who require specifically targeted work. Their work should be carefully taught by a dyslexia specialist, backed up by the teacher in the classroom to allow for maximum transfer, and other curriculum subjects suitably differentiated in the classroom setting.

When teachers are fortunate enough to have the services of "reading helpers" or paraprofessionals, they should have these extra personnel under their direction or that of the SENCO's in collaboration with them. Helpers should be advised against constant surveillance, but encouraged to provide *discreet* support when needed. Paraprofessionals in particular should be involved at the planning stage so they will have a clear idea of the teacher's aims and expectations. They need to be aware of what the child is to learn, not just what he is to do. They must know when it is appropriate to come forward to help, and when to stay back, letting the child wrestle with the problem and learn equally from his own successes and mistakes.

The National Numeracy Project (draft November 1997) advises that occasional support personnel should, among other things:

- Be involved in planning.
- Position themselves close to any children who might need help and provide that help discreetly.
- Help children interpret instructions correctly.
- Help children make frequent use of concrete aids such as counting apparatus and visual aid such as number lines, or multiplication squares.

Dyslexic children—all children—hate to fail, hate to be different, hate to be singled out as having "special needs." In the spirit of the times, teachers who focus on inclusive education can help children to feel equally able and equally worthy if they give them equal access to support in the classroom as any other child, rather than have them endure the constant and stifling presence of an overseer.

1.9. Effective Teaching

Martin Turner (1997), outlines the 20 most promising features in effective teaching, based on evidence from a large number of studies. At the interactive phase, teacher expectations, enthusiasm, clarity, organization, flexibility, and management are highlighted, together with a supportive, pleasant, democratic, and understanding climate in the classroom, as some of the main determiners of success for learners. He also states that "direct instruction (teacher-directed instruction) . . . is highly associated with increased learning gains among primary children . . . is the almost universal conclusion of recent research."

This author wishes to add to the list that in the classroom a sense of humor goes a long way.

1.10. Successful Learning

To summarize much of this chapter, these questions, which the teacher may ask herself, will help all her students, and be an absolute lifesaver for her dyslexic students:

- Has my presentation incorporated visual, auditory and kinesthetic strategies? If so could he see and hear me, and does he have a sharp pencil?
- Have I broken the material down into manageable chunks?
- Have I linked to personal–familiar material?
- Did I do enough varied repetition?
- Can I summarize the main points in a logical order, using restricted vocabulary?
- Can the student tell me what he has to do?
- Have I left him with a memory trigger to access this lesson?
- Are the main spellings available?
- Have I allowed him to record his work in an appropriate way?
- Did I ensure discreet but effective support?
- Can I grade his work positively?
- Did we all enjoy ourselves?

2. THE DYSLEXIC CHILD AT HOME

2.1. Introduction

The second part of this chapter will address the following issues:

- Why parents of dyslexic students can become anxious and demanding.
- How the emergence of dyslexic-type learning difficulties affects the young child.

- A school's responsibility to respond to parental concerns.
- Developing good communication channels between parents and school.
- Involving parents in the educational management of their dyslexic child by helping with reading, spelling, handwriting, and mathematics as well as helping with homework.
- The importance of the partnership between school, student, and home.

2.2. Supporting Parents

The parent of a dyslexic child can appear fussy, demanding, overanxious, or even confrontational. Such a parent can take up a seemingly disproportionate amount of a teacher's time. By understanding why a parent is behaving in such a way the teacher can keep their relationship with the parent from becoming strained and tainted with resentment. Having some insight into what it is like to be the parent of a dyslexic child can lead to a constructive and supportive relationship.

2.3. The Young Dyslexic Child

Most dyslexic children are similar to others in their peer group prior to their starting school. Their speech may be a little indistinct or delayed, but this is often excused by saying they are too busy being creative, or that older siblings do all the talking. In retrospect, it may be noted that they were rather clumsy, but again this is put down to their being adventurous and "into everything." Their time at nursery school may go quite smoothly, even if a little unconventionally. While being perfectly happy, they may be loners, totally absorbed in their own world. They may love building towers with bricks and constructing Lego masterpieces but may shy away from organized activities that require them to follow instructions or to remember the words of a song.

A few months after beginning school, the once happy and contented young child may not be quite so settled. Often, parents develop vague feelings of unease about their child's development, but they will probably not be able to put their finger on what is wrong. They will be baffled by their child, who seems so able and bright in some contexts, but so poorly skilled in others. He may have trouble remembering how to write his name, or he may be the only one who has not been given a reading book because he hasn't learned how to recognize the key word flash cards. Behavioral problems may appear as he rebels over having to conform to the class rules. He may start wetting the bed, having been dry for two years or more, or he may become reluctant about attending school. As he falls farther and farther behind his peer group in literacy skills, his self-esteem may suffer and poor behavior, mood swings, introversion or depression may become manifest.

2.4. Parental Concerns

At this stage, parents may start coming into school with their concerns. Whether they turn into fussy, demanding, overanxious, or confrontational parents will be determined partly by the way they are handled by the school. If they are given the impression that "the professionals" know best and that their concerns are not relevant, or if they are told that "children develop at different rates" and that "little Johnny is not ready for reading yet," but two years have passed and no progress has been made, is it any wonder they may appear to overreact?

2.5. A School's Responsibility

It is a school's responsibility to take seriously concerns a parent might have, to explore the reasons for these concerns, and to develop a constructive approach to help alleviate them. The Code of Practice (Df EE, 1994), which is in force in England and Wales, states that "the knowledge, views and experience of parents are vital. Effective assessment and provision will be secured where there is the greatest possible degree of partnership between parents and their children and schools." Throughout the Code, partnership with parents is emphasized. No matter to which educational system a school belongs, this advice seems eminently sensible.

There are a number of reasons why parents might start to worry about their child's progress at school, and the worries may not be rooted entirely in the child's problems. Dyslexia is often inherited. Ott (1997) has collated information on family history and genetic evidence in which she cites research by Finucci et al. (1976) which states that 81 percent of dyslexic students had at least one dyslexic parent, and Vogler, De Fries, and Deckler (1985) found that there is a 40 percent chance of a dyslexic boy having a dyslexic father and a 35 percent chance of his having a dyslexic mother. Girls had a 17–18 percent chance of having a dyslexic parent. Even if the parents themselves are not dyslexic, there is a strong possibility that a grandparent, aunt, or uncle may be affected. Consequently, a parent may well recognize that history is repeating itself, i.e. one of the parents or a close relative has literacy problems and has suffered at school because of it. If so, a parent will be only too aware of the ongoing frustrations, feelings of failure and inadequacies that such difficulties engender. Parents may be fearful of what the future holds in store for their child (Ostler, 1991).

A parent may have an older child with similar learning disabilities that were not identified early on. The parent might have been aware of these problems, but did not press the school for action if the teachers had stated the child was not yet ready for reading. Now that their child is older and is still not reading and has serious learning problems, and probably serious behavioral issues as well, the parent may have feelings of guilt, anger, and frustration, and a desire to not let this happen again.

It could be that their child is not dyslexic, but rather has general learning disabilities. This should make no difference to a school's response. Parents have a right to be heard, and they should be given constructive help and support so that they, in their turn, can be support their child.

The situation can be reversed. A school may identify a student's learning problems, but a parent may refuse to accept them, and may consequently become uncooperative or even hostile when asked to help at home. Again, the reasons can be quite complex and may be rooted in the parent's own negative school experience, suppressed feelings of failure, or inability to face up to their own learning disabilities. They may believe that they have become successful in spite of their schooling. In the author's experience, this reaction is more common in fathers than mothers (Ostler, 1991). Mothers often find it easy to accept that their child is struggling and is in need of learning support. They are less likely to feel their child is being lazy and not trying hard enough.

2.6. Misunderstandings

Poor relationships can occur between parents and teachers when there is a lack of communication. It is not unusual to come across a parent who is critical of a school which they believe to be doing nothing for their child. Upon investigation, it is often found that the school has made a variety of special arrangements for the student, but the parents have not been informed or have failed to appreciate the significance of what is being done. Parents may question their child about their support lessons, and the child may say "Oh, we don't do any work, we just play games!" A parent is not to know that these so-called "games" are actually highly structured activities that reinforce a particular teaching point. Likewise, in-class support may be such a part of the normal routine that a child may not realize that it is for his benefit.

2.7. Terminology

No television soap opera or talk show is without its dyslexic character these days. Some recent novels have included a dyslexic character, and comedians tell dyslexic jokes! Through extensive media coverage the term "dyslexia" has entered everyday language. The general public may not be able to give a precise definition of what is meant by the term, but most people have some kind of concept as to its meaning—that is, a dyslexic person has difficulties with reading and writing. They may also know there are famous dyslexic people who have made a success of their lives, such as Susan Hampshire and Tom Cruise.

The layman cannot be blamed for not being able to give a definition because many education experts, psychologists, neurologists, and other experts differ over their definitions. Consequently, many schools prefer to use the term "specific learning difficulty" or "learning impaired." Parents can become confused. They may think the school has not identified their child's problems if the term "dyslexia" is not used. However, with the identification of other learning difficulties such as dyspraxia, dyscalculia, and dyssemia, which are all specific in nature, there appears to be a swing back to the use of the term "dyslexia," although it may be qualified by the addition of other terms, as in "visual dyslexia" and "auditory dyslexia," which could be even more confusing for parents. So how should a school cope with this dilemma?

2.8. Communication

For there to be a true working partnership between home and school there needs to be regular and constructive communication. It is essential for the school to keep parents informed about what is being done to support their child. Assumptions should not be made that parents understand the meaning of terminology such as "inclass support," "withdrawal lessons," "peer tutoring" and so on.

Care should be taken if letters that explain what provision is being arranged are sent home with a student. A letter may not arrive home safely. Dyslexic students can be quite forgetful and some have a penchant for losing things. Parents may have reading problems themselves, or they may be quite intimidated by an official looking letter. English may not be the main language in the home. Misunderstandings occur very easily. Alternative means of communication may need to be considered. An open house night for parents, which includes a video of children receiving learning support, will help parents see clearly what is happening in school. When sending home specific information, include an audio cassette recording (after first ascertaining that the home has suitable equipment). This may need recording in the home language. If the school has a learning support unit, offer opportunities for parents to visit and observe some lessons.

Obviously, this is all time consuming. It needs to be part of a whole-school approach that can include the support of all members of staff from classroom assistants to senior management. Parents need to be kept up-to-date on their child's progress. With the record-keeping requirements of the Code of Practice, for example, this should not be difficult, since they can be shown what objectives have been set and the level their child has achieved. Above all, parents need to feel their child counts, that he is being treated as an individual. To be told there are children with far more serious problems in the class is of no comfort to a parent who lies awake at night worrying about what the future holds in store for their child. It can exacerbate the situation because the comment could imply to the parents that the teacher has little time to give their child.

2.9. Keeping Parents Informed

It is important that parents are kept informed right from the beginning if a learning support or an intervention program is arranged for their child. Some form of "start-up" meeting, which should include the teacher who is to oversee the provision and any staff who will be responsible for specific support, be it inclass or withdrawal teaching, could be arranged for the parents. The nature of the learning disabilities and the steps that will be taken to remediate these difficulties need to be explained clearly. If English is not the first language of the parents, then an interpreter's presence should be considered. An older brother or sister can sometimes help in this situation. It is probable that specific targets will be set and these should be defined as clearly as possible, e.g., "By the end of the term, John will be able to read and spell one-syllable words with the pattern vowel-consonant-final **e**." At least once a term, feedback meetings should be arranged at which a teacher can explain to parents which targets have been met and what arrangements are to be made for the following term. If it can be shown that specific objectives have been achieved it will go a long way to reassure parents their child is making progress and there is hope for the future. If parents have been instrumental in helping to achieve these objectives, then they should be praised and their importance in the school–parent partnership reiterated.

2.10. Involving Parents

One of the most effective ways of supporting parents, of showing that their worries and frustrations are taken seriously, is to involve them in the educational management of their dyslexic child. Manageable and attainable objectives, which can be worked toward at home, can be given so that parents can become involved in their child's learning. When these objectives are met, parents can see they are making a difference in the life of their child and this will help them feel more in control of their negative feelings.

2.10.1. Organizational Skills

Poor organizational skills form one of the major learning handicaps of dyslexic students. They frequently lose their books, sports clothes, and other personal possessions. They are forgetful and have difficulty taking messages, following instructions, and remembering where they have left something. They have a poor sense of time and so are late for lessons. They miss appointments and can confuse the order of the days of the week, which can result in their failure to take their musical instrument to school on the correct day because they thought Tuesday followed Wednesday! Parents can do much to help in these situations. However, it must be remembered that the parents may well be dyslexic themselves, and the whole household may be totally disorganized. Highly specific strategies will need to be introduced to parents which will help them to be better organized themselves and thus help their children become more efficient.

The following suggestions can be adapted to suit the particular needs of the school and the families concerned. A school may want to produce their own booklet. Patience and perseverance will be needed with disorganized families. A 100 percent success is highly unlikely, but any improvement will be good news!

2.10.2. Possessions

For the *beginning of each term*, supply a *checklist* (Ostler, 1996) of what equipment, clothing, etc. will be needed. The list needs to be tabulated and should include two boxes to check off after each item: one check for having the item and a second check to indicate it has been named. Information about where labels or marking pens can be obtained could be included, for example, *WHOSHOE!* (shoe labels), *NAMEMARK* (durable plastic name labels). It would be helpful to have indelible pens available at school. This procedure will not stop possessions from getting lost, but it does make it much easier to return items!

2.10.3. Equipment

A *daily checklist* is needed to make certain the student has what he needs for the day: lunch money, reading book, pencil case, art materials, sports clothes, musical instrument, books, etc.

A disorganized student may need to report daily to a tutor, special needs department or an older student to check that he has the above, but if a parent can ensure that the items were brought to school, then some measure of success can be achieved. It is also useful if a student can report back at the end of the day to verify he has what he needs to take home for his homework.

2.10.4. Time Management

By the time a student reaches secondary education he will need to organize himself in time and space. That is, he will have to be in the *right place*, at the *right time*, with the *right equipment* having done the *right work*—quite an achievement for most dyslexic students. He may find the following equipment and strategies helpful:

2.10.4.1. Schedule. At least three copies of his schedule: one taped to the inside door of his locker, one in his homework diary, and one at home *which his parents will need to remind him to check* before he leaves the house in the morning. Some schools operate a two-week schedule which is extremely difficult for the dyslexic student to cope with: A large fluorescent star or marker would be needed to indicate which schedule is in operation each week.

2.10.4.2. Year-planner. A *year-planner* to record term dates, coursework deadlines, field trips, examinations, modular tests, so that he can monitor the passing of time and anticipate what is imminent (photocopyable planners are included in *Study Skills—A Pupil's Survival Guide,* Ostler, 1996*).*

2.10.4.3. Diary. A *homework diary* to record all details of each assignment. He should also record the names of any books he needs to take home to help with the work and the date when assigned work is due. If he has trouble writing down the instructions, he could use a dictaphone in which either he or his teacher dictate the relevant information. Sensitivity would be needed in suggesting this strategy. Dyslexic students often do not like to be singled out or be made to look different. With younger students, parents should be asked to sign the diary on a daily or weekly basis to indicate they have checked their child's homework, and to add comments if there were any problems.

2.10.4.4. Organizer. Instead of a homework diary, a *personal organizer* can be customized to include a map of the school, names and responsibilities of his teachers (parents will find this particularly helpful to refer to), academic schedule, extracurricular activities schedule, syllabuses for his subjects, a year-planner to record details as already described and any other pages that are relevant to his school. Younger students may need a home–school liaison page so that parents and teachers can communicate.

2.10.4.5. Contact. The *telephone number* of a member of his class who can be relied upon to have all of the homework details is invaluable for the occasions when his homework instructions are incomplete, or when he can't read his own writing.

2.10.4.6. Clear notes. The opportunity to *photocopy* the notes of a class member who has neat handwriting if his own notes are illegible or incomplete.

2.10.4.7. Bulletin board. A *bulletin*, either in the student's bedroom or the kitchen, for displaying his schedule for easy reference, his daily checklist, year-planner with coursework deadlines, telephone number of a class member and any letters or forms that are sent home from school. This needs to be easily accessible, kept up-to-date, and referred to daily.

2.10.5. Learning Support at Home

Learning support might be given by a parent, but it can give rise to much tension and disagreement between parent and child. An older sibling, relation, neighbor or babysitter could be a viable option. Parents must be reassured that it is not unusual for support to be sometimes better when given by someone other than themselves. They should not feel guilty or inadequate. It might be that a parent feels too insecure with regard to his own literacy or arithmatic skills to help. Great tact is needed when suggesting that certain skills be practiced at home. The support can take many different forms and will vary with the student's age and home circumstances.

2.10.6. Helping with Reading

It would be helpful if a school supplied a booklet describing how they would like reading support to be given at home. Sensitivity is needed as the parents themselves may be insecure readers. The booklet needs to explain the enormous benefits to be gained from the "little-but-often" approach. Suggestions as to when, where, and how the reading sessions should be carried out need to be explained:

- "Choose a time other than when your child's favourite television program is on."
- "Find somewhere quiet and comfortable to sit, away from nondyslexic brothers and sisters, where you can both see the book."
- "Give lots of praise."
- "Don't criticize when an error is made, but give the correct word and continue reading."

Put their emphasis on reading enjoyment rather than on reading instruction.

However, parents need guidance as to what to do if their child makes a mistake or doesn't know a word. Examples of the kind of questions that can be asked to develop comprehension and predictions skills can be given, such as: "What do you think happens next?" "Why do you think she did that?" The questions need to be structured so that more than a "yes–no" answer has to be given.

A *reading record* needs to be kept (see Figure 4). The reading helper (it need not be a parent) should be encouraged to make a comment each time, such as: "This was a good session." "This book is too difficult/easy/boring: Find something more appropriate." "He's still having difficulty reading the word *said.*"

Boys often view reading as a girlish occupation, and so if an older boy could be found, either in school or out, to help with reading sessions, this could help greatly to overcome the nonmacho image.

2.10.7. Nonreading Help with Reading!

It can be explained to parents that they can help their child improve their reading without even opening a book. Any activity that increases children's vocabulary and knowledge of the world will help their prediction technique when they read. Visits to museums, exhibitions, parks, and zoos will broaden their horizons, as will watching and discussing television documentary programs. The key is for parents and children to discuss what they have seen.

DATE	TITLE	PAGES READ	COMMENTS
Monday			
Tuesday			

Figure 4. Reading record.

Encouraging a hobby or interest in which the child can derive enjoyment and, one hopes, excel, will help to build self-confidence. It can also give them status among peers. If this can be an interest that their siblings and friends know nothing about or are unskilled in, so much the better (Ostler, 1991). Feeling confident about any aspect of one's life can spill over into feeling confident in other learning situations.

2.10.8. Helping with Spelling

As with reading, an instruction booklet with plenty of illustrations needs to be given to parents so they may help their child learn spelling. It must be emphasized that the child should not just sit and stare at the words, or copy them out letter by letter. Rather, a multisensory approach is needed. For example: Look—Say—Spell Aloud—Cover—Write—Check

- Look at the word.
- Say the word.
- Say the names of the letters.
- Cover the word.
- Write the word from memory saying the letter names again.
- Check that the word is correct.
- Repeat until the word is secure.

This works best when carried out in a small vocabulary book that uses four ruled columns (see Figure 5).

2.10 9. Multisensory Learning

To give the child tactile experience, use wooden or plastic letters to practice spellings. Working with magnetic letters on a refrigerator door can also be fun. Alphabet cookie cutters or alphabet sponges that stick to the bath tiles are also

WORD	1st TRY	2nd TRY	3rd TRY

Figure 5. The vocabulary notebook should be divided to like this.

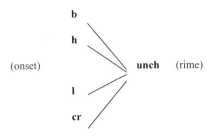

Figure 6. The "–unch" onset–rime family.

available. Tactile letters are particularly useful when teaching word families with onset and rimes (see Figure 6).

The older student can collate a notebook of subject-specific words (such as "reign," "rhythm," and "temperature") from coursework errors and learn them using the Look, Say, Spell aloud, Cover, Write, Check method.

2.10.10. Helping with Mathematics

Parents can be reluctant to help their children with math because so often the vocabulary used and the methods for calculation have changed since they were at school. A booklet explaining the methods their child is using in school, with step-by-step examples, would save a lot of frayed tempers at home (see Russell, 1996). A multiplication square could be supplied for home use. This should be displayed prominently, and when a new times-table number bond is learned, the relevant square can be colored in, e.g., $6 \times 8 = 48$ (see Figure 7).

	1	2	3	4	5	6	7	8	9	10
1	1	2	3	4	5	6	7	8	9	10
2	2	4	6	8	10	12	14	16	18	20
3	3	6	9	12	15	18	21	24	27	30
4	4	8	12	16	20	24	28	32	36	40
5	5	10	15	20	25	30	35	40	45	50
6	6	12	18	24	30	36	42	48	54	60
7	7	14	21	28	35	42	49	56	63	70
8	8	16	24	32	40	48	56	64	72	80
9	9	18	27	36	45	54	63	72	81	90
10	10	20	30	40	50	60	70	80	90	100

Figure 7. Multiplication square.

A set of multiplication flip cards is available (Parry, 1988) and there are some excellent suggestions in Steve Chinn's book *What to Do When You Can't Learn the Times Tables* (Chinn, 1996). It is also available on CD-ROM.

2.10.11. Helping with Handwriting

Daily handwriting practice is essential when a cursive, flowing hand is being established. However, students need to be watched in the early stages to ensure they form the letters in the correct way. This is where parents can help. It is important that parents are shown how to implement the school's approach, particularly with regard to entry and exit strokes, which letters join, the use of loops, or otherwise. Parents also need guidance on writing posture, pen grip, writing tools, the paper position, and, if necessary, the particular needs of the left-hander.

If the child has a protracted difficulty with handwriting, and regular practice is not helping, then this may be a dyspraxic difficulty that will require training in fine motor control and finger strengthening exercises. Suggestions are contained in Nash-Wortham and Hunt (1990).

2.10.12. Helping with Homework

The nightly homework session is a frustrating time in many households. When a dyslexic student is involved, it can be doubly difficult. He may not have remembered the instructions, or if he has written them down, he may not be able to read his own writing. He may not understand what he has to do, and he has probably forgotten to take home the relevant books anyway. Having had a frustrating and possibly humiliating time in school, he is tired. The last thing he wants to do is his homework. Parents can be advised as to how they can help their dyslexic children. The following approach is helpful for all students (Ostler, 1996).

- A *routine* needs to be established as to when the homework is to be done (not during their favorite television program!). Bribery might be needed to get this going, e.g., you can go out/watch a video/walk the dog when you have finished.
- A particular *place to work* needs to be associated with homework. This might be in their room, a corner in the kitchen or living room, but NOT in front of the television. If the home situation does not allow for this, a homework club at school would be a good option.
- The use of a *homework diary* is essential. The teachers will probably need to ensure that instructions and assignments are recorded accurately.
- Parents can help by keeping a duplicate stock of *paper and pens* so that time is not wasted at the beginning of a work session.

- Obviously, there may well be financial restraints for many families, but access to *reference books*, revision books, and *CD-ROMs* can be very useful.
- If a dyslexic child is having difficulty with his or her homework, a parent can try the following:
  1. Ask their child to read them the instructions. Reading aloud can often help make the task seem clearer, or it may become evident that the child misread the first time. Once the instructions have been read accurately, the task will be understood.
  2. Explain the instructions if they have not been understood.
  3. Look at a previous example to see if the same procedure can be used.
  4. Read other sources on the subject to obtain more information or to put the problem in context.
  5. Act as a transcriber if the writing progress is becoming too laborious. The child could then recopy the work when feeling less tired. Alternatively the teacher may accept the parent's script.
  6. Wordprocess the homework: Editing is so much less daunting on a computer.
  7. Record text onto tape for the child to refer to while answering questions.

Obviously, some parents would be able to cope with these suggestions better than others. These strategies are a few examples of what parents could employ. Careful thought would need to be given to the number of suggestions that are made to parents at any one time. It may be best to introduce just one idea at a time, while saying if this strategy is successful thus-and-such strategy will be tried next week/month. *It would be for the teacher to assess what would be appropriate to suggest to individual parents.*

2.11. Whom to Contact

In a primary or first school, regular contact and communication is usually quite easy to maintain between parents and teacher. Parents can usually visit the school at the beginning or end of the day to raise any queries or worries. However, when a student moves into secondary school, this move is often not so straightforward. Parents must know *whom* to approach, and when and where to contact a staff member who has responsibility for their child. Each school will have its own system which may involve a teacher, special education teacher, school counselor, lead teacher, principal, and so on. This is confusing and sometimes intimidating for parents. It needs to be made very clear to parents whom they can contact if they need any information or if they have a particular concern.

2.12. Involving Students

Although parental involvement is paramount, student involvement must not be overlooked. The student needs to know the nature of his learning problems, what is being planned to help him overcome and compensate for them and, most important, how the combination of his family and school working together can be a powerful force. Depending on his age and his home circumstances, it can be beneficial for the student to be involved in the discussions between teacher and parent when planning what support is to be given at home. The ultimate aim is to establish a three-way partnership between school, student, and home.

2.13. Summary

The overriding concern when considering the dyslexic child in his environment is the quality of the communication that exists between home and school. It is essential that parents be kept informed about their child's problems, the kind of support that is being given, how they can help their child at home, and what progress is being made. They must be made to feel that their concerns and anxieties are taken seriously, and that they can contact someone at school, who knows their child well, when they have problems or queries.

This places enormous demands on the teaching staff. The author acknowledges that some parents never seem to be satisfied with what is being done, but if parents are actively involved with the educational management of their child, and can see tangible proof of improvement, then this can go a long way toward ameliorating their anxiety.

Parents can play an important part in helping their dyslexic child become better organized, which is essential if students are to become confident and independent learners. Encouraging a hobby in which he or she can succeed will help build self-confidence and a feeling of worth. Due praise should be given to parents for the help they give.

It bodes well for the dyslexic student when school and home become "partners in learning" (Code of Practice, 1994).

APPENDIX

The Special Educational Needs Code of Practice (England and Wales)

The **Code of Practice** came into effect in September 1994 as a requirement of the 1993 Education Act, to provide guidance to Local Education Authorities (LEAs), schools, and other agencies in England and Wales on:

- The identification and assessment of children with special educational needs;

- The cycle of planning, teaching, assessing and reviewing to meet those needs;
- The responsibilities of LEAs, schools, Health Services and Social Services Departments, to work in partnership with each other and with parents, in their responses to children with special educational needs.

The code recommends the adoption of a staged model of special educational needs, Stages one, two, and three mainly school-based, but calling on external specialists as necessary, with responsibility for Stages 4 and 5 being shared between the school and the LEA.

Details of the school-based stages are as follows:

A child might be placed at **Stage one** as the result of a global discrepancy between that child's performance and the class average noticed in fairly general terms by the class teacher. The class teacher collects information of the need to be addressed as clues toward *basic differentiation* within the classroom setting.

A child is moved to **Stage two** if the low level Stage one intervention had little or no effect, and at this stage, a closer look at skill areas might be taken, by the class teacher, or in conjunction with the school's Special Educational Needs Coordinator (SENCO). An Individual Education Plan (IEP) is prepared to address specific weaknesses or needs and at this stage grouping is feasible with others who might have similar difficulties in related skill areas. The features of this stage then are *differentiation within class, plus a group, or general, IEP.*

If little or no progress is made by the child as a result of Stage two intervention, he or she would then be placed at **Stage three** and furnished with an IEP with narrower, more tightly defined targets and time frames. At this stage, advice might be sought from external agencies. This stage is characterized by *differentiation within class plus an IEP delineating a specific and intensive program of work.*

A multidisciplinary team at termly In-School Reviews considers each movement of stage, either up or down.

Lack of progress at Stage three triggers consideration of the need for statutory multiprofessional assessments which is covered by Stages four and five. A Statement of Special Educational Need is prepared, which carries statutory special provision and an annual review.

RESOURCES

Memory Cards, Sutton Dyslexia Association, 21 Princes Ave., Carshalton, Surrey SM5 4NZ

Parry, J. (1998), My Tables Box, Pippin Products, Bedfordshire.

WHOSHOE! (shoe labels), NAMEMARK (durable plastic name labels). P.O. Box 1792, Christchurch, Dorset BH23 4YR.

REFERENCES

Burns, R. (1982). *Self-Concept, Development and Education.* London: Holt, Rinehart and Winston.

Buzan, T. (1990). *Use Your Head.* London: BBC Books.

Chinn, S. (1996). *What to Do If You Can't Learn the Times Tables.* Herts: Egon.

Code of Practice (1994). *Code of Practice on the Identification and Assessment of Special Educational Needs.* London: Department for Education and Employment, Central Office of Information.

Condry, J. (1977). Enemies of exploration: Self-initiated versus other-initiated learning. *Journal of Personality and Social Psychology, 35.*

Conway, M., & Gathercole, S. (1990). *Paper on Translation in Quarterly Journal Educational Psychology 42.*

Csikszentmihalyi, M. *Intrinsic Rewards and Emergent Motivation* in Lepper, M.R. & Greene, D. (1978)

Deci, E.L., & Ryan, R.M. (1985). *Intrinsic Motivation and Self-Determination in Human Behaviour.* New York: Plenum.

Department for Education. (1995). The National Curriculum. London: HMSO.

Department for Education & Employment. (1998). The National Literacy Strategy. London: DfEE.

Department for Education & Employment. (1997 draft). The National Numeracy Project

Finucci, J.M., Guthrie, J.T., Childs, A.L., Abbey, H., & Child, B. (1976). The genetics of specific reading disability. *Annals of Human Genetics, 40,* 1–23.

Flavell, J.H. (1979). Metacognition and cognitive monitoring. *American Psychologist, 34,* 907–911.

Holt, J. (1991). *Learning All The Time.* Ticknell, Derbyshire: Education Now.

Kohn, A. (1993). *Punished by Rewards.* Boston and New York: Houghton Mifflin.

Kyriacou, C. (1997). *Effective Teaching in Schools.* Cheltenham: Stanley Thornes.

Lepper, M.R., & Greene, D. (1978). *The Hidden Costs of Rewards.* Hillsdale, N.J.: Erlbaum.

Moyles, J. (1997). *Organising for Learning in the Primary Classroom.* Milton Keynes: Open University Press.

Nash-Wortham, M., & Hunt, J. (1990). *Take Time.* Stourbridge: Robinswood Press.

Ostler, C.A. (1991). *Dyslexia—A Parents' Survival Guide.* Godalming: Ammonite Books.

Ostler, C.A. (1996). *Study Skills—A Pupil's Survival Guide.* Godalming: Ammonite Books.

Ott, P. (1997). *How to Detect and Manage Dyslexia.* Oxford: Heinemann.

Russell, R. (1996). *Maths for Parents.* London: Piccadilly Press.

Sawyer, D.J.(1991) Early Language Intervention: A deterrent to reading disability. *Orton Dyslexia Society Annals of Dyslexia,* XXXXI: 55–79.

Turner, M. (1997). *Psychological Assessment of Dyslexia.* London: Whurr.

Vogler, G.P., De Fries, J.C., & Deckler, S.N. (1985). Family history as an indicator of risk for reading disability. *Journal of Learning Disabilities, 18,* 419–421.

About the Authors

Janet Townend is a speech and language therapist, specialist dyslexia teacher, and teacher trainer. She established and led the Learning Centre at Eton College and is now Head of Training at the Dyslexia Institute.

Caroline Borwick is a Principal Training Tutor with the Dyslexia Institute. She is a speech and language therapist, lecturer, specialist teacher, and teacher trainer. She is the coauthor, with Janet Townend, of *Developing Spoken Language Skills* (1993).

Christine Firman has worked with dyslexic children in Malta and overseas for a number of years. She is responsible for the Specific Learning Difficulties Service in Malta. She also contributes to teacher training.

Martin Turner became Head of Psychology at the Dyslexia Institute in 1991. Prior to that, he served for many years as a Local Education Authority educational psychologist. He is the author of *Sponsored Reading Failure* (1990) and *The Psychological Assessment of Dyslexia* (1997).

Angie Nicholas is a specialist teacher and member of the Training Department at the Dyslexia Institute. She has worked in both primary and secondary schools and has been involved in specialist teacher assessments.

Jean Walker is an experienced dyslexia teacher and Training Principal based at the Dyslexia Institute in Sheffield. She is the lead author of the *Dyslexia Institute Literacy Programme* (1993 and 1996).

Wendy Goldup is a Training Principal at the Dyslexia Institute. She is responsible for short courses which aim to link Dyslexia Institute principles with mainstream practice. She is also a course director on the Dyslexia Institute Post Graduate Diploma Course.

Helen Moss was until recently a principal tutor at the Dyslexia Institute in Bath and a course director on the Dyslexia Institute Post Graduate Diploma Course. She has worked with Walter Bramley for many years on his Developing Literacy for Study and Work, Units of Sound and the Active Literacy Kit.

Mary Flecker is a specialist teacher, and a teacher trainer for the Dyslexia Institute. She teaches at City of London School. She and Jennifer Cogan run a study skills course for teachers and parents.

Jennifer Cogan is head of the Dyslexia Unit at Westminster School. She contributes to teacher training at the Hornsby International Dyslexia Centre.

Clare Elwell is a specialist dyslexia teacher. She is head of the Learning Centre at Eton College. The Learning Centre exists to support and teach boys who have dyslexia or other specific learning disabilities.

Margaret Rooms taught mathematics before specializing in teaching dyslexic students. She is Head of Teaching Development at the Dyslexia Institute and has been responsible for developing Walter Bramley's Units of Sound programme for multimedia, and the Active Literacy Kit.

Pauline Clayton is a specialist dyslexia teacher and teacher trainer. She has developed and written the Dyslexia Institute Maths Programme. She lectures in dyslexia and mathematics.

Jenny Lee is the Adult Basic Education coordinator for the southern half of County Durham. Her center, while catering for all adults with basic skills needs, specializes in dyslexia. She trained with the Dyslexia Institute. She has over 12 years of experience in working with dyslexic adults and lecturing on the subject. She has pioneered work with dyslexic employees in industry and serves as a dyslexia consultant to a local university.

Christine Ostler is director of the Susan Hampshire (dyslexia) Centre at Cobham Hall School. She is the author of *Dyslexia—A Parents' Survival Guide* and *Study Skills—a Pupil's Survival Guide.*

Author Index

Subject Index